Mathematics and Visualization

Springer-Verlag Berlin Heidelberg GmbH

Michael Jünger
Petra Mutzel (Editors)

Graph Drawing Software

With 220 Figures, 183 in Color

Springer

Michael Jünger

Universität zu Köln
Institut für Informatik
Pohligstraße 1
50969 Köln, Germany

e-mail: mjuenger@informatik.uni-koeln.de

Petra Mutzel

Technische Universität Wien
Institut für Computergraphik und Algorithmen
Favoritenstraße 9-11 E186
1040 Wien, Austria

Cataloging-in-Publication Data applied for

A catalog record for this book is available from the Library of Congress.

Bibliographic information published by Die Deutsche Bibliothek
Die Deutsche Bibliothek lists this publication in the Deutsche Nationalbibliografie; detailed bibliographic data is available in the Internet at http://dnb.ddb.de

Mathematics Subject Classification (2000): I14002; I230044; W26007; W27003; T24035; T26003; M17009; M26008; M1400X; M14042; M14026; M14018; M13003; M13046; M13046; M13038

ISBN 978-3-642-62214-4 ISBN 978-3-642-18638-7 (eBook)
DOI 10.1007/978-3-642-18638-7

http://www.springer.de

Originally published by Springer-Verlag Berlin Heidelberg New York in 2004
Softcover reprint of the hardcover 1st edition 2004

Typeset in TEX by the authors
Cover design: *design & production* GmbH, Heidelberg

Printed on acid-free paper 46/3142db - 5 4 3 2 1 0 –

Preface

This book presents a collection of state-of-the-art graph drawing software tools whose purpose is to generate layouts of objects and their relationships. It covers fourteen software packages presented at the software exhibition during GD 2001, the *Ninth International Symposium on Graph Drawing* that took place in Vienna in September 2001, organized by the Vienna University of Technology, the Austrian Academy of Sciences, and the University of Cologne. The Graph Drawing Symposium is held annually, alternating between North America and Europe. GD 2001 hosted the first software exhibition that gave participants and guests the opportunity for hands-on experience with state-of-the-art graph drawing software tools.

Even though software demonstrations have a long tradition in graph drawing conferences, it is our feeling that graph drawing software has not yet received the recognition that it deserves. The graph drawing discipline is motivated by visualizing discrete structures that have, to a large extent, their origins outside the graph drawing community. The impact of graph drawing research for these application areas is mainly perceived via user-friendly software tools.

In view of the low quality graph drawing tools in some popular software environments we find it important that scientists from other disciplines and practitioners are exposed to state-of-the-art graph drawing software. We hope that this book will contribute towards achieving this goal.

May 2003

Cologne *Michael Jünger*
Vienna *Petra Mutzel*

Cover

The book cover shows an eigenvector-based 3D layout of a 5-regular graph constructed from the truncated cuboctohedron graph by replacing each vertex by a triangle and each edge by a pair of triangles. The coloring of the vertices represents the distance partition from a selected (cyan) vertex. The graph belongs to the Vega collection of graphs (`http://vega.ijp.si`). Its layout has been produced by Vladimir Batagelj and Andrej Mrvar with the `Pajek` system described in this book and rendered by Merijam Percan using PovRay.

Acknowledgements

We would like to thank Merijam Percan for her help in the technical editing of this book and Christoph Buchheim for careful proofreading. We gratefully acknowledge the pleasant cooperation with Martin Peters, Ute McCrory, and Daniela Brandt of Springer Verlag.

Contents

Introduction

Michael Jünger[1] and Petra Mutzel[2]

[1] University of Cologne, Department of Computer Science, Pohligstraße 1, D-50969 Köln, Germany

[2] Vienna University of Technology, Institute of Computer Graphics and Algorithms, Favoritenstraße 9–11, A-1040 Wien, Austria

Social networks, computer networks, business processes, biochemical reactions, data base schemas, software systems, and the world wide web have in common that they can be modeled as graphs and that visualization is crucial. A graph is a discrete structure consisting of vertices and edges, where the vertices correspond to the objects, and the edges to the relations of the structure to be modeled. Graph drawing is the task of the design, analysis, implementation, and evaluation of algorithms for automatically generating graph layouts that are easy to read and understand.

The history of graph drawing started in 1963 with the paper by Bill Tutte: *How to draw a graph* [16] in which he suggested an algorithm that places each vertex into the center of its neighbors. Intuition says that a layout satisfying this criterion is desirable, although it seems to be difficult to model the *niceness* of a layout. However, there are some criteria, supported by perceptual psychology studies (e.g., [11,12]), that are widely understood as important for *nice* layouts. E.g., the vertices displaying the objects should not overlap each other or the lines representing the edges.

An important criterion for many applications is a small number of edge crossings. E.g., consider Figure 1 displaying the network of the electric power industry as it appeared in a German newspaper [15]. Because of the large number of crossings in the diagram, it is very hard to get an overview over the dependency network. Moreover, it is not easy to answer specific questions of the kind: *"Is there a direct relation between VEAG and RWE?"* — This question can immediately be answered by looking at Figure 2, which shows a better layout of the same network.

Both diagrams are drawn in an *orthogonal style*, i.e., the lines representing the edges consist of a series of horizontal and vertical segments only. In many applications, an orthogonal style is desirable. Here, it is essential to keep the number of bends small so that it is easier to follow the edges. This is also achieved by keeping the length of the edge segments short. Drawings in which the edges are displayed as a series of straight lines are called *polyline drawings*. Sometimes, edges are also displayed as *curved lines*.

The *vertex resolution* of a drawing is the minimum distance between a pair of vertices in this drawing. In connection with the width and height of a drawing, it essentially determines the smallest possible size of the draw-

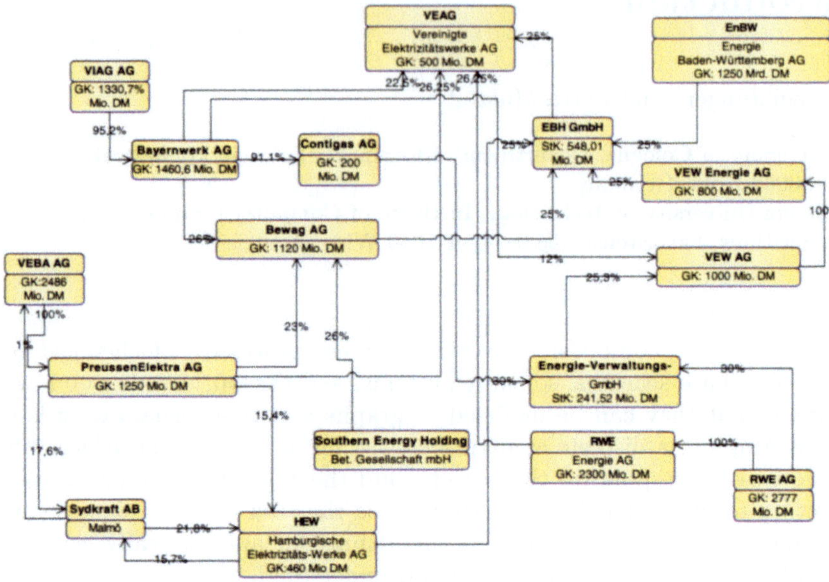

Fig. 1. A newspaper diagram displaying the dependencies of energy companies.

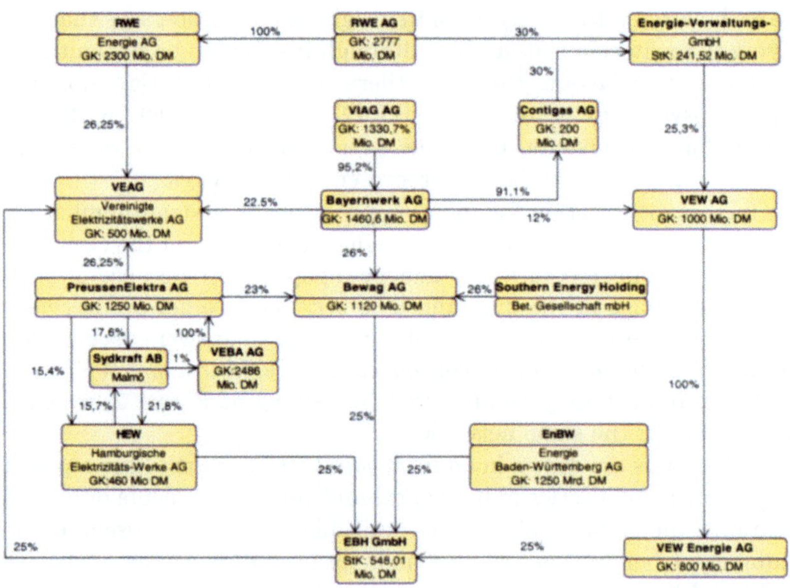

Fig. 2. A better layout of the diagram shown in Figure 1 in orthogonal style.

ing without loosing information. A small area allows for large magnification within a desired maximum width or height. A common drawing convention is to only use integer coordinates, i.e., to use a grid, for placing the vertices.

In many applications, the data contains some flow or hierarchical structure, such as, e.g., organization diagrams or PERT (program evaluation and review technique) diagrams. In these cases, the layout should reflect this. In our example, a flow is induced by the hierarchy of dependencies. A drawing highlighting this in so-called *layered* style is shown in Figure 3.

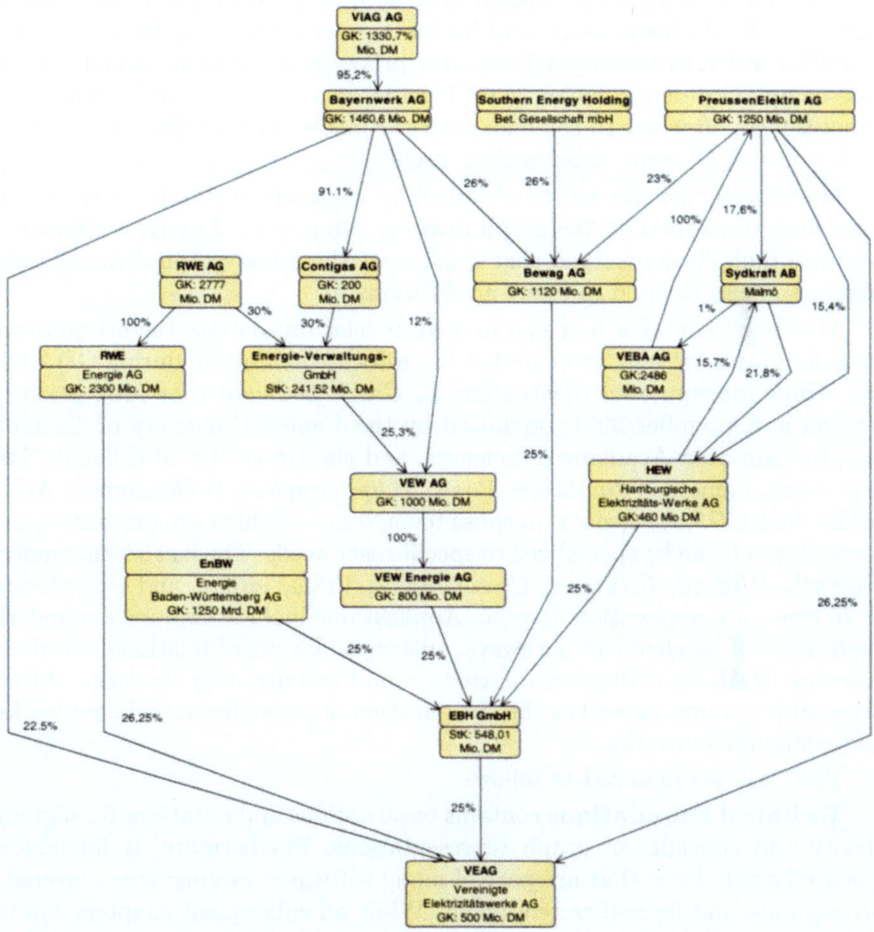

Fig. 3. A layout of the diagram shown in Figure 1 that highlights the dependency hierarchy of the energy companies.

More application specific requirements deal with symmetries, grouping of vertices, and annotations. If there are symmetries in the data, they should be displayed in the layout. Groups of vertices shall stay together in the drawings, and annotations should be placed close to the corresponding vertices and edges, respectively.

Since the seminal paper by Tutte [16], many papers about graph drawing have been published. In 1992, there was so much interest in graph drawing that the researchers decided to start an Annual International Symposium on Graph Drawing. Since then, a strong graph drawing community has been established, which did not only produce theoretical results, but also practical tools for graph layout, see [4,6,13,14,2,10,3,17,7–9,5].

Recently, visualization of discrete structures is getting increasing attention. E.g., UML diagrams [1] and business process modeling have been suggested in order to understand complex processes of software and business. The complexity of producing good layout tools is usually underestimated. Practitioners often try to come up with self-made solutions that do — at the end — not at all come close to their needs.

Much better results can be obtained by using one of the techniques that have been developed by the graph drawing community. Lately, a number of software tools have emerged that implement the latest graph drawing techniques and can be used in many applications.

This book contains fourteen invited articles on state-of-the-art software tools for graph drawing presented at the software exhibition during GD 2001, the *Ninth International Symposium on Graph Drawing* that took place in Vienna in September 2001, organized by the Vienna University of Technology, the Austrian Academy of Sciences, and the University of Cologne. The first seven, namely *WilmaScope*, *Pajek*, *Tulip*, *Graphviz & Dynagraph*, *AGD*, *yFiles*, and *GDS*, are general purpose tools, some of which are extendible and some of which can be specialized to specific user needs. The last seven, namely *BioPath*, *DBdraw*, *GoVisual*, *CrocoCosmos*, *ViSta*, *visone*, and *Polyphemus & Hermes*, are application specific. Applications include exploration and visualization of biochemical pathways, automatic layout of relational database schemas, UML class diagrams, structure and metrics data for large object-oriented programs, as well as the visualization of statecharts, social networks, and computer networks.

The book is organized as follows.

Technical Foundations contains basic notions and notations from graph theory and concepts of graph representations. Furthermore, it introduces generic layout styles that are part of many software systems: tree-, layered-, orthogonal-, and force-directed layout. While all subsequent chapters can be read independently, they all refer to the material presented in the Technical Foundations.

The remaining chapters contain a description of a software tool each. These chapters are organized in a uniform way. They all contain an introduction and sections on applications, algorithms, implementation issues, examples of application as well as instructions on how to obtain the software.

WilmaScope is a three-dimensional graph visualization system. Emphasis is on flexibility, interactivity, and extensibility. The implemented algorithms include a variety of force-directed layout methods as well as a method which uses the external DOT program from the AT&T Graphviz toolkit (see below) to produce a Sugiyama style layout. WilmaScope features clustering of related groups of nodes, and an interface for editing graphs and adjusting layout parameters.

Pajek is a tool for the analysis and visualization of large networks with hundreds of thousands of vertices. It supports recursive factorization of such big graphs into several smaller networks, which are then visualized. In addition to standard layout algorithms such as force-directed and hierarchical algorithms in two and three dimensions, Pajek contains eigenvector methods, block matrix representations, and supports user constraints.

Tulip is a huge graphs visualization framework, and here this means graphs with up to 1.000.000 elements. This software focuses on clustering in two and three dimensions, metrics algorithms, and visual attribute mapping algorithms for the purpose of information visualization. Special emphasis is put on the running time and the memory consumption of the algorithms.

Graphviz and **Dynagraph** are graph drawing tools for static and dynamic layouts, respectively. Graphviz provides various layout utilities for force-directed and hierarchical layouts. Dynagraph is a sibling of Graphviz, with algorithms and interactive programs for incremental layout. At the library level, it provides an object-oriented interface for graphs and graph algorithms.

AGD is a library of algorithms (and data structures) for graph drawing. It aims at bridging the gap between theory and practice in the area of graph drawing. The library contains a large number of drawing algorithms, including orthogonal and planarity-based algorithms, for many of which implementations can only be found in AGD, and which can be used as a tool-box for creating own implementations of graph drawing algorithms.

yFiles is a library for the visualization and automatic layout of graphs. Included features are data structures, graph algorithms, a graph viewer component and diverse layout and labeling algorithms. The main layout styles are orthogonal, tree, circular-radial, layered and force-directed. Emphasis is on flexibility, extensibility, and reuseability.

GDS is a graph drawing server on the internet. Users interact with the server by sending a request consisting of the graph to be drawn, the algorithm to be run and values for its parameters, the format of the input, and the desired output format. Emphasis is on ease-of-use, platform independence, flexibility, authoring, data protection, code protection, and security.

BioPath is a web-based dynamical tool for exploration and visualization of biochemical pathways. The layout algorithms are based on layered drawing including clustering and constraints. The system preserves the mental map of the user in sequences of related drawings. Emphasis is on dynamic visualization and interactive navigation through biochemical pathways.

DBdraw provides automatic layout of relational database schemas. Such schemas are drawn as tables with boxes, and table attributes with distinct stripes inside each table. Links connecting attributes of two different tables represent referential constraints or join relationships. The used drawing technique is inspired by the topology-shape-metrics approach via planarization.

GoVisual is a diagramming software for UML class diagrams whose purpose is to display class hierarchies (generalizations), associations, aggregations, and compositions within software systems in one picture. The combination of hierarchical and non-hierarchical relations poses the special challenge addressed by this software.

CrocoCosmos provides three-dimensional visualization of large object-oriented programs. The nodes represent structure entities like classes or packages. They are visualized by simple geometric objects with geometrical properties (as color or size) representing software metrics values. Relations are displayed as straight lines colored according to their relation type (method usage, inheritance). The large resulting graphs are visualized using specially tailored spring-embedder approaches.

ViSta is a tool for visualizing statecharts. Statecharts are widely used for the requirements specification of reactive systems. This notation captures the requirements attributes that are concerned with the behavioral features of a system, and models these features in terms of a hierarchy of diagrams and states. The techniques are based on layered drawing methods, inclusion drawings, labeling, and floor-planning methods.

visone is a tool for the analysis and visualization of social networks. Social network analysis is a methodological approach in the social sciences using graph-theoretic concepts to describe, understand and explain social structure. The visone software is an attempt to integrate analysis and visualization of social networks and is intended to be used in research and teaching. Methods are based on force-directed, spectral, layered, and radial layout methods.

Polyphemus and **Hermes** provide exploration and visualization of computer networks in the context of autonomous systems, i.e., networks under a single administrative authority. Polyphemus implements interaction techniques and algorithms to visually navigate a clustered graph representing an open shortest path first protocol network. Hermes allows users to interactively explore the autonomous system interconnection graph facing the problem to visualize very dense graphs in which vertices may have very high degree.

References

1. Booch, G., Rumbaugh, J., Jacobson, I. (1999) Unified Modeling Language User Guide. Addison Wesley Longman
2. Brandenburg, F.-J. (ed.) Graph Drawing '95. Lecture Notes in Computer Science 1027, Springer-Verlag, 1995
3. Di Battista, G. (ed.) Graph Drawing '97. Lecture Notes in Computer Science 1353, Springer-Verlag, 1997
4. Di Battista, G., Eades, P., Tamassia, R., Tollis, I. G. (1999) Graph Drawing: Algorithms for the visualization of graphs. Prentice Hall, New Jersey

5. Goodrich, M., Kobourov, S. (eds.) Graph Drawing '02. Lecture Notes in Computer Science 2528, Springer-Verlag, 2002
6. Kaufmann, M., Wagner, D. (eds.) Drawing Graphs: Methods and Models. Lecture Notes in Computer Science 2025, Springer-Verlag, 2001
7. Kratochvíl, J. (ed.) Graph Drawing '99. Lecture Notes in Computer Science 1731, Springer-Verlag, 1999
8. Marks, J. (ed.) Graph Drawing '00. Lecture Notes in Computer Science 1984, Springer-Verlag, 2000
9. Mutzel, P, Jünger, M., Leipert, S. (eds.) Graph Drawing '01. Lecture Notes in Computer Science 2265, Springer-Verlag, 2001
10. North, S. (ed.) Graph Drawing '96. Lecture Notes in Computer Science 1190, Springer-Verlag, 1996
11. Purchase, H. (1997) Which aesthetic has the greatest effect on human understanding? In: G. Di Battista (ed.) Graph Drawing '97, Lecture Notes in Computer Science 1353, Springer-Verlag, 248–261
12. Purchase, H., Allder, J.-A., Carrington, D. (2001) User preference of graph layout aesthetics: A UML study. In: J. Marks (ed.) Graph Drawing '00, Lecture Notes in Computer Science 1984, Springer-Verlag, 5–18
13. Rosenstiehl, P., de Fraysseix, H. (eds.) Graph Drawing '93. Abstract Book, 1993, unpublished.
14. Tamassia, R., Tollis, I. G.(eds.) Graph Drawing '94. Lecture Notes in Computer Science 894, Springer-Verlag, 1994
15. TAZ, November 2, 1999, 24
16. Tutte, W.T. (1963) How to draw a graph. Proc. London Math. Society **13**, 743–768
17. Whitesides, S. H. (ed.) Graph Drawing '98. Lecture Notes in Computer Science 1547, Springer-Verlag, 1998

Technical Foundations*

Michael Jünger[1] and Petra Mutzel[2]

[1] University of Cologne, Department of Computer Science, Pohligstraße 1, D-50969 Köln, Germany

[2] Vienna University of Technology, Institute of Computer Graphics and Algorithms, Favoritenstraße 9–11, A-1040 Wien, Austria

1 Introduction

Graph drawing software relies on a variety of mathematical results, mainly in *graph theory*, *topology*, and *geometry*, as well as computer science techniques, mainly in the areas *algorithms and data structures*, *software engineering*, and *user interfaces*. Many of the core techniques used in automatic graph drawing come from the intersection of mathematics and computer science in combinatorial and continuous optimization.

Even though automatic graph drawing is a relatively young scientific field, a few generic approaches have emerged in the graph drawing community. They allow a classification of layout methods so that most software packages implement variations of such approaches.

The purpose of this chapter is to lay the foundations for all subsequent chapters so that they can be read independently from each other while referring back to the common material presented here. This chapter has been written based on the requirements and the contributions of all authors in this book. This chapter is *not* an introduction to automatic graph drawing, because it is neither complete nor balanced. In order to avoid repetitions, we only explain subjects that are basic or used in at least two subsequent chapters. The following chapters contain a lot of additional material. For introductions into the field of automatic graph drawing we recommend the books "Graph Drawing" by Di Battista, Eades, Tamassia, and Tollis [23] and "Drawing Graphs" edited by Kaufmann and Wagner [52]. Nevertheless, this book is self-contained in the sense that after this chapter has been read, every subsequent chapter can be read without referring to external sources.

* We gratefully acknowledge the many contributions of the authors of the subsequent chapters. In particular, Gabriele Barbagallo, Andrea Carmignani, Giuseppe Di Battista, Walter Didimo, Carsten Gutwenger, Sebastian Leipert, Maurizio Patrignani, and Maurizio Pizzonia have contributed text fragments and figures that were very helpful to us. In addition, the constructive remarks on earlier drafts by David Auber, Vladimir Batagelj, Ulrik Brandes, Christoph Buchheim, Tim Dwyer, Michael Kaufmann, Gunnar W. Klau, Stephen C. North, Merijam Percan, Georg Sander, and Ioannis G. Tollis were very helpful for corrections and improvements.

Section 2 contains basic notions and notations from graph theory concerning graphs and their representations including undirected and directed graphs, layered graphs, and hierarchical and clustered graphs. It closes with some remarks on the storage of graphs in computer memory. Section 3 discusses concepts of graph planarity and graph embeddings including planar graphs, upward planarity, and cluster planar graphs. Section 4 introduces generic layout styles: tree-, layered-, planarization-, orthogonal-, and force-directed-layout.

2 Graphs and Their Representation

2.1 Undirected Graphs

A *graph* $G = (V, E, \lambda)$ consists of a finite set $V = V(G)$ of *vertices* or *nodes*, a finite set $E = E(G)$ of *edges*, and a function λ that maps each edge to a subset $V' \subseteq V$ with $|V'| \in \{1, 2\}$. An edge e for which $|\lambda(e)| = 1$ is called a *loop* and if for two edges $e_1, e_2 \in E$ we have $\lambda(e_1) = \lambda(e_2)$ we say that e_1 and e_2 are multi-edges. Figure 1 shows a graph with a loop and a pair of multi-edges.

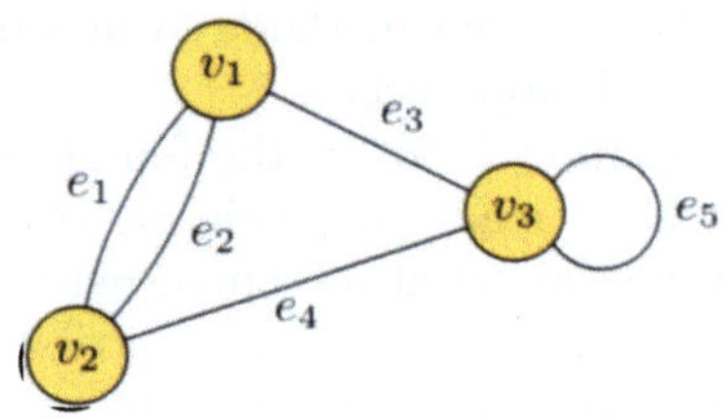

Fig. 1. A graph with a loop and two multi-edges.

A graph with no loops and no multi-edges is characterized by a finite set V of vertices and a finite set $E \subseteq \{\{u, v\} \mid u, v \in V, u \neq v\}$ of edges and called a *simple graph*. In the sequel, we deal mostly (unless stated otherwise) with simple graphs, but non-simple graphs are important in automatic graph drawing and for ease of notation, we use the simplified $G = (V, E)$ notation with the understanding that multi-edges and loops are distinguishable elements of the multi-set E. E.g., for the non-simple graph in Figure 1, the notation $G(V, E, \lambda) = (\{v_1, v_2, v_3\}, \{e_1, e_2, e_3, e_4, e_5\}, \lambda(e_1) = \{v_1, v_2\}, \lambda(e_2) = \{v_1, v_2\}, \lambda(e_3) = \{v_1, v_3\}, \lambda(e_4) = \{v_2, v_3\}, \lambda(e_5) = \{v_3, v_3\})$ becomes simplified to $G(V, E) = (\{v_1, v_2, v_3\}, \{e_1, e_2, e_3, e_4, e_5\}) = (\{v_1, v_2, v_3\}, \{\{v_1, v_2\}, \{v_1, v_2\}, \{v_1, v_3\}, \{v_2, v_3\}, \{v_3, v_3\}\})$.

For an edge $e = \{u, v\}$, the vertices u and v are the *end-vertices* of e, and e is *incident* to u and v. An edge $\{u, v\} \in E$ *connects* the vertices u and v. Two vertices $u, v \in V$ are *adjacent* if $\{u, v\} \in E$. By $\text{star}(v) = \{e \in E \mid v \in e\}$ we denote the set of edges incident to a vertex $v \in V$ and $\text{adj}(v) = \{u \in V \mid$

$\{u, v\} \in E\}$ is the set of vertices adjacent to a vertex $v \in V$. By $\deg(v) = |\operatorname{star}(v)| + |\operatorname{loop}(v)|$, where $\operatorname{loop}(v)$ is the set of edges of the form $\{v, v\}$, we denote the *degree* of a vertex $v \in V$, $\operatorname{mindeg}(G) = \min\{\deg(v) \mid v \in V\}$ is the *minimum degree* and $\operatorname{maxdeg}(G) = \max\{\deg(v) \mid v \in V\}$ is the *maximum degree* of G. E.g., in Figure 1, $\operatorname{star}(v_1) = \{e_1, e_2, e_3\}$, $\operatorname{star}(v_3) = \{e_3, e_4, e_5\}$, whereas $\operatorname{adj}(v_1) = \{v_2, v_3\}$ and $\operatorname{adj}(v_3) = \{v_1, v_2, v_3\}$. The degrees of these two vertices are $\deg(v_1) = 3$ and $\deg(v_3) = 4$, the minimal degree of the graph is $\operatorname{mindeg}(G) = 3$ and the maximum degree is $\operatorname{maxdeg}(G) = 4$. A vertex v with $\deg(v) = 0$ is called an *isolated vertex*.

For $W \subseteq V$ let $E[W] = \{\{u, v\} \in E \mid u, v \in W\}$ and for $F \subseteq E$ let $V[F] = \{v \in V \mid v \in e \text{ for some } e \in F\}$. A graph $G' = (V', E')$ is a *subgraph* of $G = (V, E)$ or *contained* in G if $V' \subseteq V$ and $E' \subseteq E$. For a vertex set $W \subseteq V$ we call $G[W] = (W, E[W])$ a *vertex-induced subgraph* of G and for an edge set $F \subseteq E$ we call $G[F] = (V[F], F)$ an *edge-induced subgraph* of G.

A *walk* W of *length* k in a graph G is an alternating sequence of vertices and edges $v_0, e_1, v_1, e_2, v_2, \ldots, e_k, v_k$, *beginning* and *ending* with the vertices v_0 and v_k, respectively, and $e_i = \{v_{i-1}, v_i\}$ for $i = 1, 2, \ldots, k$. This walk *connects* v_0 and v_k and may also be denoted by $W = (v_0, v_1, \ldots, v_k)$, when the edges are evident by context. A walk W is called a *path* if all vertices are distinct, and it is called a *trail* if all edges are distinct. The *distance* of two vertices u and v in $G = (V, E)$, denoted by $\operatorname{dist}(u, v)$, is the number of edges in a shortest path connecting u and v in G, and the *diameter* of G is defined by $\operatorname{diam}(G) = \max\{\operatorname{dist}(u, v) \mid u, v \in V\}$. A walk is called a *cycle* if all vertices are distinct except for $v_0 = v_k$ and $k \geq 2$. A graph that does not have any cycles is called a *forest*.

A graph G is *connected* if every pair of vertices is connected by a path, otherwise it is called *disconnected*. A *component* of G is a maximal connected subgraph of G. Thus a disconnected graph has at least two components. A connected forest G is called a *tree*.

A graph $G = (V, E)$ is *k-connected* if at least k vertices must be removed from V in order to make the resulting vertex-induced subgraph disconnected. By $\kappa(G) = \max\{k \mid G \text{ is } k\text{-connected}\}$ we denote the *(vertex-)connectivity* of G.

Of special interest in automatic graph drawing are 1, 2, and 3-connected graphs, also called *connected*, *biconnected*, and *triconnected* graphs, respectively. A vertex whose removal disconnects the graph is called a *cut-vertex*, i.e., a graph is biconnected if it has no cut-vertex. The maximal biconnected components of a graph G are called the *blocks* of G. The blocks intersect in cut-vertices, see Figure 2 for an illustration.

Two vertices whose removal disconnects a biconnected graph are called a *separating vertex pair*, i.e., a graph is triconnected if it has no separating vertex pair.

An edge whose removal disconnects the graph is called a *bridge*. The graph in Figure 2 contains exactly one bridge.

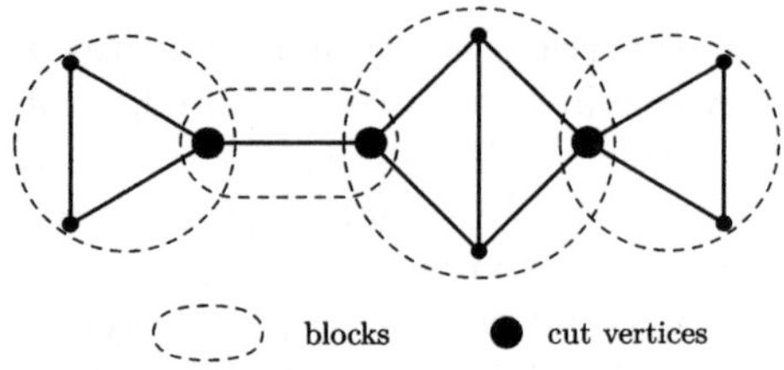

Fig. 2. The cut-vertices and the blocks of a graph.

A graph $G = (V, E)$ is *k-edge-connected* if at least k edges must be removed from E in order to make the resulting edge-induced subgraph disconnected. By $\lambda(G) = \max\{k \mid G \text{ is } k\text{-edge-connected}\}$ we denote the *edge-connectivity* of G.

A *vertex-k-coloring* of a loop-less graph $G = (V, E)$ is an assignment $c : V \to \{1, 2, \ldots, k\}$ such that $c(u) \neq c(v)$ whenever $\{u, v\} \in E$. By $\chi(G) = \min\{k \mid G \text{ has a vertex-}k\text{-coloring}\}$ we denote the *chromatic number* of G. Graphs G with $\chi(G) \leq 2$ are called *bipartite graphs*. Their vertex set can be partitioned into two subsets (corresponding to the two color classes, one of them possibly empty) such that all edges connect vertices of different subsets of the bipartition. A graph is bipartite if and only if it does not contain a cycle of odd length.

2.2 Directed Graphs

A *directed graph* or *digraph* $G = (V, E)$ consists of a finite set $V = V(G)$ of *vertices* and a finite multi-set $E \subseteq V \times V = \{(u, v) \mid u, v \in V\}$ of (*directed*) *edges* or *arcs* that are ordered pairs of vertices. Ignoring for every edge the order of its vertices, we get an undirected graph that is called the *underlying graph* of G. Thus, concepts like subgraph, walk, path, trail, cycle, forest, component, or tree, naturally carry over to directed graphs. In addition, for a *directed walk* we require that the involved edges are ordered pairs (v_{i-1}, v_i) and so we get *directed trails*, *directed paths*, and *directed cycles*. If a digraph $G = (V, E)$ is *simple*, i.e., contains no loops or multi-arcs, it determines a relation $R \subseteq V \times V$ defined by $uRv \iff (u, v) \in E$.

A digraph G is *strongly connected* if each pair of vertices $u, v \in V$ is connected by a directed path from u to v. An *acyclic digraph (directed acyclic graph: dag)* is a digraph with no directed cycle or loop. If $e = (u, v)$ then e is an *outgoing* or *leaving* edge of u and an *incoming* or *entering* edge of v. By $\text{instar}(v) = \{(u, v) \in E \mid u \in V\}$ we denote the set of incoming edges of a vertex $v \in V$ and by $\text{outstar}(v) = \{(v, u) \in E \mid u \in V\}$ we denote the set of outgoing edges of a vertex $v \in V$. Accordingly, we define $\text{inadj}(v) = \{u \in V \mid (u, v) \in E\}$ and $\text{outadj}(v) = \{u \in V \mid (v, u) \in E\}$. Then $\text{indeg}(v) = |\,\text{instar}(v)|$ is the *in-degree* and $\text{outdeg}(v) = |\,\text{outstar}(v)|$ is the *out-degree* of a vertex $v \in V$.

A *source* is a vertex with no incoming edges and a *sink* is a vertex with no outgoing edges. An acyclic digraph G with exactly one source is called a *single source directed graph* digraph. If, in addition, its underlying graph is connected and has no loop and no (undirected) cycle, the graph is called a *rooted tree* whose *root* is the only vertex $v = \text{root}(T) \in V$ with $\text{indeg}(v) = 0$ and whose *leaves* are vertices $v \in V$ with $\text{outdeg}(v) = 0$. The *depth* $\text{depth}(v)$ of a vertex v in a rooted tree $T = (V, E)$ is the length of the (unique) directed path from the root of T to v. All vertices of depth k constitute *tree level* k. Furthermore, for each $v \in V$ that is not a leaf, the vertices in $\text{outadj}(v)$ are called *children* of v, and for each $v \in V$ other than the root, the vertex in $\text{inadj}(v)$ is called *parent* of v. Children of the same parent are called *siblings*. An acyclic digraph with exactly one sink is called a *single sink* digraph. An acyclic digraph with exactly one source s and exactly one sink t and an edge (s, t) is called an *st-digraph*.

A *topological numbering* of G is an assignment of numbers $\text{topnumber}(v)$ to the vertices v of G such that for every edge (u, v) of G the number assigned to v is greater than the one assigned to u (i.e., $\text{topnumber}(v) > \text{topnumber}(u)$). A *topological sorting* of G is a topological numbering of G such that every vertex is assigned a distinct integer between 1 and $|V|$. It is easy to see that G admits a topological numbering or sorting if and only if G is acyclic.

2.3 Representation of Graphs

There are several ways to represent an (undirected or directed) graph. Here, we restrict our attention to the classical representation in graph drawing. A graph $G = (V, E)$ is generally visualized by a *drawing* in 2 or 3-dimensional space with the vertices drawn as points or boxes of a pre-specified width and height, and the edges drawn as closed Jordan curves, connecting their incident vertices. Layouts in which the coordinates of the vertex representations are restricted to integer values are called *grid layouts*.

In this book, we describe software for generating graph drawings in 2 or 3-dimensional space. In this chapter, however, we restrict our attention mainly to drawings in 2-dimensional space.

2.4 Layered Graphs

Let $\langle L_1, L_2, \ldots, L_h \rangle$ denote an ordered set of elements, called the *layers* of the graph. A *layered graph* $H = (G, \Lambda)$ consists of a (directed or undirected) graph $G = (V, E)$ and a function $\Lambda : V \to \langle L_1, L_2, \ldots, L_h \rangle$ assigning each vertex $v \in V$ to exactly one layer L_i, $i \in \{1, \ldots, h\}$.

Layered graphs are often represented "top-to-bottom" as follows: For $i = 1, \ldots, h$, the vertices belonging to layer L_i are drawn on a horizontal line with y-coordinate y_i, satisfying the condition $y_1 > y_2 > \cdots > y_h$. A popular alternative is a "left-to-right" representation with vertical lines at x_i and $x_1 < x_2 < \cdots < x_h$.

In graph drawing, layered graphs occur in the context of directed acyclic graphs. For these graphs, a layering is generated based on a topological numbering, i.e., the function Λ satisfies $\Lambda(v) > \Lambda(u)$ for each edge $(u, v) \in E$. In this context it is common to draw all the edges as curves monotonically decreasing in vertical direction in a top-to-bottom representation and monotonically increasing in horizontal direction in a left-to-right representation.

2.5 Clustered Graphs

Clustered graphs are graphs with recursive clustering structures over the vertices. A *clustered graph* $C = (G, T)$ consists of an undirected graph $G = (V, E)$ and a rooted tree T such that the leaves of T are exactly the vertices of G. Each vertex ν of T represents a *cluster* $V(\nu)$ of the vertices of G that are the leaves of the subtree rooted at ν. The root of T is called *root cluster*. The tree T is called the *inclusion tree* of C because it describes an inclusion relation between clusters. The graph G is called the *underlying graph* of C. The tree $T(\nu)$ represents the subtree of T rooted at the vertex ν, and $G(\nu)$ denotes the subgraph of G induced by the cluster associated with vertex ν. We define $C(\nu) = (G(\nu), T(\nu))$ to be the *sub-clustered graph* associated with vertex ν. An edge $\{v, w\} \in E$ with $v \in V(G(\nu))$ and $w \in V \setminus V(G(\nu))$ is said to be *incident* to cluster ν. Figure 3 shows a drawing of a clustered graph $C = (G, T)$ and the corresponding tree T.

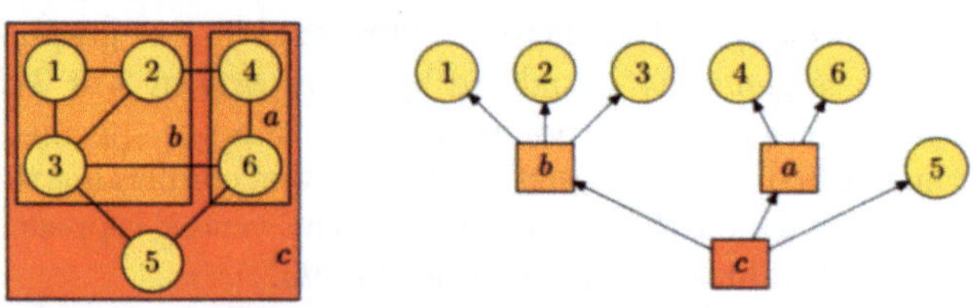

Fig. 3. A drawing of a clustered graph and its defining tree.

In a *drawing of a clustered graph* $C = (G, T)$, the graph G is drawn with points and curves as usual. For each vertex ν of T, the cluster is drawn as a simple closed region R (i.e., a region without holes) that contains the drawing of $V(G(\nu))$, such that the following three conditions hold.

(i) The regions for all sub-clusters of ν are completely contained in the interior of R.
(ii) The regions for all other clusters are completely contained in the exterior of R.
(iii) If there is an edge e between two vertices of $V(\nu)$ then the drawing of e is completely contained in R.

2.6 Compound Graphs

Compound graphs have been introduced for representing graphs with both inclusion and adjacency relationships [63]. A *compound graph* $C = (G, T)$ is defined as an (undirected or directed) graph $G = (V, E_G)$ and a rooted tree $T = (V, E_T)$ that share the same vertex set V. There is a one to one correspondence between the structure of the tree and the set of inclusions between the vertices, namely, a vertex u is in direct inclusion relation to v if and only if u is a child of v in the tree. If the end-vertices u and v of all edges $\{u, v\} \in E_G$ belong to different root-leaf paths in T, C is called a *simple compound graph*. In a simple compound graph, a pair of vertices (u, v) cannot be in an adjacency and in an inclusion relation at the same time. Figure 4 shows an example of a simple compound graph.

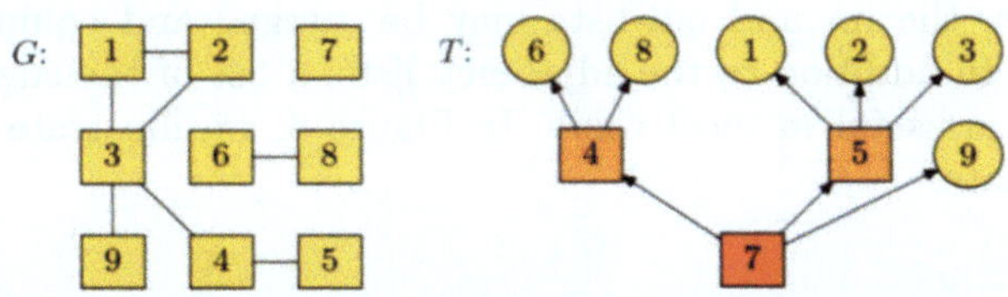

Fig. 4. A compound graph defined by a graph and a tree.

Edges connecting vertices of different tree levels are called *inter-level edges*. If a compound graph does not contain inter-level edges, we call it a *nested graph*.

A further restriction allowing only edges between the leaves of the tree leads to an alternative definition of clustered graphs (see Section 2.5).

In a *drawing of a compound graph* $C = (G, T)$, the vertices of the graph G are drawn as closed regions so that a vertex u is included in the region representing the vertex parent(u) in T, and the edges in E_G are drawn as curves connecting the regions associated with its end-vertices. Figure 5 shows a drawing of the compound graph defined in Figure 4.

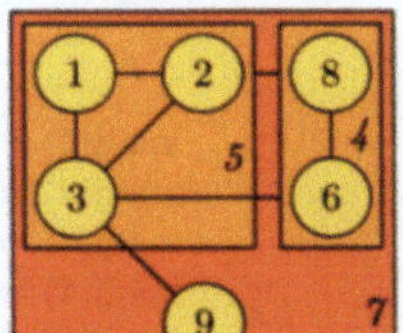

Fig. 5. A drawing of the compound graph defined in Figure 4.

2.7 Storage of Graphs and Digraphs

Common data structures for storing graphs and digraphs $G = (V, E)$ are adjacency matrices and adjacency lists. An *adjacency matrix* for an undirected graph is a $|V|$ by $|V|$ matrix $A(G) = (a_{uv})_{u,v \in V}$ where a_{uv} is the number of edges connecting the vertices u and v, i.e., $a_{uv} \in \{0, 1\}$ for simple graphs. For a digraph, a_{uv} is the number of edges leaving u and entering v, again, $a_{uv} \in \{0, 1\}$ for simple digraphs. Adjacency matrices are, due to their storage requirement of $|V|^2$, independently of $|E|$, unattractive for *sparse graphs*, i.e., graphs in which E contains only a small subset of all possible edges.

In automatic graph drawing, usually sparse graphs are considered. In fact, we often have $|E| \leq c|V|$ for some constant c. Therefore a different data structure is usually more appropriate. Most common are *star*- and/or *adjacency-lists* that give (in-/out-)star(v) and/or (in-/out-)adj(v) for each $v \in V$ as linear, linked, or doubly linked lists, depending on the application. For digraphs, the in- and out-lists may be merged and equipped with an in-/out-flag. In addition to the adjacency lists, a list of the edges with their end-vertices is useful in most cases. In Figure 6, we illustrate the different storage formats.

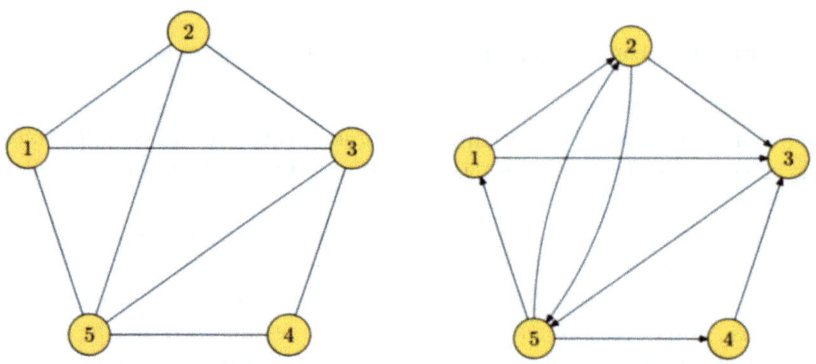

Adjacency matrix

$$\begin{array}{c|ccccc} & 1 & 2 & 3 & 4 & 5 \\ \hline 1 & 0 & 1 & 1 & 0 & 1 \\ 2 & 1 & 0 & 1 & 0 & 1 \\ 3 & 1 & 1 & 0 & 1 & 1 \\ 4 & 0 & 0 & 1 & 0 & 1 \\ 5 & 1 & 1 & 1 & 1 & 0 \end{array}$$

Adjacency lists

adj(1) = $\langle 2, 3, 5 \rangle$
adj(2) = $\langle 3, 5, 1 \rangle$
adj(3) = $\langle 4, 5, 1, 2 \rangle$
adj(4) = $\langle 5, 3 \rangle$
adj(5) = $\langle 1, 2, 3, 4 \rangle$

Adjacency matrix

$$\begin{array}{c|ccccc} & 1 & 2 & 3 & 4 & 5 \\ \hline 1 & 0 & 1 & 1 & 0 & 0 \\ 2 & 0 & 0 & 1 & 0 & 1 \\ 3 & 0 & 0 & 0 & 0 & 1 \\ 4 & 0 & 0 & 1 & 0 & 0 \\ 5 & 1 & 1 & 0 & 1 & 0 \end{array}$$

Adjacency lists

inadj(1) = $\langle 5 \rangle$ outadj(1) = $\langle 2, 3 \rangle$
inadj(2) = $\langle 1, 5 \rangle$ outadj(2) = $\langle 5, 3 \rangle$
inadj(3) = $\langle 2, 1, 4 \rangle$ outadj(3) = $\langle 5 \rangle$
inadj(4) = $\langle 5 \rangle$ outadj(4) = $\langle 3 \rangle$
inadj(5) = $\langle 2, 3 \rangle$ outadj(5) = $\langle 1, 2, 4 \rangle$

Fig. 6. Storage of graphs and digraphs.

3 Graph Planarity and Embeddings

This section deals with drawings and embeddings of a graph onto the plane unless otherwise stated. A drawing of a graph G on the plane yields an *embedding* Π of G, i.e., a clockwise ordering of the incident edges for every vertex with respect to the drawing. Such an embedding can be conveniently stored by ordering the star- or adjacency-lists of Section 2.7 accordingly.

3.1 Planar Graphs

A graph $G = (V, E)$ is called *planar* if it can be drawn in the plane such that no two edges cross each other except at common endpoints. An intersection of two edges in a drawing other than at their endpoints is called a *crossing*. A *planar* or *combinatorial embedding* Π of a planar graph G is an embedding with respect to a planar drawing. A graph with a given fixed planar embedding Π is also called a *plane graph*. Given a drawing of a plane graph G, a *face* of G is a topologically connected region in the drawing bounded by the (Jordan curves corresponding to the) edges of G. A face of a plane graph is uniquely described by its boundary edges. The degree $\deg(f)$ of a face f is defined as the number of its boundary edges, where each boundary edge with both sides on the boundary of f is counted twice. The faces of a plane graph are already described by the planar embedding. Two faces are *adjacent* if their boundaries share an edge. The one unbounded face of a plane graph is called the *outer face* or *exterior face*. All other faces are called *interior faces*. An equivalent definition of a planar embedding is an ordered list of the boundary edges for each face, clockwise for interior faces and counter-clockwise for the exterior face.

A famous result of Euler [34] for polytopes relates the number of vertices, edges, and faces in any planar embedding of a connected planar graph:

Theorem 1 (Euler's Formula [34]). *Let Π be a planar embedding of a connected planar graph $G = (V, E)$ and let F be the set of faces in Π. Then $|V| - |E| + |F| = 2$.*

From Euler's formula, an upper bound on the number of edges of a planar graph with a given number of vertices is easily derived:

Theorem 2. *For any simple planar graph $G = (V, E)$ with at least 3 vertices we have $|E| \leq 3|V| - 6$.*

The bound is attained for *triangulated* planar graphs, i.e., planar graphs in which every face is a triangle.

While, in general, the number of different planar embeddings of a planar graph is exponential in $|V|$, a triconnected planar graph has only two different planar embeddings, which are mirror-images of each other, see Figures 7 and 8 for illustrations.

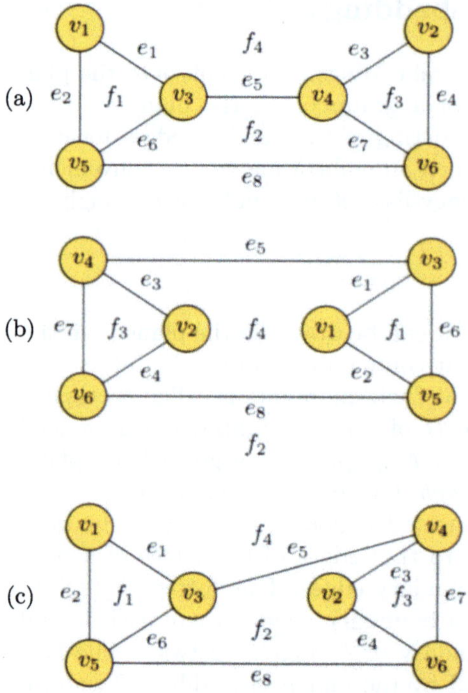

planar embedding

v_1: $\langle v_3, v_5 \rangle$ f_1: $\langle e_1, e_6, e_2 \rangle$
v_2: $\langle v_4, v_6 \rangle$ f_2: $\langle e_6, e_5, e_7, e_8 \rangle$
v_3: $\langle v_1, v_4, v_5 \rangle$ f_3: $\langle e_3, e_4, e_7 \rangle$
v_4: $\langle v_2, v_6, v_3 \rangle$ f_4: $\langle e_1, e_2, e_8, e_4, e_3, e_5 \rangle$
v_5: $\langle v_1, v_3, v_6 \rangle$
v_6: $\langle v_2, v_5, v_4 \rangle$

same planar embedding as (a), i.e., combinatorially equivalent to (a)

different planar embedding

v_1: $\langle v_3, v_5 \rangle$ f_1: $\langle e_1, e_6, e_2 \rangle$
v_2: $\langle v_4, v_6 \rangle$ f_2: $\langle e_3, e_4, e_8, e_6, e_5 \rangle$
v_3: $\langle v_1, v_4, v_5 \rangle$ f_3: $\langle e_4, e_3, e_7 \rangle$
v_4: $\langle v_2, v_3, v_6 \rangle$ f_4: $\langle e_1, e_2, e_8, e_7, e_5 \rangle$
v_5: $\langle v_1, v_3, v_6 \rangle$
v_6: $\langle v_2, v_4, v_5 \rangle$

Fig. 7. Combinatorial embeddings.

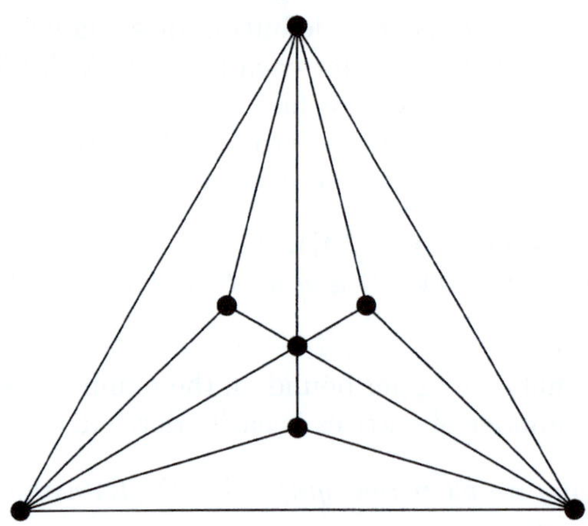

$|V| = 7, \quad |E| = 3|V| - 6 = 15$

Fig. 8. A triconnected graph has a unique embedding up to reflection.

Given a planar embedding $\Pi(G)$ of a planar graph $G = (V, E)$ with face set F, the *dual graph* $G' = (V', E')$ is constructed as follows: $V' = F$ and E' contains an edge $\{f_i, f_j\}$ for each $e \in E$ such that e is on the boundary of both f_i and f_j. (f_i and f_j may be identical.) By definition, the degree $\deg(f)$ of a face f of G agrees with the degree of f as a vertex of G'. The dual graph of a planar graph is in general a non-simple graph (i.e., contains loops and multi-edges) as can be seen in the example shown in Figure 9. Loops in G' correspond to bridges in G.

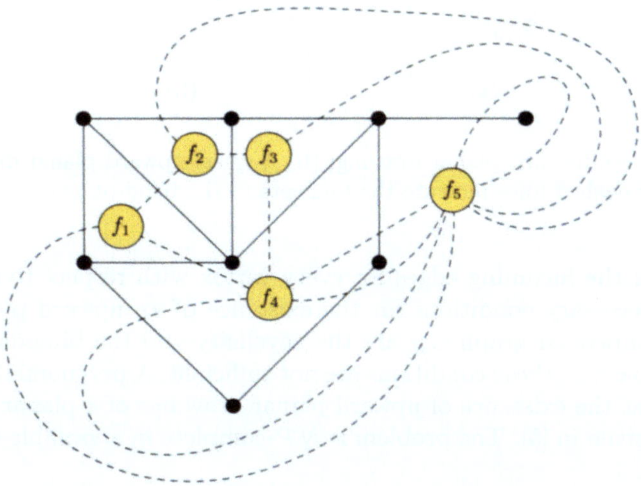

f_5 has a loop and there are three copies of $\{f_4, f_5\}$

Fig. 9. A planar graph and its non-simple dual graph.

Planarity of a graph $G = (V, E)$ can be tested in $O(|V|)$ time by, e.g., the algorithm of Hopcroft and Tarjan [45], or an approach of Lempel *et al.* [55] using the special data structure PQ-tree introduced by Booth and Lueker [7]. For a planar graph G, an embedding Π of G can be determined in linear time by, e.g., the algorithms of Chiba *et al.* [17] or Mehlhorn and Mutzel [57].

3.2 Upward Planarity

Let G be an embedded digraph. A vertex v of G is called *bimodal* if the circular list of the edges incident to v can be partitioned into two (possibly empty) linear lists of edges, one consisting of the incoming edges and the other consisting of the outgoing edges. An embedding is called a *bimodal embedding* if every vertex is bimodal. A planar graph is said to be *bimodal* if it admits a planar bimodal embedding.

A drawing of G such that all the edges are curves monotonically increasing in a given direction is known as an *upward drawing*. Figure 10(a) shows an example of an upward planar drawing in the left-to-right direction. An *upward embedding* $\mathcal{U}$ is a representation of G that consists of the clockwise

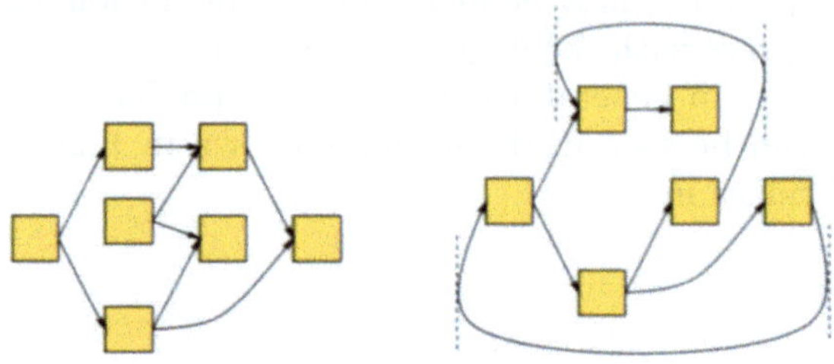

(a) (b)

Fig. 10. (a) An upward planar drawing; (b) A quasi-upward planar drawing with 4 bends; the dashed lines indicate the tangents to the bend-points.

orderings of the incoming edges for every vertex with respect to an upward drawing. Necessary conditions for the existence of an upward planar drawing of an embedded graph G_Π are the acyclicity and the bimodality of G_Π itself [5]. However, these conditions are not sufficient. A polynomial time algorithm to test the existence of upward planar drawings of a planar embedded digraph is given in [5]. The problem is $\mathcal{NP}$-complete in a variable embedding setting [41].

The quasi-upward drawing convention extends the upward drawing convention [3]. A *quasi-upward drawing* of a digraph in the left-to-right direction is such that the vertical line through each vertex v "locally" splits the incoming edges from the outgoing edges of v. The term locally is used to identify a sufficiently small connected region properly containing v.

A *bend* of a quasi-upward drawing in the left-to-right direction is a point on an edge such that the vertical line through this point is tangent to the edge. Intuitively, a bend is a point in which an edge inverts its left-to-right direction. In Figure 10(b) a quasi-upward planar drawing with four bends is shown. In [3] it is proven that a quasi-upward planar drawing of a digraph exists if and only if the digraph is planar bimodal, and a polynomial time algorithm for computing quasi-upward planar drawings with the minimum number of bends of an embedded bimodal digraph is described.

A directed acyclic graph $G = (V, E)$ is called *upward planar* if it has an upward drawing without edge crossings. An *upward planar embedding* is an upward embedding with respect to an upward planar drawing.

Upward planarity testing of directed acyclic graphs is $\mathcal{NP}$-complete as has been shown by Garg and Tamassia [41]. Acyclic digraphs with a single source can be tested for upward planarity:

Theorem 3 (Bertolazzi *et al.* [6]). *There is an $O(|V|)$ time algorithm using SPQR-trees to test whether a single source acyclic digraph $G = (V, E)$ is upward planar, and if so, it outputs an upward planar embedding.*

3.3 Cluster Planarity

In Section 2.5 we have already discussed clustered graphs and their representation. Here, we adapt the concept of planarity to clustered graphs.

In a drawing of a clustered graph, an edge e and a region R have an *edge-region crossing* if the drawing of e crosses the boundary of R more than once. A drawing of a clustered graph is *c-planar* if there are no edge crossings or edge-region crossings. A graph that admits a c-planar drawing is called *c-planar*. Notice that the planarity of the underlying graph does not imply the existence of a c-planar drawing of a clustered graph, see Figure 11.

A c-planar drawing of C induces a c-planar embedding. A *c-planar embedding* of C fixes the planar embedding of the underlying graph G and contains the circular ordering of all edges crossing the boundary of each non-trivial cluster region.

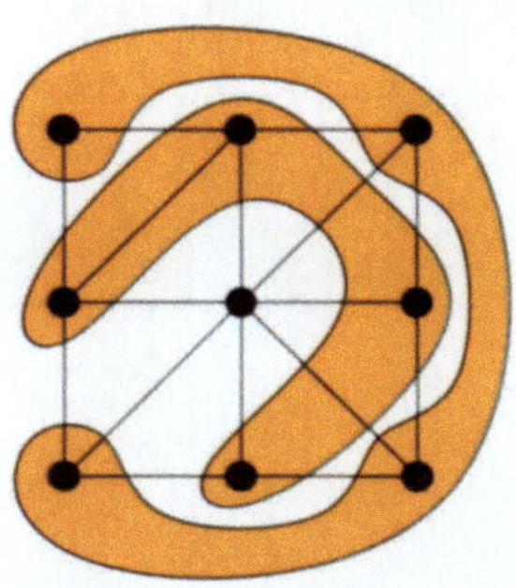

Fig. 11. A clustered graph that is not c-planar.

Unfortunately, so far no polynomial time algorithm is known for c-planarity testing. However, c-planarity can be tested for a subclass of clustered graphs. A clustered graph $C = (G, T)$ is called *c-connected* if each cluster induces a connected subgraph of G.

Theorem 4 (Feng *et al.* [35], Dahlhaus [21]). *The c-planarity of a c-connected clustered graph $C = (G, T)$ can be tested in linear time.*

The algorithm of [35] is based on the following theorem that gives a necessary and sufficient condition for c-planarity of c-connected graphs.

Theorem 5 (Feng *et al.* [35]). *A c-connected clustered graph $C = (G, T)$ is c-planar if and only if G is planar, and there exists a planar drawing of G such that for each vertex ν of T, all vertices and edges of $G \setminus G(\nu)$ are in the outer face of the drawing of $G(\nu)$.*

4 Graph Drawing Methods

4.1 Tree Layout

In automatic graph drawing, the notion "Tree Layout" refers to drawing rooted trees. Before a general (undirected) tree can be processed, a root must be chosen and all edges must be directed away from the root. Forests are processed by drawing each connected component separately. Since for a tree $T = (V, E)$, we have $|E| = |V| - 1$, running times are given as functions of $|V|$. For a typical tree layout, see Figure 12.

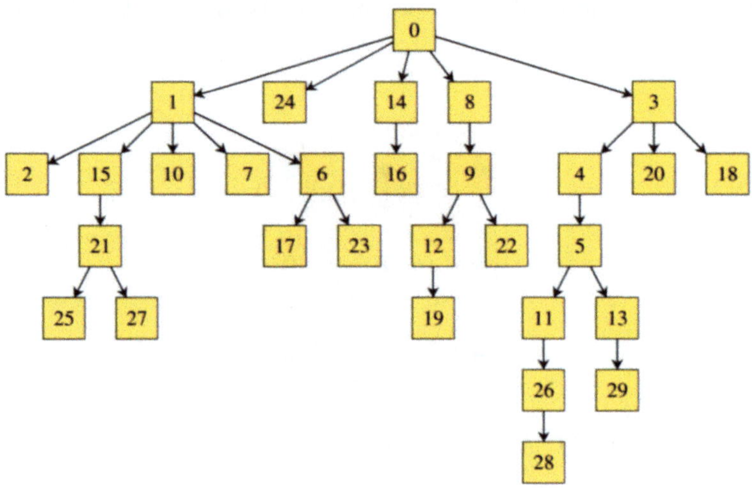

Fig. 12. A typical tree layout.

We start by treating an important special case, namely *binary trees*, in which each vertex has 0, 1, or 2 children. If a vertex has two children, one is a *left* and the other is a *right* child, and if it has one child, this is either a left or a right child. We describe a beautiful $O(|V|)$ algorithm of Reingold and Tilford [60] whose grid layout satisfies the following æsthetic criteria:

(A1) All vertices $v \in V$ of the same depth are drawn on a straight horizontal line whose y-coordinate is $-\operatorname{depth}(v)$.
(A2) A left child is placed to the left (smaller x-coordinate), a right child is placed to the right (bigger x-coordinate) of its parent.
(A3) If a parent has two children, it is centered above its children.
(A4) A tree and its mirror image are drawn identically up to reflection.
(A5) Isomorphic subtrees are drawn identically up to translation.

For a vertex $v \in V$ let $T_l(v)$ be the subtree rooted at the left child of v, if it exists, else $T_l(v) = (\emptyset, \emptyset)$, and let $T_r(v)$ be the subtree rooted at the right child of v, if it exists, else $T_r(v) = (\emptyset, \emptyset)$. Basic traversal orders for the vertices of a binary tree $T = (V, E)$ are defined by the following recursive functions:

```
preorder(T)
{
  if V(T) ≠ ∅  {
    v = root(T);
    visit(v);
    preorder(T_l(v));
    preorder(T_r(v));
  }
}

inorder(T)
{
  if V(T) ≠ ∅  {
    v = root(T);
    inorder(T_l(v));
    visit(v);
    inorder(T_r(v));
  }
}

postorder(T)
{
  if V(T) ≠ ∅  {
    v = root(T);
    postorder(T_l(v));
    postorder(T_r(v));
    visit(v);
  }
}
```

The algorithm of Reingold and Tilford follows the divide and conquer principle implemented in the form of a postorder traversal of $T = (V, E)$. Namely, for each $v \in V$ the algorithm computes layouts for $T_l(v)$ and $T_r(v)$ up to horizontal translation, and when v is visited, the two drawings are horizontally shifted together up to a minimum vertex separation of 2 or 3 grid points so that v can be centered above the roots of $T_l(v)$ and $T_r(v)$ at an integer grid coordinate. If one of $T_l(v)$ and $T_r(v)$ is empty, v is placed one grid unit to the left or right, respectively, of the root of the other.

For a tree T, the left contour of T consists of the vertices with minimum x-coordinate at each depth in the tree, and the right contour is defined analogously. The contour information can be stored and updated efficiently with additional flags at each vertex. Whenever the subtrees $T_l(v)$ and $T_r(v)$ are shifted together, the amount of shift is calculated by traversing the right contour of $T_l(v)$ and the left contour of $T_r(v)$ in order to determine the first point of contact. See Figure 13 for an illustration.

Linear running time is achieved by delaying all shifts of subtrees to a second phase. Rather than performing the shifts directly, the necessary displacements for subtrees are stored at their respective roots. In a second phase, this information is processed in a preorder traversal of T in order to compute the final x-coordinates of all vertices.

While the Reingold-Tilford algorithm is very efficient and delivers æsthetically pleasing drawings, the width of the drawing may be arbitrarily far from the minimum width subject to the five æsthetic criteria, more precisely, there is a family of binary trees $T = (V, E)$ that can be drawn on a grid of width 2, yet the Reingold-Tilford algorithm delivers a drawing of width $(|V| + 2)/3$. It has been shown by Supowit and Reingold [65] that achieving minimum grid width is $\mathcal{NP}$-hard, and, even worse, that, unless $\mathcal{P} = \mathcal{NP}$, there is no polynomial time algorithm for achieving a width that is smaller than $\frac{25}{24}$ times the minimum width. On the other hand, if continuous coordinates (rather

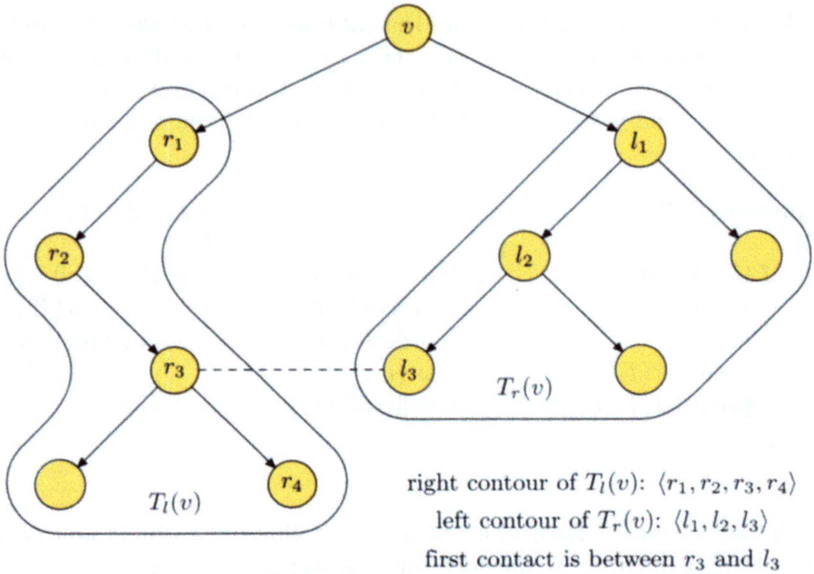

Fig. 13. The Reingold-Tilford algorithm for binary tree drawing.

than integral grid coordinates) are allowed, Supowit and Reingold [65] have shown that minimum width drawings can be found with the help of a linear programming technique in polynomial time.

In practice, the Reingold-Tilford algorithm is generally accepted as the method of choice for drawing binary trees. Walker [70] has generalized this algorithm to general rooted trees, and Buchheim *et al.* [15] have improved the running time of Walker's algorithm to $O(|V|)$ time. An easy modification involving basic trigonometry allows for planar tree drawings in which the vertices are placed on concentric circles around the root rather than on parallel lines, see Eades [29].

4.2 Layered Layout

In the previous section, we have already seen a special case of layered layout: all vertices of a rooted tree $T = (V, E)$ were drawn on parallel horizontal lines, i.e., assigned to parallel horizontal layers, and all directed tree edges $(u, v) \in E$ were drawn as straight lines between two consecutive layers such that the y-coordinate of u was one grid unit bigger than the y-coordinate of v. Conceptually, this drawing style easily extends to general acyclic digraphs $G = (V, E)$ by stipulating that, again, all vertices are drawn on parallel horizontal lines such that for each directed edge $(u, v) \in E$ the y-coordinate of u is bigger than the y-coordinate of v. This idea has been worked out in an automatic graph drawing cornerstone paper by Sugiyama *et al.* [62]. Therefore, this drawing style is commonly referred to as *Sugiyama-style layout*, see Figure 14 for a typical Sugiyama-style layout on five layers.

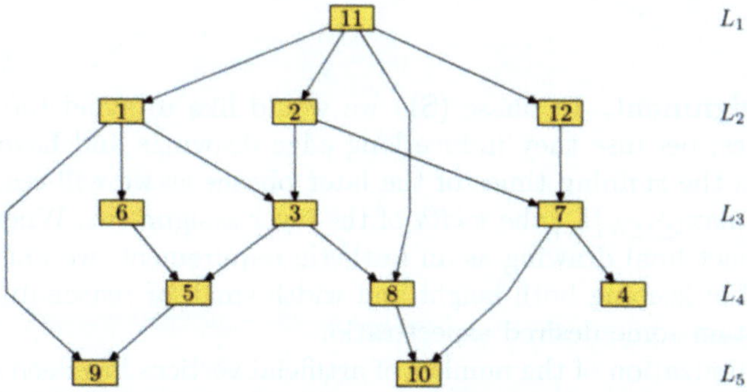

Fig. 14. A typical Sugiyama-style layout.

The great popularity of Sugiyama-style layout is boosted by the fact that any directed or undirected graph can be converted into an acyclic digraph either by reversing directed edges in the case of a digraph or assigning appropriate directions to the edges in the case of an undirected graph. We will first describe layered layout for acyclic digraphs and then discuss the conversion of any graph into an acyclic digraph.

Sugiyama-style layout for an acyclic digraph $G = (V, E)$ decomposes into three phases:

(S1) **Layer Assignment:** Compute a layering of the graph via a topological numbering (see Section 2.4). I.e., assign all vertices to disjoint nonempty subsets $L_1, L_2, \ldots, L_h$ of V called *layers* such that for each edge (u, v) the following holds: If the end-vertex u is assigned to layer L_i and the end-vertex v is assigned to layer L_j then $j > i$. If $j > i+1$, i.e., the edge traverses intermediate layers, we call e a *long* edge and replace it by a directed path from u to v with $j - i - 1$ artificial intermediate vertices for each traversed layer. In Figure 14, the artificial vertices coïncide with the edge bends.

(S2) **Crossing Minimization:** For each layer L, determine permutations of the vertices in L with the goal of obtaining few crossings under the following assumptions: (1) The layers are parallel horizontal lines. (2) Each vertex is drawn on the line corresponding to its layer with x-coordinate compatible with its position in the layer permutation. (3) All edges are drawn as straight line segments between consecutive layers.

(S3) **Coordinate Assignment:** Turn the topological layout of (S2) into a geometric layout by assigning to each $v \in V$ the y-coordinate $-i$ if $v \in L_i$ and an x-coordinate compatible with the vertex permutation of L_i. Finally, suppress the artificial vertices in the drawing.

For each of the three phases, there is a variety of possibilities for implementation. We restrict ourselves to complexity considerations and the discussion of a selection of ideas that are widely used in the practice of automatic graph drawing.

Layer Assignment. In phase (S1) we would like to avoid too many artificial vertices, because they induce long edge drawings and have a negative influence on the running times of the later phases as we will see. Call h the *height* and $\max_{1 \le i \le h} |L_i|$ the *width* of the layer assignment. When we postulate a compact final drawing as an æsthetic requirement, we must deal with the tradeoff of keeping both height and width small or reasonably related in order to obtain some desired aspect ratio.

The minimization of the number of artificial vertices has been successfully addressed by Gansner *et al.* [40]. If y_v denotes the vertical coordinate of vertex $v \in V$, then the problem can be formulated as the integer linear programming problem

$$\begin{aligned} \text{minimize} \sum_{(u,v) \in E} y_u - y_v & \\ \text{subject to } y_u - y_v \ge 1 & \text{ for all } (u,v) \in E \\ y_v \ge 0 & \text{ and integral for all } v \in V \end{aligned}$$

that can be solved efficiently in polynomial time with network flow techniques. (For network flow algorithms, see, e.g., Cook *et al.* [18].)

It is quite simple to compute a layer assignment with minimum height by observing that the length of a longest directed path in G is a lower bound on the height of the layer assignment, and that an easy modification of a topological sorting algorithm, called *longest path layering* can be used to find a layer assignment with this height. The method uses a first-in-first-out-queue Q of vertices initialized with all vertices $v \in V$ with $\text{indeg}(v) = 0$. Starting with $i = 1$, each vertex $v \in Q$ is removed from Q, assigned to L_i, and all edges in $\text{outstar}(v)$ are deleted. When a deletion operation leads to $\text{indeg}(w) = 0$ for a vertex $w \in \text{outadj}(v)$, then w is inserted as a new vertex at the end of Q. Finally, i is increased by one as soon as all old vertices have been processed and then the new vertices in Q become old vertices. This procedure takes $O(|V| + |E|)$ time and space. Its drawback is that it has no control over the width of the layer assignment.

Unfortunately, it is $\mathcal{NP}$-hard to minimize the height for a given width $w \ge 3$. This can be proved via a simple transformation from a well-known $\mathcal{NP}$-hard multiprocessor scheduling problem in which $|V|$ unit-time jobs with $|E|$ precedence constraints between pairs of jobs must be processed on w parallel machines so as to minimize the completion time. This relation suggests the application of a very popular polynomial time approximative algorithm by Coffman and Graham [19] for this multiprocessor scheduling problem to the layer assignment problem. We refrain from explaining the method but only state that if h is the height attained by the algorithm and $h_{\min}$ is the minimum possible height given width w, then we have $h \leq (2 - \frac{2}{w})h_{\min}$, i.e., the algorithm computes the optimum solution for $w = 2$ and has a decent performance guarantee for larger w.

From now on, let $G = (V, E)$ be the acyclic digraph *after* the addition of artificial vertices and their incident edges.

Crossing Minimization. The crossing minimization problem is $\mathcal{NP}$-hard even when restricted to 2-layer instances. Nevertheless, it has been attacked with a *branch-and-cut algorithm* that produces an optimum solution in exponential running time, see Healy and Kuusik [44]. (For an introduction to branch-and-cut algorithms see, e.g., Elf *et al.* [33].) However, such methods have not yet reached the maturity and practical efficiency to be used in software systems for automatic graph drawing. Instead, most systems apply a *layer by layer sweep* as follows: Starting from some initial permutation of the vertices on each layer, such heuristics consider pairs of layers $(L_{\text{fixed}}, L_{\text{free}}) = (L_1, L_2), (L_2, L_3), \ldots, (L_{h-1}, L_h), (L_h, L_{h-1}), \ldots, (L_2, L_1), (L_1, L_2), \ldots$ and try to determine a permutation of the vertices in L_{free} that induces a small bilayer cross count for the subgraph induced by the two layers, while keeping L_{fixed} temporarily fixed. These down and up sweeps continue until no improvement is achieved.

Thus the problem is reduced to the *2-layer crossing minimization problem* in which a vertex permutation on one layer is fixed and the other is computed so as to induce the minimum (or at least a small) number of pairwise interior edge crossings among the edges connecting vertices of the two layers. Eades and Wormald [31] have shown that the 2-layer crossing minimization problem with one fixed layer is $\mathcal{NP}$-hard as well, nevertheless, in this case, the optimum can be found efficiently in practice for instances with up to about 60 vertices on the free layer, albeit with a rather complicated branch-and-cut algorithm by Jünger and Mutzel [49]. Experimental studies in the same article have shown that certain efficient heuristics perform very well in practice. We describe two of them: the *barycenter heuristic* of Sugiyama *et al.* [62] and the *median heuristic* by Eades and Wormald [31].

In the 2-layer crossing minimization problem with one fixed layer we have a bipartite graph $G = (V, E)$ with bipartition $V = N \dot{\cup} S$ such that all edges $(u, v) \in E$ have $u \in N$ (the "northern layer") and $v \in S$ (the "southern layer"). Given a permutation $\langle n_1, n_2, \ldots, n_p \rangle$ of all $n_i \in N$, $i \in \{1, 2, \ldots, p\}$ we wish to find a permutation $\langle s_1, s_2, \ldots, s_q \rangle$ of all $s_j \in S$, $j \in \{1, 2, \ldots, q\}$ that induces a small number of interior edge crossings when the edges are drawn as straight line segments connecting the positions of their end-vertices which are placed on two parallel lines according to the permutations. We use the example in Figure 15 for illustration. The permutations given in this figure induce 12 crossings.

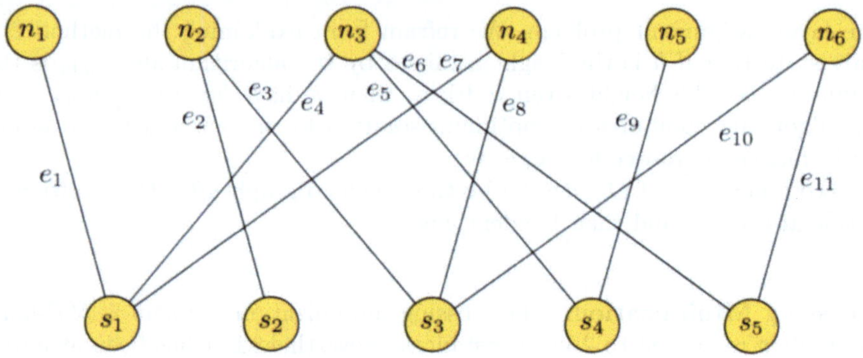

Fig. 15. A two layer graph.

For ease of exposition, we assume without loss of generality that there are no isolated vertices. For each vertex $s \in S$, let

$$\text{barycenter}(s) = \frac{1}{\text{indeg}(s)} \sum_{n_i \in \text{ inadj}(s)} i$$
$$\text{median}(s) = \text{med}\{i \mid n_i \in \text{inadj}(s)\}$$

where med(M) denotes the *median*, i.e., the element in position $\lfloor \frac{|M|}{2} \rfloor$ when the finite multi-set $M \subseteq \mathbb{N}$ is sorted in ascending order.

The medians and barycenters can be computed for all $s \in S$ in $O(|E|)$ time and space. The two heuristics return S sorted by barycenters or medians, respectively, as the southern vertex permutation. In our example, the barycenter permutation is $\langle s_2, s_1, s_3, s_4, s_5 \rangle$ with barycenter values $\langle 2, 2.\bar{6}, 4, 4, 4.5 \rangle$ and the median permutation is $\langle s_2, s_1, s_4, s_5, s_3 \rangle$ with median values $\langle 2, 3, 3, 3, 4 \rangle$. In this case the barycenter permutation induces 11 crossings and the median permutation stays at 12 crossings.

The sorting step takes $O(|S| \log |S|)$ time in the barycenter heuristic and $O(|N|)$ time in the median heuristic, so that the total running time is $O(|E| + |S| \log |S|)$ for the former and $O(|E|)$ for the latter, with $O(|E|)$ space for both.

The heuristics have been analyzed theoretically and an interesting result (shown by Eades and Wormald [31]) is that for any given northern permutation, if c is the number of crossings induced by the result of the median heuristic and $c_{\min}$ is the minimum possible number of crossings, then $c \leq 3\, c_{\min}$ when a certain tie breaking rule in the sorting step is obeyed.

Finally, we discuss an innocent looking problem, namely counting the number of crossings once crossing minimization heuristics have been performed, in order to decide if the layer by layer sweep should be continued or terminated. Since all crossings occur between consecutive layer pairs, the problem reduces to the *2-layer cross counting problem*: Given permutations

π_N of N and π_S of S, determine the number of pairwise interior edge crossings in the above setting.

Of course, it is easy to determine if two given edges in a 2-layer graph with given permutations π_N and π_S cross or not by simple comparisons of the relative orderings of their end vertices on L_N and L_S. This leads to an obvious algorithm with running time $O(|E|^2)$. This algorithm can even output the crossings rather than only count them, and since the number of crossings is $\Theta(|E|^2)$ in the worst case, there can be no asymptotically better algorithm. However, we do not need a list of all crossings, but only their number.

The best known approaches to the 2-layer cross counting problem, both in theory and in practice, are by Waddle and Malhotra [69] and by Barth *et al.* [1] and run in $O(|E| \log |E|)$ and $O(|E| \log(\min\{|N|, |S|\}))$ time, respectively. The former is a sweep line algorithm and the latter uses a reduction of the cross counting problem to the counting of the inversions of a certain sequence. We refrain from a detailed description and only mention that an experimental evaluation by Barth *et al.* [1] shows that a combination of the median heuristic for crossing minimization and cross counting with any of the $O(|E| \log |E|)$ algorithms can be performed for very large graphs very fast.

Coordinate Assignment. After the topology of the layout has been fixed by the previous two phases (S1) and (S2), the purpose of phase (S3) is the assignment of coordinates to the vertices. Since each artificial vertex introduced in phase (S1) gives rise to a possible edge bend in the final layout, a careless implementation of phase (S3) usually leads to the so-called "spaghetti effect" as shown in Figure 16(a).

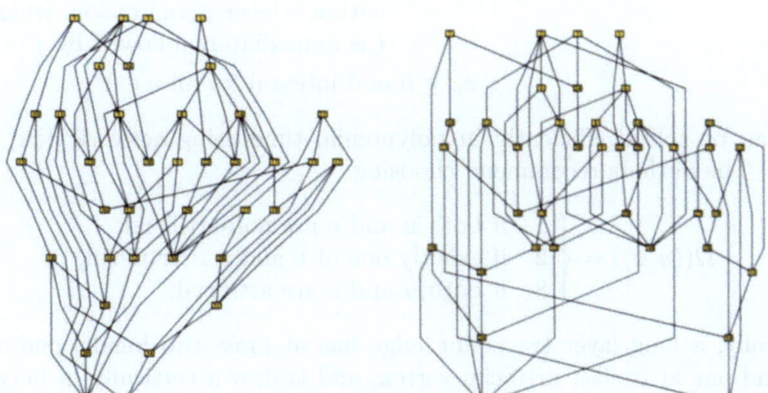

(a) (b)

Fig. 16. The spaghetti effect and a remedy.

The goal is to avoid this effect by "straightening" the long edges that traverse layers in the layout so as to obtain results as shown in Figure 16(b). A landmark paper on layered layout by Gansner *et al.* [40] treats this problem in much detail. In addition to a layer by layer sweep heuristic similar in spirit to the one described in the previous subsection for crossing reduction, the authors give an integer linear programming formulation as follows.

For each $e \in E$, let $\Omega(e)$ be a priority for edge e to be drawn as a vertical line segment. We wish to assign integer x-coordinates within a grid drawing in which the vertices are separated by at least one grid unit. If x_v is the x-coordinate to be assigned to $v \in V$, then the spaghetti avoidance problem can be formulated as the integer non-linear program

$$\begin{aligned} \text{minimize} \sum_{(u,v)\in E} \Omega((u,v))\,|x_v - x_u| & \\ \text{subject to } x_j - x_i \geq 1 & \text{ for all pairs } i \text{ and } j \text{ of vertices} \\ & \text{ within a layer permutation, where} \\ & \text{ } i \text{ is immediately followed by } j \\ x_v \geq 0 & \text{ and integral for all } v \in V \end{aligned}$$

which can be transformed via additional variables to the integer linear program

$$\begin{aligned} \text{minimize} \sum_{(u,v)\in E} \Omega((u,v))\, z_{uv} & \\ \text{subject to } z_{uv} \geq x_v - x_u & \text{ for all } (u,v) \in E \\ z_{uv} \geq x_u - x_v & \text{ for all } (u,v) \in E \\ x_j - x_i \geq 1 & \text{ for all pairs } i \text{ and } j \text{ of vertices} \\ & \text{ within a layer permutation, where} \\ & \text{ } i \text{ is immediately followed by } j \\ x_v \geq 0 & \text{ and integral for all } v \in V \end{aligned}$$

that can be solved efficiently in polynomial time using network flow techniques. The authors recommend choosing

$$\Omega((u,v)) = \begin{cases} 1 & \text{if both } u \text{ and } v \text{ are non-artificial,} \\ 2 & \text{if exactly one of } u \text{ and } v \text{ is artificial,} \\ 8 & \text{if both } u \text{ and } v \text{ are artificial.} \end{cases}$$

Ideally, a long layer traversing edge has at most two bends, one at its first and one at its last artificial vertex, and is drawn vertically in between. The optimum of the above optimization problem cannot guarantee this. With certain additional requirements on the outcome of the crossing minimization phase (S2), two fast heuristics overcome this problem by trying to obtain near optimum solutions to the above optimization problem under the additional restriction that all long edges indeed have at most two bends and the internal parts are drawn vertically, the first by Buchheim *et al.* [14] runs in $O(|E|\log^2|E|)$ time, and the second by Brandes and Köpf [10] runs in $O(|E|)$ time. Both produce visually pleasing results very efficiently.

Making any Graph Acyclic and Directed. If we want to apply Sugiyama-style layout to a non-acyclic digraph, a natural way to make it acyclic is reversing the directions of edges in order to obtain an acyclic digraph. In many cases, such as the drawing of flowcharts, the input data can be expected to determine the choice of such reversals. In the absence of such input data, we would like to reverse as few edges as possible. Thus we can guarantee that, in the final layout, a minimum number of edges point upward rather than downward. This problem is equivalent to the *feedback arc set problem*, also known as the *acyclic subdigraph problem*. It is $\mathcal{NP}$-hard yet can be solved in many reasonably sized cases to optimality by branch-and-cut, see Jünger *et al.* [50]. When more than the minimum number of edges are reversed, the equivalence is lost. Fortunately, there are fast heuristics for finding a small number of edges whose reversal makes the digraph acyclic, most notably a heuristic by Eades *et al.* [30] that runs in $O(|E|)$ time and guarantees a solution in which at most $\frac{|E|}{2} - \frac{|V|}{6}$ edges must be reversed in order to obtain an acyclic digraph.

If we want to apply a Sugiyama-style method to an undirected graph, various application-dependent considerations may guide the assignment of directions to the edges so as to obtain an acyclic digraph. In the absence of such guidance, or in addition to it, it is reasonable to assign the directions to the edges with the goal of obtaining a compact final layout. Sander [61] discusses various heuristics, among them a force-directed layout (see Section 4.5) from which the layer assignment, and thus the edge direction assignment, is extracted. This practically successful idea saves phase (S1) and tends to produce uniform edge lengths. See [24] for an experimental study of the many alternative ways to draw directed graphs.

4.3 Planarization

There are many interesting drawing methods for planar graphs that yield plane drawings as we will discuss in Section 4.4. Such a method can be applied to a non-planar graph G after transforming G into a planar graph G'. The basic idea of the planarization method was introduced by Tamassia *et al.* [67].

There are different ways of *planarizing* a given non-planar graph. The most widely used method in graph drawing is to construct an embedding of G with a small number of crossings, and then to substitute each crossing and its involved pair of edges $(\{u_1, v_1\}, \{u_2, v_2\})$ by an artificial vertex w and four incident edges $\{w, u_1\}, \{w, u_2\}, \{w, v_1\}$, and $\{w, v_2\}$. We call the resulting planar graph $G_P = (V_P, E_P)$ a *planarized* graph from G.

After the *planarization phase*, the resulting planar graph G' is drawn using a planar drawing algorithm, and then the artificial vertices are re-substituted by crossings.

The *crossing minimization problem* searches for a drawing with the minimum number of crossings. Unfortunately, this problem is $\mathcal{NP}$-hard [39]. A classical approach for generating a drawing with a small number of crossings is to compute a planar subgraph P of G by temporarily removing edges. Then the removed edges are re-inserted while trying to keep the number of crossings small. In practice, this method usually leads to drawings with few crossings.

Further restrictions of planarity, such as upward or c-planarity, lead to similar planarization methods. Under the restriction that upward planarity and c-planarity can only be tested for a subset of directed and clustered graphs, respectively, approaches for *upward planarization* and *cluster planarization* can be developed by using the corresponding testing algorithms.

In the sequel we will explain the two steps, namely edge removal and edge re-insertion, in more detail.

Edge Removal. We consider the *maximum planar subgraph problem* which is the problem of removing the minimum number of edges of a non-planar graph so that the resulting graph P is planar. This problem is $\mathcal{NP}$-hard [56]. However, Jünger and Mutzel suggest a branch-and-cut algorithm which is able to solve small problem instances to provable optimality in short computation time [48]. Since this algorithm has exponential running time in the worst case, heuristics are often used for solving this problem in practice.

A subgraph $P = (V, E')$ of a graph $G = (V, E)$ is called a *maximal planar subgraph* of G if there is no edge $e \in E \setminus E'$ so that the graph $(V, E' \cup e\}$ is planar.

A simple algorithm for computing a maximal planar subgraph of a given graph G is to start with the empty graph and successively add the edges of G if their addition results in a planar graph. Edges destroying the planarity are discarded (see Algorithm 1). The incremental algorithm can be implemented in time $O(|V||E|)$ by simply calling a linear planarity testing algorithm. Di Battista and Tamassia have suggested an incremental planarity testing algorithm which can test in $O(\log |V|)$ time whether an edge can be added to a graph without destroying planarity, thus leading to a total running time of $O(|E| \log |V|)$. The best theoretical algorithm for incremental planarity testing has been suggested by Djidjev [27] and runs in time $O(|E| + |V|)$. It is based on the SPQR-tree data structure and special dynamic data structures that allow union and splits for sets in constant amortized time.

Another method based on the planarity testing algorithm by Hopcroft and Tarjan has been suggested by Cai *et al.* [16] and runs in time $O(|E| \log |V|)$.

An algorithm based on PQ-trees has been suggested by Jayakumar *et al.* [46] and runs in time $O(|V|^2)$. The peculiarities of this algorithm are

Algorithm 1: Incremental maximal planar subgraph

Input : Graph $G = (V, E)$
Output: Maximal planar subgraph $P = (V, F)$ of G
Set $F = \emptyset$
for *all edges* $e \in E$ **do**
  if $P = (V, F \cup \{e\})$ *is planar* **then**
    Set $P = (V, F \cup \{e\})$
  end
end

discussed in various subsequent papers, see, e.g., [47], and it turns out that algorithms based on PQ-trees are not appropriate for finding maximal planar subgraphs in general. Despite the fact that this algorithm does not compute a maximal planar subgraph, it leads to larger subgraphs than the naïve method in general. Ziegler has shown that the results improve if the algorithm is applied several times to the same graph with perturbed input data [71].

Edge Re-Insertion. Given a planar subgraph P of $G = (V, E)$, our task is to re-insert the removed edges so that the number of edge crossings is small. More formally, the problem is to create a drawing with the minimum number of crossings in which the planar subgraph is drawn crossing-free. Without the latter restriction, the problem would be equivalent to the crossing minimization problem.

The most widely used edge re-insertion method is shown in Algorithm 2. It chooses a planar embedding of P and successively inserts the edges of F. After each re-insertion step, the crossings are substituted by artificial vertices, thus providing a planar graph after each step. For a fixed planar embedding, an edge $e = \{u, v\}$ can be inserted with the minimum number of crossings by computing a shortest path in an extended dual graph. The extension is necessary to connect the primal vertices u and v with the dual graph. This is done by adding u^* and v^* inside the faces F_u and F_v that correspond to u and v in the primal graph, respectively, and by adding artificial edges from the new vertices to the dual vertices bounding the faces F_u and F_v. The new edge creates a crossing in G_P whenever a (real) dual edge in G_P^* is used, which corresponds to crossing the boundary of two adjacent faces. Figure 17 shows a plane graph, its extended dual graph, and an edge e to be inserted. The algorithm can be implemented in time $O(|F|(|E'| + |C|))$, where $|C|$ is the number of generated crossings.

Clearly, the number of generated crossings highly depends on the chosen embedding Π at the beginning. Gutwenger *et al.* [43] have presented an algorithm which solves the one-edge insertion problem optimally over the set of all embeddings of G in linear time, thus overcoming this problem. Since the embedding of G_P is changed after substituting the crossings dur-

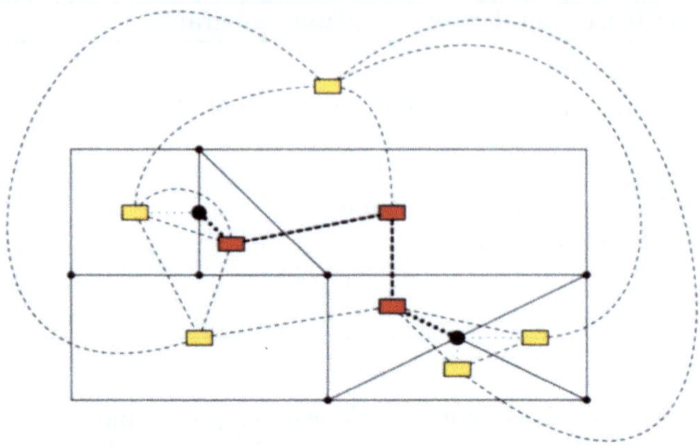

Fig. 17. The edge re-insertion step for one edge.

Algorithm 2: Classical edge re-insertion algorithm

Input : Planar graph $P = (V, E')$ of $G = (V, E)$ and edge set $F = E \setminus E'$
Output: Planarized graph $G_P = (V_P, E_P)$ of G

Set $G_P = (V, E')$
Compute a planar embedding Π of G_P
Compute the dual graph G_P^* of G_P with respect to Π
for *all edges* $e = \{u, v\} \in F$ **do**
    Extend the dual graph G_P^* at the end-vertices of e
    Compute a shortest path from u to v in G_P^*
    Update $G_P = (V_P, E_P)$ by substituting all crossings by new vertices
    Update the dual graph G_P^*
end

---

ing the run of the algorithm, it may happen that some of the crossings are not needed anymore in the final drawing, and this leads to further crossing reduction. The edge re-insertion is specified in Algorithm 3, whose running time is $O(|F|(|E'| + |C|))$.

Algorithm 3: Optimal embedding re-insertion algorithm

Input : Planar graph $P = (V, E')$ of $G = (V, E)$ and edge set $F = E \setminus E'$
Output: Planarized graph $G_P = (V_P, E_P)$ of G

Set $G_P = (V, E')$
for *all edges* $e = \{u, v\} \in F$ **do**
    Call the optimal 1-edge re-insertion algorithm for e and G_P
    Update $G_P = (V_P, E_P)$ by substituting all crossings by new vertices
end
Reduce superfluous crossings in the planarized graph G_P

The number of generated crossings can be further decreased by a remove-and-reinsert post-processing step (see, e.g., Ziegler [71] for experimental results). A typical drawing using planarization in combination with a planar orthogonal layout method is shown in Figure 18.

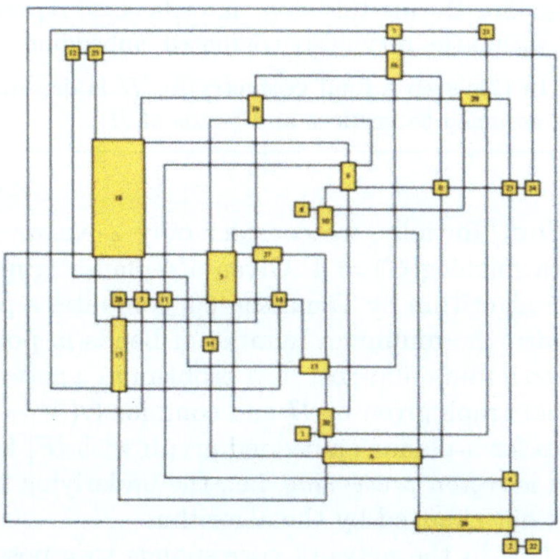

Fig. 18. A typical drawing in planarization style.

4.4 Orthogonal Layout

A popular style in graph drawing is orthogonal drawing. In an *orthogonal drawing* each edge is represented as a chain of horizontal and vertical segments. A point where a horizontal and a vertical segment of an edge meet is called a *bend*.

A popular orthogonal drawing method is the *topology-shape-metrics approach* of Batini *et al.* [2], which we will discuss now. The topology-shape-metrics method focuses on the æsthetic criteria crossings, bends, and area of the drawing and tries to keep these numbers small while fixing the topology, the shape, and the edge lengths, in this order. It deals with topology, shape, and geometry of the drawing separately, allowing for each æsthetic criterion to be addressed in the corresponding step, avoiding the complexity of a global optimization. Experimental results have shown that minimization in all these steps does in fact lead to better drawings (see, e.g., [25]). Algorithm 4 gives an overview of the topology-shape-metrics method.

The topology is fixed using the planarization method based on planar subgraphs (see Section 4.3). Then, a planar orthogonal drawing method is used for planar graphs, which we will discuss in the sequel.

Algorithm 4: The topology-shape-metrics method

Input : Graph $G = (V, E)$;
Output: Orthogonal drawing of $G = (V, E)$

Planarization. If G is planar, then a planar embedding for G is computed. If G is not planar, a set of artificial vertices is added to replace crossings.

Orthogonalization. During this step, an orthogonal representation H of G is computed within the previously computed embedding.

Compaction. In this step a final geometry for H is determined. Namely, coordinates are assigned to vertices and bends of H.

Orthogonalization. Initially, we consider only *4-planar* graphs, i.e., planar graphs G with $\text{maxdeg}(G) = 4$. Given a 4-planar graph G with planar embedding Π, the algorithm by Tamassia [66] computes a planar orthogonal grid embedding with the minimum number of bends in polynomial time by transforming it into a minimum-cost flow problem in a network. The network is based on the dual graph given by Π and contains $O(|V|+|F|)$ vertices and $O(|V|+|E|)$ edges for a planar embedded graph with $|F|$ faces.

The algorithm is *region preserving*, i.e., the underlying topological structure given in Π is not changed by the algorithm.

Each feasible flow in the network corresponds to a possible shape of G. In particular, the minimum cost flow leads to the orthogonal shape with the lowest number of bends since each unit of cost is associated with a bend in the drawing. The flow is used to build a so-called *orthogonal!representation* H that describes the shape of the final drawing in terms of bends occurring along the edges and angles formed by the edges. Formally, H is a function from the set of faces F to lists of triples $r = (e_r, s_r, a_r)$ where e_r is an edge, s_r is a bit string, and a_r is the angle formed with the following edge inside the appropriate face. The bit string s_r provides information about the bends along edge e_r, and the kth bit describes the kth bend on the right side of e_r where a zero indicates a 90° bend and a one a 270° bend. The empty string ε is used to characterize straight line edges. Figure 19 shows an example.

There are four necessary and sufficient conditions for an orthogonal representation H to be a valid shape description of some 4-planar graph:

(P1) There is a 4-planar graph whose planar embedding Π is identical to that given by H restricted to the e-fields. We say that H *extends* Π.
(P2) Let r and r' be two elements in H with $e_r = e_{r'}$. Since each edge is contained twice in H these pairs always exist. Then string $s_{r'}$ can be obtained by applying bitwise negation to the reversion of s_r.
(P3) Let $|s|_0$ and $|s|_1$ denote the numbers of zeroes and ones in string s, respectively. Define for each element r in H the value

$$\rho(r) = |s_r|_0 - |s_r|_1 + (2 - \frac{a_r}{90}).$$

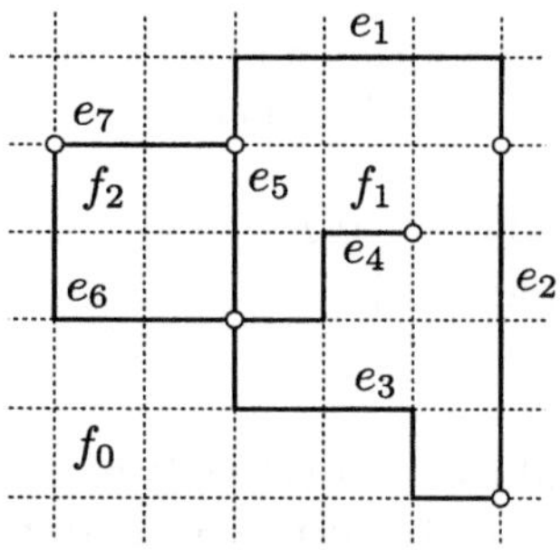

$$H(f_1) = ((e_1, 00, 180), (e_2, \varepsilon, 90), (e_3, 010, 90), (e_4, 10, 360), (e_4, 10, 90), (e_5, \varepsilon, 180))$$
$$H(f_2) = ((e_6, 0, 90), (e_7, \varepsilon, 90), (e_5, \varepsilon, 90))$$
$$H(f_0) = ((e_7, \varepsilon, 270), (e_6, 1, 90), (e_3, 101, 270), (e_2, \varepsilon, 180), (e_1, 11, 90))$$

Fig. 19. Orthogonal grid drawing with corresponding orthogonal representation of a 4-planar graph

Then for each face f

$$\sum_{r \in H(f)} \rho(r) = \begin{cases} +4 & \text{if } f \text{ is an internal face} \\ -4 & \text{if } f \text{ is the external face } f_0. \end{cases}$$

(P4) For each vertex $v \in V$ we have

$$\sum_{e_r=(u,v)} a_r = 360 \qquad \forall u \in V,$$

i.e., the angles around v given by the a-fields sum up to 360°.

We say that a drawing Γ *realizes* H if H is a valid description for the shape of Γ. Figure 19 shows an orthogonal representation H and a grid embedding realizing H. Note that the number of bends in any drawing that realizes H is

$$b(H) = \frac{1}{2} \sum_{f \in F} \sum_{r \in H(f)} |s_r|.$$

Let $G = (V, E)$ be the input graph with planar embedding Π defining the face set F. The construction of the underlying network N follows [42]: Let $U = U_F \cup U_V$ denote its vertex set. Then for each face $f \in F$ there is a vertex in U_F and for each vertex $v \in V$ there is one in U_V. Vertices $u_v \in U_V$ supply $b(u_v) = 4$ units of flow and vertices $u_f \in U_F$ consume

$$-b(u_f) = \begin{cases} 2\deg(f) - 4 & \text{if } f \text{ is an internal face} \\ 2\deg(f) + 4 & \text{if } f \text{ is the external face } f_0 \end{cases}$$

units of flow. Thus, the total supply is $4|V|$ and the total demand is

$$\sum_{f \neq f_0} (2\deg(f) - 4) + 2\deg(f_0) + 4 = 4|E| - 4|F| + 8$$

which is equal to the total supply, according to Euler's formula (Theorem 1). The arc set A of network N consists of two sets A_V and A_F where

$$\begin{aligned} A_V &= \{(u_v, u_f) \mid u_v \in U_V,\ u_f \in U_F,\ v \text{ is adjacent to } f\} \quad \text{and} \\ A_F &= \{(u_f, u_g) \mid u_f \neq u_g \in U_F,\ f \text{ is adjacent to } g\} \\ &\quad \cup \{(u_f, u_f) \mid f \text{ contains a bridge}\}. \end{aligned}$$

Arcs in A_V have lower bound 1, capacity 4, and cost 0. Each unit of flow represents an angle of 90°, so a flow in an arc $(u_v, u_f) \in A_V$ corresponds to the angles formed at vertex v inside face f. Note that there can be more than one angle, see for example Figure 19 where the vertex common to edges e_6, e_5, e_4, and e_3 builds two angles in f_1. Precisely, the flow in (u_v, u_f) corresponds to the sum of the angles at v inside f. Following this interpretation, flow in arcs $(u_f, u_g) \in A_F$ find their analogy in bends occurring along edges separating f and g that form a 90° angle in f. Naturally their lower bound is 0, their capacity unbounded, and they have unit cost.

The conservation rule at vertices $u_v \in U_V$ expresses that the angle sum around the corresponding vertex v is equal to 360°. The vertices in U_F consume flow; here, the conservation rule states that every face has the shape of a rectilinear polygon. A planar graph and the transformation into a network is shown in Figure 20(a)–(d).

It is easy to see that there is always a feasible flow in network N: Flow produced by vertices in U_V can be transported to vertices in U_F where it satisfies their demand. In case it is not possible to satisfy every vertex in U_F by exclusively using arcs in A_V, units of flow can be shifted without restriction between vertices in U_F because of their mutual interconnection by arcs in A_F. Every feasible flow can be used to construct an orthogonal representation for the input graph G, in particular the minimum cost flow, leading to the orthogonal representation with the minimum number of bends. The following lemma states the analogy between flows in the network and orthogonal representations.

Lemma 1 (Tamassia [66]). *Let G be the input graph, Π its planar embedding, and N the constructed network. For each integer flow χ in network N, there is an orthogonal representation H that extends Π and whose number of bends is equal to the cost of χ. The flow χ can be used to construct the orthogonal representation.*

Figure 21 completes the example from Figure 20, showing the minimum cost flow in the constructed network and a realizing grid embedding for the derived orthogonal representation.

Vice versa, it can be shown that the number of bends in each orthogonal grid embedding of a graph with planar embedding Π is equal to the cost of some feasible flow in network N. This result and Lemma 1 lead to the following theorem, combining the basic results of [66] and [42]:

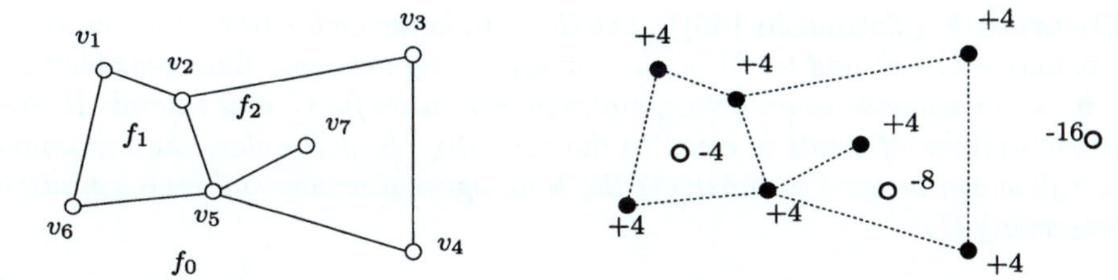

(a) Planar embedding P

(b) Nodes in network N. Supply/demand shown

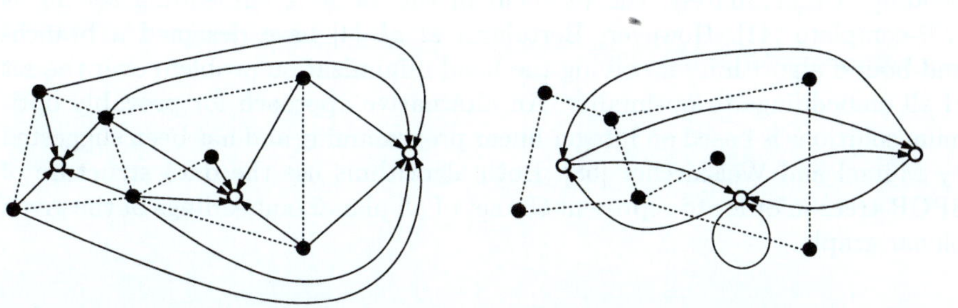

(c) Arcs in A_V. Capacity 4, lower bound 1, cost 0

(d) Arcs in A_F. Capacity ∞, lower bound 0, cost 1

Fig. 20. Network construction.

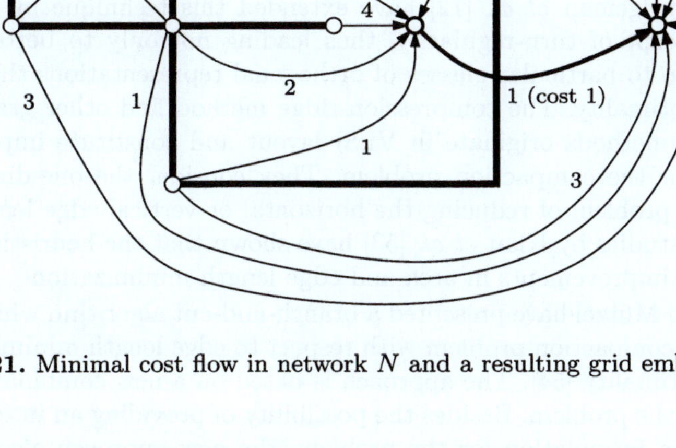

Fig. 21. Minimal cost flow in network N and a resulting grid embedding.

Theorem 6 (Tamassia [66]). *Let Π be a planar embedding of a connected 4-planar graph G and let N be the corresponding network. Each feasible flow χ in N corresponds to an orthogonal representation for G that extends Π and whose number of bends is equal to the cost of χ. In particular, the minimum cost flow can be used to construct the bend optimal orthogonal representation preserving Π.*

Garg and Tamassia [42] have shown that the minimum cost flow problem in this specific network can be solved in $O(|V|^{7/4}\sqrt{\log|V|})$ time.

Obviously, the number of bends is highly dependent on the chosen embedding. Unfortunately, the problem in the variable embedding setting is $\mathcal{NP}$-complete [41]. However, Bertolazzi *et al.* [4] have designed a branch-and-bound algorithm for solving the bend minimization problem over the set of all embeddings to optimality. An alternative approach for provably optimum solutions is based on integer linear programming and has been suggested by Mutzel and Weiskircher [58]. Both algorithms use the data structure of SPQR-trees in order to represent the set of all planar embeddings of the given planar graph.

Compaction. After the orthogonalization phase, the description is dimensionless, and coordinates need to be assigned to the vertices and bends. The problem of computing the edge lengths of an orthogonal representation minimizing the area or the total edge length of the drawing is called the *compaction problem*. This problem is $\mathcal{NP}$-hard [59].

There is a vast amount of literature concerning the compaction problem, since it has played an important role not only in graph drawing, but also in the context of circuit design. The heuristic methods can be categorized into constructive and improvement methods. Tamassia has suggested the first approach in the context of graph drawing. In [66], he provides a linear time algorithm based on rectilinear dissection of the orthogonal representation. Recently, Bridgeman *et al.* [12] have extended this technique by introducing the concept of turn-regularity, thus leading not only to better heuristics, but also to particular classes of orthogonal representations that can be solved to optimality. The compression-ridge method and other graph-based compaction methods originate in VLSI layout and constitute improvement heuristics for the compaction problem. They consider the one-dimensional compaction problem of reducing the horizontal or vertical edge lengths. Experimental studies by Klau *et al.* [53] have shown that the heuristics lead to tremendous improvements in area and edge length minimization.

Klau and Mutzel have presented a branch-and-cut algorithm which is able to solve the compaction problem with respect to edge length minimization to provable optimality [54]. The approach is based on a new combinatorial formulation of the problem. Besides the possibility of providing an integer linear programming formulation for the problem, the new approach also provides new classes of orthogonal representations that can be solved in polynomial time [54].

High Degree Orthogonal Drawings. As already discussed above, the bend minimization algorithm by Tamassia only works for graphs with vertex degree bounded by four. In order to generate orthogonal drawings for graphs of arbitrary vertex degree, different drawing conventions have been introduced in the literature. Here we introduce the basic Kandinsky drawing convention, defined by Fößmeier and Kaufmann [36].

A *basic Kandinsky drawing* (see Figures 22(a) and (b)) is an orthogonal drawing such that:

1. Segments representing edges may not cross, with the exception that two segments that are incident on the same vertex may overlap. Observe that the angle between such segments has zero degree. Roughly speaking, a basic Kandinsky drawing is "almost" planar: it is planar everywhere but in the possible overlap of segments incident on the same vertex. Observe in Figure 22(b) the overlap of segments incident on vertices 1, 2, and 3.
2. All the polygons representing the faces have an area strictly greater than zero.

Basic Kandinsky drawings are usually visualized by representing vertices as boxes with equal size and representing two overlapping segments as two very near segments. See Figure 22(c).

In [36] an algorithm is presented that computes a basic Kandinsky drawing of an embedded planar graph with the minimum number of bends. Furthermore, the authors conjecture that the drawing problem becomes $\mathcal{NP}$-hard when condition 2 is omitted. Basic Kandinsky drawings generalize the concept of orthogonal representation, allowing angles between two edges incident to the same vertex to have zero degree. The consequence of the assumption that the polygons representing the faces have area strictly greater than zero is that the angles have specific constraints. Namely, because of conditions 1 and 2, each zero degree angle is in correspondence with exactly one bend [36]. An orthogonal representation corresponding to the above definition is a *basic Kandinsky orthogonal representation.*

Figure 23 shows a typical planar orthogonal drawing in basic Kandinsky style.

The basic Kandinsky model has been extended in [26] to deal with drawings in which the size (width and height) of each single vertex is assigned by the user. We refer to this extended model as the Kandinsky model. A *Kandinsky drawing* has the following properties (see also Figure 22(d)):

1. Each vertex is represented by a box with its specific width and height (width and height are assigned to each single vertex by the user).

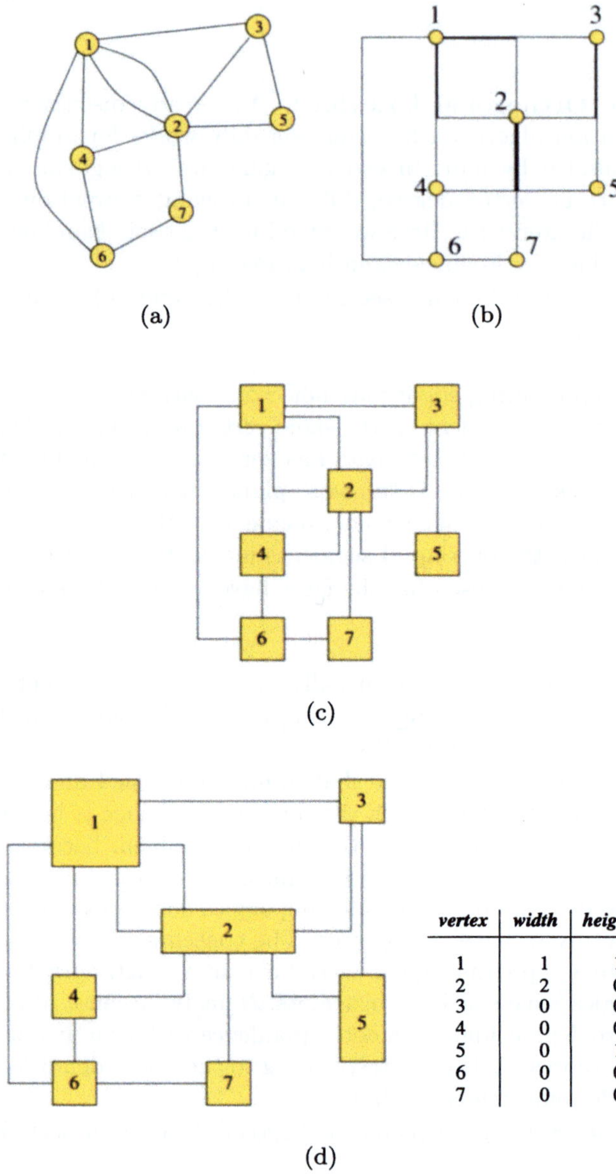

vertex	*width*	*height*
1	1	1
2	2	0
3	0	0
4	0	0
5	0	1
6	0	0
7	0	0

Fig. 22. (a) A planar graph and (b) one of its basic Kandinsky drawings; (c) A more effective visualization of the basic Kandinsky drawing in (b); (d) A Kandinsky drawing with the same shape as the drawing in (b); the sizes of the vertices are specified in the table.

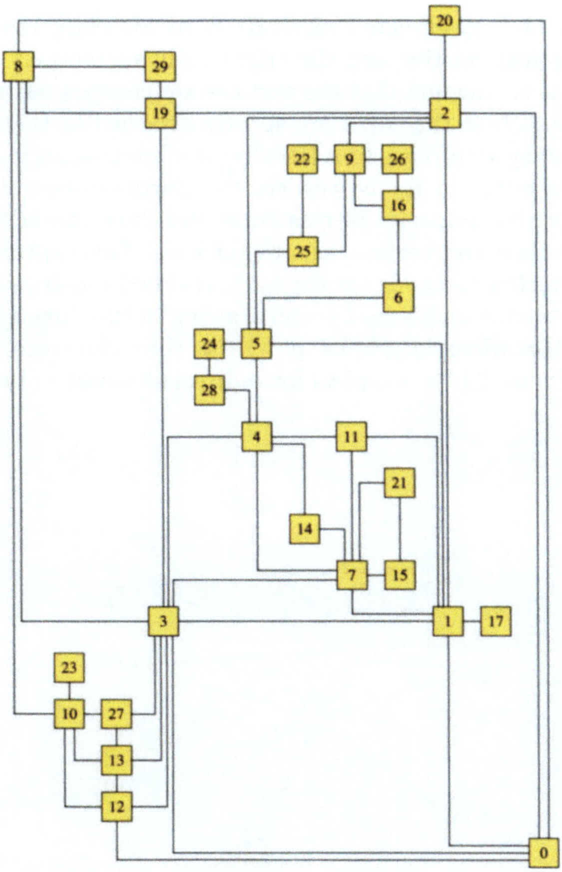

Fig. 23. A typical planar orthogonal drawing in basic Kandinsky style.

2. Consider any side of length $l \geq 0$ of a vertex v and consider the set I of arcs that are incident on such a side.
   (a) If $l+1 \geq |I|$ then the edges of I may not overlap.
   (b) If $l+1 < |I|$ then the edges of I are partitioned into $l+1$ non-empty subsets such that all the edges of the same subset overlap.
3. The orthogonal representation constructed from a Kandinsky drawing by contracting each vertex into a single point is a basic Kandinsky orthogonal representation.

Di Battista *et al.* [26] suggest a polynomial time algorithm for computing Kandinsky drawings of an embedded planar graph that have the minimum number of bends over a wide class of Kandinsky drawings.

4.5 Force Directed Layout

The basic idea of force-directed methods is to associate the vertices of a graph with physical entities and the edges with interactions between their end-vertex entities. Imagine that the vertices are charged particles with mutual repulsion and that the edges are springs attached at their end-vertices. Let this physical system relax to a (locally) minimum energy state in three-dimensional space, assign to the vertices the Cartesian coordinates of their corresponding vertex particles in this state and draw the edges connecting the positions of their end-vertices as straight lines. This captures the general idea of force-directed methods for three-dimensional graph drawing. We apply this idea to simple undirected graph drawing in two dimensions and treat non-simple and/or directed graphs as well as three-dimensional layouts afterwards. See Figure 24 for a typical force-directed layout in two dimensions.

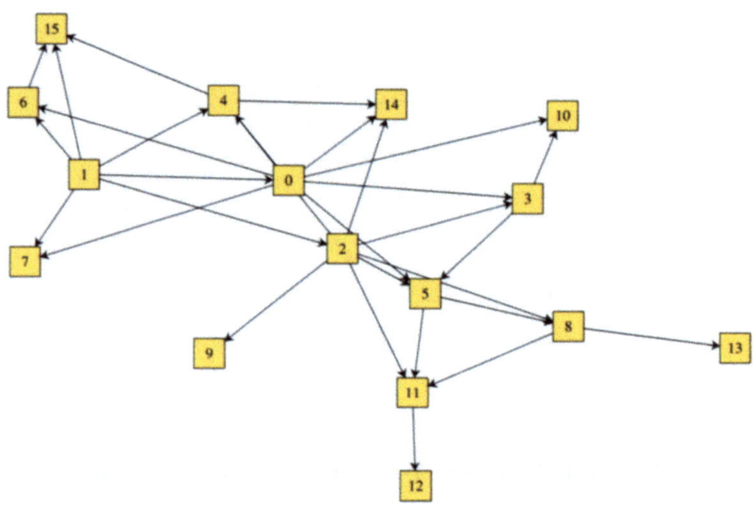

Fig. 24. A typical force-directed layout.

It should be stressed that the title of this section is a concession to the short tradition of automatic graph drawing and the title "Drawing on Physical *Analogies*" of a recommended survey of Brandes [9] would be much more appropriate, because what follows has little to do with what physicists do when they study ground states of physical systems and relaxation dynamics.

Two-Dimensional Force-Directed Layout of Undirected Graphs. For ease of notation, we identify vertices and edges with their physical counterparts. In approaching the charged particles and spring model, the force acting on a vertex $v \in V$ depends on the locations $p_v = (x_v, y_v) \in \mathbb{R}^2$ of the vertices $v \in V$ and is composed of the repulsive forces by the other vertices and the forces by the edges in star(v), i.e.,

$$F(p_v) = \sum_{u \in V \setminus \{v\}} \text{repulsionforce}(p_u, p_v) + \sum_{\{u,v\} \in \mathtt{star}(v)} \text{springforce}(\{p_u, p_v\}).$$

For $p = (x, y) \in \mathbb{R}^2$ let $\|p\| = \sqrt{x^2 + y^2}$ denote the Euclidean norm of p and let $\overrightarrow{p_u p_v} = \frac{p_v - p_u}{\|p_v - p_u\|}$ be the normalized difference vector of p_v and p_u. We may choose the repulsion force between vertices u and v to follow an inverse square law, i.e.,

$$\text{repulsionforce}(p_u, p_v) = \frac{R}{\|p_u - p_v\|^2} \cdot \overrightarrow{p_u p_v}$$

where R is a repulsion constant, and the spring force of edge $\{u, v\}$ according to Hooke's law, i.e.,

$$\text{springforce}(p_u, p_v) = S_{\{u,v\}} \cdot (\|p_u - p_v\| - l_{\{u,v\}}) \cdot \overrightarrow{p_u p_v}$$

where $S_{\{u,v\}}$ is the stiffness and $l_{\{u,v\}}$ is the natural length of the spring between u and v such that springforce(u, v) is proportional to the difference between the distance of u and v and the natural length of the spring. The natural spring lengths $l_{\{u,v\}}$ reflect the desirable lengths of the edges in the drawing and can be passed together with the stiffnesses $S_{\{u,v\}}$ as additional input to a force-directed method.

Force-directed methods try to compute vertex positions p_v for which the physical system attains an equilibrium state in which $F(p_v) = 0$ for all $v \in V$. Such a state is approximated in practice by iterative algorithms that, starting with some initial (possibly random) positions p_v for the vertices $v \in V$, compute $F(p_v)$ for all $v \in V$ and then update the positions $p_v \longleftarrow p_v + \mu \cdot F(p_v)$ where the step length μ is a small number, either given as a parameter or chosen dynamically depending on the number of iterations already performed. The (dynamic) choice of μ, a stopping criterion, and whether all moves are parallel or sequential are among the many choices an implementor of a force-directed method must make. For the dynamic choice of μ, all kinds of iterative improvement schemes, e.g., simulated annealing or genetic algorithms, can be used.

Inspired by previous usage of force-directed methods in VLSI layout algorithms, this method that is usually referred to as *spring embedder* was introduced into automatic graph drawing by Eades [28] with a modified force model that replaces the definition of springforce(p_u, p_v) with a logarithmic counterpart

$$\text{springforce}_{\text{Eades}}(p_u, p_v) = S_{\{u,v\}} \cdot \log\left(\frac{\|p_u - p_v\|}{l_{\{u,v\}}}\right) \cdot \overrightarrow{p_u p_v} .$$

A very early paper on automatic graph drawing by Tutte [68] can be interpreted as a spring embedder method for the special case $R = 0$, $S_e = 1$ and $l_e = 0$ for all $e \in E$ so that $F(p_v)$ is replaced by

$$F_{\text{Tutte}}(p_v) = \sum_{\{u,v\} \in \text{star}(v)} (p_v - p_u)$$

and the positions of at least three vertices are fixed in advance. (If no vertices are fixed, the solution $p_v = (0,0)$ for all $v \in V$ is an undesired optimum.) Here, the problem of coordinate assignment is reduced to the solution of a (sparse) system of linear equations. The resulting coordinates have the nice property that each non-fixed vertex position is at the barycenter of its neighbor vertex positions. If Tutte's method is applied to a 3-connected planar graph and the coordinates of the vertices of a face of some planar embedding are fixed to their positions in a strictly convex planar drawing of this face, it produces a planar straight line drawing.

Many variants closer to the generic model have been proposed and experimentally evaluated in the literature, the modifications concern various redefinitions of the forces in order to facilitate their evaluation and/or obtain faster convergence of the iterative method, and speeding up the iterative process by evaluating only a subset of the repulsion force terms in $F(p_v)$. E.g., Fruchterman and Reingold [38] replace repulsionforce(p_u, p_v) by

$$\text{repulsionforce}_{\text{FG}}(p_u, p_v) = \frac{l^2_{\{u,v\}}}{\|p_u - p_v\|} \cdot \overrightarrow{p_u p_v}$$

and springforce(p_u, p_v) by

$$\text{springforce}_{\text{FG}}(p_u, p_v) = \frac{\|p_u - p_v\|^2}{l_{\{u,v\}}} \cdot \overrightarrow{p_v p_u}$$

whereas Frick *et al.* [37] use

$$\text{repulsionforce}_{\text{FLM}}(p_u, p_v) = \frac{l^2_{\{u,v\}}}{\|p_u - p_v\|^2} \cdot (p_u - p_v)$$

$$\text{springforce}_{\text{FLM}}(p_u, p_v) = \frac{\|p_u - p_v\|^2}{l^2_{\{u,v\}} \cdot \Phi(v)} \cdot (p_v - p_u)$$

where $\Phi(v) = 1 + \frac{\deg(v)}{2}$. They also add an additional gravitational component

$$\text{gravitationforce}_{\text{FLM}}(p_v) = \Phi(v) \cdot \gamma \cdot \left(\frac{\sum_{w \in V} p_w}{|V|} - p_v \right)$$

to $F(p_v)$, where γ is a gravitational constant, and perform all calculations in (fast) integer arithmetic. Together with more refinements, a substantial reduction in running time without visible compromises in layout quality can be achieved.

We have not yet discussed the choice of the stiffness and the natural length parameters that can be used to control the behavior of a force-directed method. An interesting suggestion has been made by Kamada and Kawai [51]. For a connected graph $G = (V, E)$ and $u, v \in V$ let $\delta(u, v)$ denote the length of a shortest path connecting u and v. The idea is to aim at a final layout in which the distance $\|p_u - p_v\|$ is approximately proportional to $\delta(u, v)$. To this end, Kamada and Kawai use springs between all $\binom{|V|}{2}$ vertex pairs so that the force between vertices u and v can be written as

$$\text{springforce}_{\text{KK}}(p_u, p_v) = S_{uv} \cdot (\|p_u - p_v\| - \delta(u, v)).$$

They choose the stiffness parameters so that they are strong for graph-theoretically near vertices and decay according to an inverse square law with increasing distance $\delta(u, v)$, namely

$$S_{uv} = \frac{S}{\delta(u, v)^2}$$

for some constant S.

The potential energy of the spring between u and v is

$$\begin{aligned} E(u, v) &= \int \text{springforce}_{\text{KK}}(p_u, p_v)\, d(\|p_u - p_v\| - \delta(u, v)) \\ &= \frac{1}{2} S_{uv} (\|p_u - p_v\| - \delta(u, v))^2 \\ &= \frac{S}{2} \left(\frac{\|p_u - p_v\|}{\delta(u, v)} - 1 \right)^2 \end{aligned}$$

and the potential energy of the whole drawing becomes

$$E = \sum_{u,v \in V,\, u \neq v} E(u, v) = \frac{S}{2} \sum_{u,v \in V,\, u \neq v} \left(\frac{\|p_u - p_v\|}{\delta(u, v)} - 1 \right)^2.$$

Necessary conditions for the optimality of vertex positions $p_v = (x_v, y_v)$ are

$$\frac{\partial E}{\partial x_v} = 0 \text{ and } \frac{\partial E}{\partial y_v} = 0 \text{ for all } v \in V.$$

For finding an approximate solution to this nonlinear system of equations, Kamada and Kawai use an iterative algorithm that in each iteration chooses a vertex $w \in V$ on which the largest force is acting, i.e.,

$$w = \text{argmax} \left\{ \sqrt{\left(\frac{\partial E}{\partial x_v} \right)^2 + \left(\frac{\partial E}{\partial y_v} \right)^2} \;\middle|\; v \in V \right\}$$

and a line search to move it to an energy minimizing position while the positions of the vertices $v \in V \setminus \{w\}$ are temporarily fixed.

Two-Dimensional Force-Directed Layout of Directed Graphs. For directed graphs, force-directed layout methods can accommodate a preferred direction within the drawing such that each directed edge is penalized proportionally to the angle φ its drawing deviates from the preferred direction. In a more general context, Sugiyama and Misue [64] propose the following amendment to basic force-directed methods: If $\overrightarrow{p_u p_v}^{\perp}$ is the unit length vector perpendicular to $\overrightarrow{p_u p_v}$ and pointing towards a decrease of φ, they add a rotation force

$$\text{rotationforce}(p_u, p_v) = M \cdot \|p_u - p_v\|^{\alpha} \cdot \varphi^{\beta} \cdot \overrightarrow{p_u p_v}^{\perp}$$

to springforce(p_u, p_v), where M is a constant for the strength of an exterior magnetic field and the parameters α and β control the relative influence of the exterior field on vertex distance and angle deviation, respectively.

Other Extensions. Eades *et al.* [32] propose a method for the layout of hierarchical (clustered) graphs with force-directed methods. For simplicity, let us assume that the vertex set of $G = (V, E)$ is partitioned into disjoint subsets V_i, $i \in \{1, 2, \ldots, k\}$ for some $k \in \mathbb{N}$, i.e., we have a hierarchy of depth one. For each V_i they introduce an additional artificial vertex v_i that is equipped with strong attractive forces with respect to the vertices $v \in V_i$ (realized by the appropriate artificial edges) and repulsive forces with respect to the artificial vertices v_j representing the other clusters $V_j \neq V_i$.

Davidson and Harel [22] propose general energy functions that try to capture various æsthetic requirements in automatic graph drawing. They try to

$$\text{minimize} \quad \eta = \lambda_1\eta_1 + \lambda_2\eta_2 + \lambda_3\eta_3 + \lambda_4\eta_4$$

where

$$\begin{aligned}
\eta_1 &= \sum_{u,v \in V} \frac{1}{\|p_u - p_v\|^2} \\
\eta_2 &= \sum_{v \in V} \left(\frac{1}{r_v^2} + \frac{1}{l_v^2} + \frac{1}{t_v^2} + \frac{1}{b_v^2} \right) \\
\eta_3 &= \sum_{\{u,v\} \in E} \|p_u - p_v\|^2 \\
\eta_4 &= \text{number of edge crossings}
\end{aligned}$$

and r_v, l_v, t_v, and b_v are the distances of vertex v to the right, left, top, and bottom boundary of the drawing area, respectively. Thus, η_1 contributes the repulsion between vertices, η_2 the respect for the drawing area, η_3 the preference for short edges, and η_4 the number of crossings (that can be easily calculated for any given vertex positions p_v). The parameters λ_i $(i \in \{1, 2, 3, 4\})$ in the objective function control the relative emphasis on each of the four criteria. Davidson and Harel use a simulated annealing procedure to find an approximation to an energy minimal state of the system.

Brandes and Wagner [11] show how the layout of curved edge representations with Bézier curves can be reduced to the straight line case by placing Bézier curve control points instead of vertices.

Final Remarks on Force-Directed Methods. In the discussion above, there is no hidden assumption on the dimension of the drawing space, so everything presented can be applied for three-dimensional force-directed layout as well with the obvious modifications. E.g., Bruß and Frick [13] present an extension of the method of Frick *et al.* [37] while Cruz and Twarog [20] present an extension of the method of Davidson and Harel [22] in which the cross counting component that is irrelevant in a three-dimensional drawing is replaced by an edge-edge repulsion term.

Due to their general applicability and the lack of special structural assumptions as well as for the ease of their implementation, force-directed methods play a central role in automatic graph drawing. Just like layered drawing methods they are included in many graph drawing software packages. An experimental comparison of various force-directed approaches is presented by Brandenburg *et al.* [8].

References

1. Barth, W., Jünger, M., Mutzel, P. (2002) Simple and efficient bilayer cross counting. In: M. Goodrich and S. Kobourov (eds.) Graph Drawing '02, Lecture Notes in Computer Science 2528, Springer-Verlag, 130–141
2. Batini, C., Nardelli, E., Tamassia, R. (1986) A layout algorithm for data flow diagrams. IEEE Transactions on Software Engineering **SE-12** (4), 538–546
3. Bertolazzi, P., Di Battista, G., Didimo, W. (1998) Quasi-upward planarity. In: S. H. Whitesides (ed.) Graph Drawing '98, Lecture Notes in Computer Science 1547, Springer-Verlag, 15–29
4. Bertolazzi, P., Di Battista, G., Didimo, W. (2000) Computing orthogonal drawings with the minimum number of bends. IEEE Transactions on Computers **49** (8), 826–840
5. Bertolazzi, P., Di Battista, G., Liotta, G., Mannino, C. (1994) Upward drawings of triconnected digraphs. Algorithmica **6** (12), 476–497
6. Bertolazzi, P., Di Battista, G., Mannino, C., Tamassia, R. (1998) Optimal upward planarity testing of single-source digraphs. SIAM Journal on Computing **27**, 132–169
7. Booth, K., Lueker, G. (1976) Testing for the consecutive ones property, interval graphs, and graph planarity using PQ-tree algorithms. Journal of Computer and System Sciences **13**, 335–379
8. Brandenburg, F. J., Himsolt, M., Rohrer, C. (1996) An experimental comparison of force-directed and randomized graph drawing algorithms. In: F.-J. Brandenburg (ed.) Graph Drawing '95, Lecture Notes in Computer Science 1027, Springer-Verlag, 76–87

9. Brandes, U. (2001) Drawing on Physical Analogies. In: M. Kaufmann and D. Wagner (eds.) Drawing Graphs, Lecture Notes in Computer Science 2025, Springer-Verlag, 71–86
10. Brandes, U., Köpf, B. (2002) Fast and simple horizontal coordinate assignment. In: P. Mutzel, M. Jünger, S. Leipert (eds.) Graph Drawing '01, Lecture Notes in Computer Science 2265, Springer-Verlag, 31–44
11. Brandes, U., Wagner, D. (2000) Using graph layout to visualize train interconnection data. J. Graph Algorithms and Applications **4** (3), 135–155
12. Bridgeman, S., Di Battista, G., Didimo, W., Liotta, G., Tamassia, R., Vismara, L. (2000) Turn-regularity and optimal area drawings of orthogonal representations. Computational Geometry: Theory and Applications, **16**, 53–93
13. Bruß, I., Frick, A. (1996) Fast interactive 3-D graph visualization. In: F.-J. Brandenburg (ed.) Graph Drawing '95, Lecture Notes in Computer Science 1027, Springer-Verlag, 99–110
14. Buchheim, C., Jünger, M., Leipert, S. (2001) A fast layout algorithm for k-level graphs. In: J. Marks (ed.) Graph Drawing '00, Lecture Notes in Computer Science 1984, Springer-Verlag, 229–240
15. Buchheim, C., Jünger, M., Leipert, S. (2002) Improving Walker's algorithm to run in linear time. In: M. Goodrich and S. Kobourov (eds.) Graph Drawing '02, Lecture Notes in Computer Science 2528, Springer-Verlag, 344–353
16. Cai, J., Han, X., Tarjan, R. E. (1993) An $O(m \log n)$-time algorithm for the maximal planar subgraph problem. SIAM Journal on Computing **22**, 1142–1164
17. Chiba, N., Nishizeki, T., Abe, S., Ozawa T. (1985) A linear algorithm for embedding planar graphs using PQ-trees. Journal of Computer System Science **30** (1), 54–76
18. Cook, W. J., Cunningham, W. H., Pulleyblank, W. R., Schrijver, A. (1998) Combinatorial Optimization. John Wiley & Sons
19. Coffman, E. G., Graham, R. L. (1972) Optimal scheduling for two processor systems. Acta Informatica **1**, 200–213
20. Cruz, I. F., and Twarog, J. P. (1996) 3D graph drawing with simulated annealing. In: F.-J. Brandenburg (ed.) Graph Drawing '95, Lecture Notes in Computer Science 1027, Springer-Verlag, 162–165
21. Dahlhaus, E. (1998) A linear time algorithm to recognize clustered graphs and its parallelization. In: C. L. Lucchesi and A. V. Moura (eds.) Latin '98, Lecture Notes in Computer Science 1380, Springer-Verlag, 239–248
22. Davidson, R., Harel, D. (1996) Drawing graphs nicely using simulated annealing. ACM Transactions on Graphics **15**, 301–331
23. Di Battista, G., Eades, P., Tamassia, R., Tollis, I. G. (1999) Graph Drawing: Algorithms for the visualization of graphs. Prentice Hall, New Jersey
24. Di Battista, G., Garg, A., Liotta, G., Parise, A., Tamassia, R., Tassinari, E., Vargiu, F., Vismara, L. (1997) Drawing Directed Graphs: an Experimental Study. In: S. North (ed.) Graph Drawing '96, Lecture Notes in Computer Science 1190, Springer-Verlag, 76–91
25. Di Battista, G., Garg, A., Liotta, G., Tamassia, R., Tassinari, E., Vargiu, F. (1997) Computational Geometry: Theory and Applications **7**, 303–316
26. Di Battista, G., Didimo, W., Patrignani, M., Pizzonia M. (1999) Orthogonal and quasi-upward drawings with vertices of arbitrary size. In: J. Kratochvíl (ed.) Graph Drawing '99, Lecture Notes in Computer Science 1731, Springer-Verlag, 297–310

27. Djidjev, H. N. (1995) A linear algorithm for the maximal planar subgraph problem. In: Proceedings of the 4th Workshop Algorithms Data Struct., Lecture Notes in Computer Science, Springer-Verlag
28. Eades, P. (1984) A heuristic for graph drawing. Congressus Numerantium **42**, 149–160
29. Eades, P. (1992) Drawing free trees. Bulletin of the Institute for Combinatorics and its Applications **5**, 10–36
30. Eades, P., Lin, X., Smyth, W. F. (1993) A fast and effective heuristic for the feedback arc set problem. Information Processing Letters **47**, 319–323
31. Eades, P., Wormald, N. (1994) Edge crossings in drawings of bipartite graphs. Algorithmica **11**, 379–403
32. Eades, P., Cohen, R. F., Huang, M. L. (1997) Online animated graph drawing for web animation. In: G. Di Battista (ed.) Graph Drawing '97, Lecture Notes in Computer Science 1353, Springer-Verlag, 330–335
33. Elf, M., Gutwenger, C., Jünger, M., Rinaldi, G. (2001) Branch-and-cut algorithms and their implementation in ABACUS. In: M. Jünger and D. Naddef (eds.) Computational Combinatorial Optimization, Lecture Notes in Computer Science 2241, Springer-Verlag, 157–222
34. Euler, L. (1750) Demonstratio nonnullarum insignium proprietatum quibus solida hedris planis inclusa sunt praedita. Novi Comm. Acad. Sci. Imp. Petropol. **4** (1752-3, published 1758), 140–160, also: Opera Omnia (1) **26**, 94–108
35. Feng, Q. W., Cohen, R. F., Eades, P. (1995) Planarity for clustered graphs. In: P. Spirakis (ed.) Algorithms – ESA '95, Lecture Notes in Computer Science 979, Springer-Verlag, 213–226
36. Fößmeier, U., Kaufmann, M. (1996) Drawing high degree graphs with low bend numbers. In: F. J. Brandenburg (ed.) Graph Drawing '95, Lecture Notes in Computer Science 1027, Springer-Verlag, 254–266
37. Frick, A., Ludwig, A., Mehldau, H. (1995) A fast adaptive layout algorithm for undirected graphs. In: R. Tamassia and I. G. Tollis (eds.) Graph Drawing '94, Lecture Notes in Computer Science 894, Springer-Verlag, 388–403
38. Fruchtermann, T. M. J., Reingold, E. M. (1991) Graph drawing by force-directed placement. Software – Practice and Experience **21**, 1129–1164
39. Garey, M. R., Johnson, D. S. (1983) Crossing number is NP-complete. SIAM J. Algebraic Discrete Methods **4**, 312–316
40. Gansner, E. R., Koutsofios, E., North, S. C., Vo, K. P. (1993) A technique for drawing directed graphs. IEEE Transactions on Software Engineering **19**, 214–230
41. Garg, A., Tamassia, R. (1995) On the computational complexity of upward and rectilinear planarity testing. In: R. Tamassia and I. G. Tollis (eds.) Graph Drawing '94, Lecture Notes in Computer Science 894, Springer-Verlag, 286–297
42. Garg, A., Tamassia, R. (1997) A New Minimum Cost Flow Algorithm with Applications to Graph Drawing. In: S. North (ed.) Graph Drawing '96, Lecture Notes in Computer Science 1190, Springer-Verlag, 201–216
43. Gutwenger, C., Mutzel, P., Weiskircher, R. (2001) Inserting an edge into a planar graph. In: Proceedings of the Ninth Annual ACM-SIAM Symposium on Discrete Algorithms (SODA 2001), ACM Press, 246-255
44. Healy, P., Kuusik, A. (1999) The vertex-exchange graph: a new concept for multi-level crossing minimization. In: J. Kratochvíl (ed.) Graph Drawing '99, Lecture Notes in Computer Science 1731, Springer-Verlag, 205–216

45. Hopcroft, J., Tarjan, R. E. (1974) Efficient planarity testing. Journal of the ACM **21**, 549–568
46. Jayakumar, R., Thulasiraman, K., Swamy, M. N. S. (1989) $O(n^2)$ algorithms for graph planarization. IEEE Transactions on Computer Aided Design **8**, 257–267
47. Jünger, M., Leipert, S., Mutzel, P. (1998) A note on computing a maximal planar subgraph using PQ-trees. IEEE Transactions of Computer-Aided Design and Integrated Circuits and Systems **17**, 609–612
48. Jünger, M., Mutzel, P. (1996) Maximum planar subgraphs and nice embeddings: practical layout tools. Algorithmica **16**, 33–59
49. Jünger, M., Mutzel, P. (1997) 2-layer straight line crossing minimization: performance of exact and heuristic algorithms. Journal of Graph Algorithms and Applications **1**, 1–25
50. Jünger, M., Reinelt, G., Thienel, S. (1995) Practical Problem Solving with Cutting Plane Algorithms in Combinatorial Optimization. In: W. Cook, L. Lovász, P. Seymour (eds.), DIMACS Series in Discrete Mathematics and Theoretical Computer Science, 111-152
51. Kamada, T., and Kawai, S. (1989) An algorithm for drawing general undirected graphs. Information Processing Letters **31**, 7–15
52. Kaufmann, M., Wagner, D. (eds.) (2001) Drawing Graphs: Methods and Models. Lecture Notes in Computer Science 2025, Springer-Verlag
53. Klau, G. W., Klein, K., Mutzel P. (2001) An Experimental Comparison of Orthogonal Compaction Algorithms. In: J. Marks (ed.) Graph Drawing '00, Lecture Notes in Computer Science 1984, Springer-Verlag, 37–51
54. Klau, G. W., Mutzel P. (1999) Optimal compaction of orthogonal grid drawings. In: G. Cornuejols, R. E. Burkard, and G. J. Woeginger (eds.), Integer Programming and Combinatorial Optimization (IPCO '99), Lecture Notes in Computer Science 1610, Springer-Verlag, 304–319
55. Lempel, A., Even, S., Cederbaum, I. (1967) An algorithm for planarity testing of graphs. Theory of Graphs: International Symposium: Rome, July 1966, Gordon and Breach, New York, 215–232
56. Liu, P.C., Geldmacher, R. C. (1977) On the deletion of nonplanar edges of a graph. Proceedings of the 10th S-E Conference on Comb., Graph Theory, and Comp., Boca Raton, FL, 727–738
57. Mehlhorn K., Mutzel, P. (1996) On the embedding phase of the Hopcroft and Tarjan planarity testing algorithm. Algorithmica **16**, 233–242
58. Mutzel, P., Weiskircher, R. (2002) Bend Minimization in Orthogonal Drawings Using Integer Programming. In: O. Ibarra and L. Zhang (eds.) Computing and Combinatorics, Eighth Annual International Conference (COCOON 2002), Lecture Notes in Computer Science 2387, Springer-Verlag, 484-493
59. Patrignani, M. (2001) On the complexity of orthogonal compaction. Computational Geometry: Theory and Applications **19** (1), 47–67
60. Reingold, E., Tilford, J. (1981) Tidier drawing of trees. IEEE Transactions on Software Engineering **7**, 223–228
61. Sander, G. (1996) Visualisierungstechniken für den Compilerbau. Pirrot Verlag & Druck, Saarbrücken
62. Sugiyama, K., Tagawa, S.,Toda, M. (1981) Methods for visual understanding of hierarchical system structures. IEEE Transactions on Systems, Man, and Cybernetics **11**, 109–125

63. Sugiyama, K., Misue, K. (1991) Visualization of structural information: automatic drawing of compound digraphs. IEEE Transactions on Systems, Man, and Cybernetics **4** (21), 876–893
64. Sugiyama, K., Misue, K. (1995) A simple and unified method for drawing graphs: magnetic-spring algorithm. In: R. Tamassia and I. G. Tollis (eds.) Graph Drawing '94, Lecture Notes in Computer Science 894, Springer-Verlag, 364–375
65. Supowit, K. J., Reingold, E. M. (1983) The complexity of drawing trees nicely. Acta Inform. **18**, 377–392
66. Tamassia, R. (1987) On embedding a graph in the grid with the minimum number of bends. SIAM Journal on Computing **16** (3), 421–444
67. Tamassia, R., Di Battista, G., Batini, C. (1988) Automatic graph drawing and readability of diagrams. IEEE Transactions on Systems, Man, and Cybernetics **18**, 61–79
68. Tutte, W. T. (1963) How to draw a graph. Proceedings of the London Mathematical Society, Third Series **13**, 743–768
69. Waddle, V., Malhotra, A. (1999) An E log E line crossing algorithm for levelled graphs. In: J. Kratochvíl (ed.) Graph Drawing '99, Lecture Notes in Computer Science 1731, Springer-Verlag, 59–70
70. Walker II, J. Q. (1990) A node-positioning algorithm for general trees. Software – Practice and Experience **20**, 685–705
71. Ziegler, T. (2001) Crossing minimization in automatic graph drawing. Doctoral Thesis, Technische Fakultät der Universität des Saarlandes

WilmaScope – A 3D Graph Visualization System

Tim Dwyer[1] and Peter Eckersley[2]

[1] School of Information Technologies, Madsen Building F09, University of Sydney, NSW 2006, Australia. E-mail: dwyer@cs.usyd.edu.au
[2] Department of Computer Science & Software Engineering, University of Melbourne, Victoria 3010, Australia. E-mail: pde@cs.mu.oz.au

1 Introduction

Despite, or perhaps because of, the extensive research literature on graph drawing techniques, there is a lack of state-of-the-art, general purpose visualization systems, particularly for application to three-dimensional embeddings.

Graph drawing problems are, of course, existent within an enormous range of fields; a key motivation for creating a general purpose 3D visualization system is to provide easy-to-use components which can be employed by future software across these application domains.

Within the graph drawing community itself a system may also aspire to streamline, elucidate and beautify the work of algorithm design, comparison and optimization. Achieving these benefits requires software that is flexible, interactive and easily extensible.

In order to provide these benefits as widely as possible and to guarantee a culture of user participation, a serious graph visualization system should also be *Free Software* [18].

In this chapter we describe WilmaScope (or "Wilma" for short), a sophisticated graph visualization infrastructure, which attempts to meet these goals. Particularly, it is intended to provide an extensible framework for use in experimentation and exploration of 3D graph applications.

In Section 2 we describe the motivation for WilmaScope with reference to applications to which it is well suited. Section 3 covers the main Graph Drawing algorithms which are available in the Wilma system. Section 4 goes into some of the implementation details including architecture, modular subsystems, and facilities for control by human users and other software. Section 5 gives a gallery of domain specific applications. In Section 6 we describe the specific software platform used and discuss Wilma's availability on the Internet.

1.1 Related Work

Where relevant, related work is referred to in later sections. However, before going on we will briefly review some 3D graph visualization systems. Each of these has introduced features which are now part of WilmaScope.

Hendley *et al.* [10] describe Narcissus, a 3D graph visualization system featuring "ball and stick" representations of nodes and edges, clusters represented by transparent spheres and force-directed layout. The layout parameters are configurable and the user can fly around the model but the layout is not animated and no facility to interact with the graph elements is mentioned.

NestedVision3D [15] is a similar system but also allows the user to interact with the graph by expanding and collapsing clusters. They use a hierarchical layout which is again not animated (apart from smoothly growing and shrinking the clusters as they are expanded and collapsed).

Brandes *et al.* [1] demonstrate a step towards a fully animated dynamic 3D graphing system by smoothly animating the transitions between a sequence of changing graphs. However, the visualization is rendered as a movie so that no interaction with the scene is possible.

Sprenger *et al.* [17] describe a VRML based system which allows the user to directly edit data parameters associated with nodes in the scene, however no animation is supported. A nice feature of this system is transparent cluster hulls which more tightly fit around their constituent nodes than simple spheres.

The WilmaScope system's main contribution over these systems is its support of a variety of animated layout algorithms, its level of interactivity and its availability under an open source license.

2 Applications

3D graph visualization has not yet found the degree of acceptance that graph drawing in 2D has found. Probably since 2D graph drawing's "killer app" is the printed page or poster[1]. Although 3D graphics technology is improving very quickly it may be that 3D visualization will have to await the advent of cheap, ubiquitous holographic, augmented or virtual reality environments before it gains universal acceptance. However, clever research into this embryonic area will hopefully produce examples which demonstrate some benefits of 3D visualization even using current hardware. User studies such as [22] and [16] claim there are certain benefits to 3D graph visualization with the caveat that the correct hardware is available and that the third dimension is used effectively. It is this latter problem that we hope a tool like Wilma can help explore. Section 5.2 provides an example of an application that we believe makes effective use of the third dimension by using it to represent time.

[1] Certainly the screen-shots of Wilma's 3D graphics display included in this chapter do not do 3D visualization much justice. Due to their small size and without the ability to rotate or zoom the scenes the labels are difficult to read and their structure is sometimes obscured.

It was with the hope of supporting such research that Wilma was conceived and offered as open source to researchers and experimenters under the Lesser GNU General Public License (LGPL). Its extensibility and broad base of features make it ideal for rapid prototyping of novel 3D graph visualizations.

This flexibility and potential is demonstrated by the number of different applications that have already been explored using Wilma including:

- software visualization using a 3D interpretation of the Unified Modeling Language
- a novel visual metaphor for visualizing fund manager movement in capital markets
- visualization of clustering in web structure
- general concept map visualization

In Section 5 we describe these domain specific applications more fully with examples of graphical results.

3 Algorithms

Four layout algorithms have so far been implemented in Wilma:

- a classic force-directed layout supporting clustered graphs
- a simulated annealing based method which attempts to reduce the algorithmic complexity of layout following a physical metaphor.
- a faster algorithm based on multi-scale force-directed layout.
- a method which uses the external DOT program from the AT&T Graphviz toolkit to produce a Sugiyama-style layout.

We refer to the implementations of these algorithms as "layout engines" and describe them in more detail below.

3.1 Force-Directed

The first layout algorithm implemented in Wilma was force-directed layout the basic principles of which are described in Section 4.5 of the Technical Foundations. There were several factors that motivated us to implement this algorithm first, notably:

- it is relatively easy to obtain good results for most types of graphs by application of the basic attractive spring force and repulsive inter-node force.
- it is easy to animate the layout process in a dynamic graph visualization to preserve a user's "mental map" [14] between changes in the graph structure. We can animate simply by redrawing the graph between each iteration of the algorithm.

- since the algorithm is iterative and does not require any special pre- or post-processing it is easy to use in a dynamic graph editor where the graph structure may be changed by the user even before the layout has stabilized.
- different layout æsthetics can be enhanced by adding extra forces such as the Sugiyama and Misue [19] directed-field force (see Section 4.5 in the Technical Foundations) for aligning directed edges to emphasize flow.
- the force-directed approach can be easily extended to support clustered graphs [13].
- the approach works just as well in three dimensions as in two.

The Wilma implementation of the force-directed algorithm attempts to make the most of these assorted advantages. Firstly it offers a user interface which allows the user to control all the parameters of the layout algorithm even while the layout is still in progress. The user can control the number of iterations of the algorithm that are executed between frames of animation, choosing to run the algorithm to convergence as fast as possible or to watch the layout unfold, and if necessary tweak the controls to adjust the embedding or to help it converge.

Different forces, such as the directed field force or a gravitational force which keeps the graph centered, may be added or removed at any time to achieve different æsthetic effects. Since each of the different forces implements a common interface (as the UML Class Diagram in Figure 6(a) illustrates), new forces can be added or removed at any time.

The force-directed layout engine fits well into Wilma's object-oriented clustered graph model described in Section 4. Our design allows for each cluster to be arranged by its own layout engine but, when the force-directed engine is used, edges connecting nodes in different clusters exert a force on the nodes inside these clusters. The nodes inside a cluster are attracted to the centroid of the cluster by a "gravitational force". The gravitational force then balances the inter-cluster forces, the net result is shown in Figure 1. This achieves a net result similar to the "dummy node" approach of Huang and Eades [13], however, repulsive forces do not need to be calculated between nodes inside different clusters.

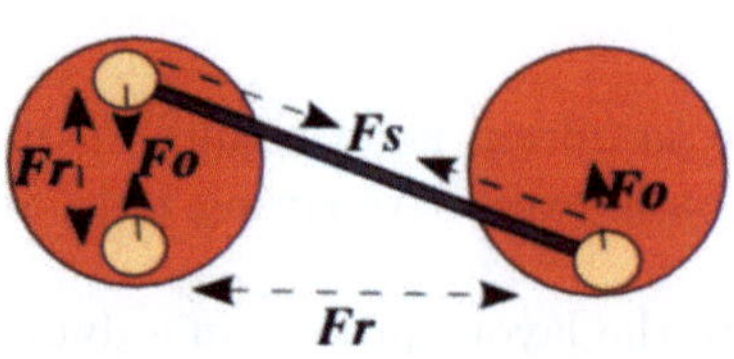

Fig. 1. The forces used in Wilma's force-directed layout engine: *Fr* is the repulsive force between nodes, *Fo* is the force attracting nodes to the origin of a cluster (the gravity force) and *Fs* is the spring force between nodes connected by an edge.

All nodes and clusters are assigned a mass. By default nodes have unit mass though a user may specify a different mass if necessary. A cluster's mass is the sum of the masses of all its children. The repulsive force used varies with the mass of nodes so that nodes with large mass, such as clusters with many descendents, will exert a strong repulsive force on their neighbors, i.e.,

$$\text{repulsionforce}(p_u, p_v) \equiv \frac{m_u m_v}{\|\overrightarrow{p_u} - \overrightarrow{p_v}\|} \cdot \overrightarrow{p_u p_v}$$

This ensures that clusters have plenty of space and avoids overlaps. It also helps to give the user a feeling for the size of collapsed clusters. That is, even though their contents are elided, the space around them gives an indication as to the number of nodes they contain.

A novel extension that has been added to our force-directed layout engine is the ability for the contents of clusters to be constrained to a plane. The orientation of this plane can then be rotated in order to help minimize the spring force of inter-cluster edges. This is illustrated in Figure 2. Restricting the contents of clusters to planes, but then allowing the clusters themselves to be arranged in three dimensions, allows certain types of clustered graphs to be more clearly displayed. For example, a graph which is not *c-planar* [6] but which has planar clusters may be best displayed in this way, showing planarity where possible but avoiding intersecting edges.

3.2 Fast Simulated Annealing

As stated in Section 1, a major design goal for Wilma was to provide a platform upon which algorithmic experimentation could be conducted elegantly and efficiently.

As we have argued, force-directed layout algorithms are well suited to a wide range of graph visualization problems. One variation on these algorithms, advocated by Fruchtermann & Reingold [8] and Davidson *et al.* [3], attempts to avoid calculation of repulsion force vectors, which is $O(|V|)$ for each node i, and $O(|V|^2)$ for the whole graph:

$$\overrightarrow{R_i} \equiv \sum_{j \in V \setminus \{i\}} \overrightarrow{p_{ij}} \tag{1}$$

Where $\overrightarrow{p_{ij}} = \overrightarrow{p_i} - \overrightarrow{p_j}$ is the displacement of node i relative to j.

To avoid this expense it is possible to approximate scalar energy potential values, caching this information at grid points throughout space. Iterated updates to the potential well then cost only $O(|V|)$ time per iteration. On the downside, the cache array itself takes $O(v \cdot \rho)$ memory, where v is the m-dimensional volume (or area) of the embedded graph and ρ is the density of stored grid points.

Cowling [2] has implemented a fast layout engine for WilmaScope which employs simulated annealing with potential energy caching to achieve graph

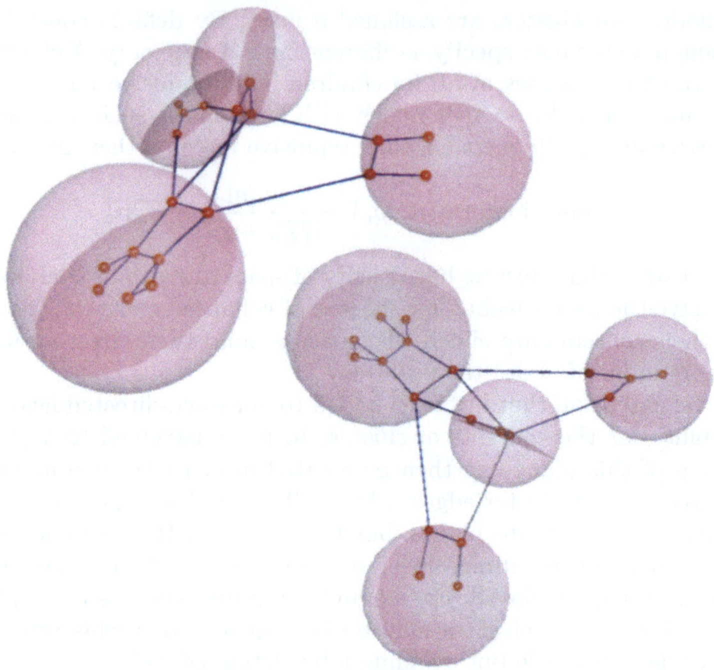

Fig. 2. A screen-shot showing a clustered graph with planar clusters. The clusters are rotated to minimize the lengths of the edges between clusters.

embeddings in time linear to the number of vertices. Cowling was able to demonstrate that the algorithms of [3] do appear to achieve linear time results. However, when the grid size $v \cdot \rho$ must be adjusted to prevent folding in large graphs, space and time complexity are no longer linear. Figure 3 shows before and after screen-shots of the algorithm's effects.

Cowling's work serves to demonstrate the utility of Wilma as an empirical platform; with the WilmaScope rendering and navigation system, and the availability of convenient data structures for input and dataset management, algorithmic experiments can be set up quickly.

3.3 Multi-Scale Force-Directed

Although the fast simulated annealing approach described above did not prove perfect as a universal replacement for iterated, force-directed layout, there are other algorithms in the literature which might be brought to bear.

We have implemented one of these – the "Multi-Level Force-Directed" approach of Walshaw [21]. This multi-scaled approach incorporates two main innovations over the common force-directed algorithm – hierarchical layout, and short-range-only repulsion forces.

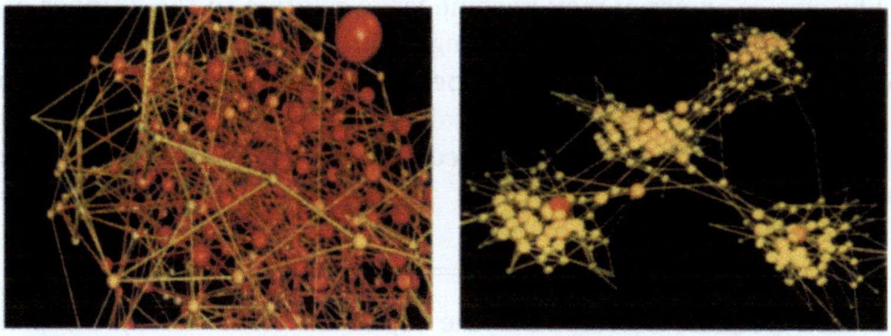

(a) After only a few iterations.

(b) After a complete run of the algorithm.

Fig. 3. These screen-shots demonstrate the effects of the simulated annealing algorithm with potential caching. Note that the color of the nodes indicates the force potential at that location.

Instead of laying out the entire graph from singular or random initial conditions, the algorithm creates a series of simplified approximations of the graph, and embeds each of these with increasingly fine detail.

The simplified approximations are generated by applying matching algorithms, which select at each iteration as many edges as possible such that no node is connected to two of these edges. Each edge is then "collapsed" so that the two nodes at either end are combined, and the process is repeated.

In order to perform these simplifications rapidly the stochastic matching approach of Hendrickson & Leland [11] is employed. This takes $O(|E|) = O(|V| \cdot \frac{|E|}{|V|})$ time and is linear for sparse graphs (where $\frac{|E|}{|V|}$ is bounded).

After each level of force-directed layout has stabilized the aggregated nodes are replaced by their pairs of matched children and the layout process is re-initialized. This process repeats until the entire graph has been embedded.

The multi-level process provides a number of benefits over single-pass force-directed layout. Notably, these include avoidance of local energy minima which may result from the arbitrary initial position of a large set of nodes; and the ability to tune layout parameters to correct for pathologies which become apparent to the user as the level of detail increases.

Walshaw's algorithm also addresses the $O(|V|^2)$ cost of calculating the repulsion force (see Equation 1). As with the fast simulated annealing strategy this involves storing information about the repulsion in a spatial data structure although the details are different.

Instead of trying to approximate the potential field of the force the spatial structure simply allows nodes to be addressed by their locality (or "cell"). A naïve method for doing this is to keep lists of nodes in a complete spatial array. The size of an array may become large relative to the number of nodes (especially for spacious 3D embeddings) but, if this is problematic, space usage can be made linear in the number of nodes in exchange for a constant slowdown through the use of a hash table.

If the repulsion force is constructed so that it cuts off beyond a certain distance d_∞, that is:

$$\exists\, d_\infty \forall i,j : ||\overrightarrow{p_i} - \overrightarrow{p_j}|| > d_\infty \Longrightarrow \text{repulsionforce}(p_i, p_j) = \overrightarrow{0} \qquad (2)$$

It is then possible to calculate the repulsion force on a particular node i with reference solely to the positions of nearby nodes. If the cells for the spatial data structure are of a size greater than or equal to d_∞ then all such nodes may be addressed through the cell containing i and those adjacent to it. In this algorithm the cost of calculating the repulsion force is $O(|V| \cdot \rho)$, where ρ is the average of the embedding density around each node.

The multi-level force-directed layout engine provides WilmaScope with an efficient mechanism for handling large graphs. Figure 4 gives six screen shots showing the progressive addition of detail as a large graph is embedded using the Wilma multi-scale layout engine. Figure 10(b) on page 69 shows the full control panel for the multi-scale layout engine. Each of these parameters may be adjusted as the layout progresses and the effect instantly seen on screen.

3.4 DOT: Layered Layout

DOT is a program included in the Graphviz (`http://www.graphviz.org`) open source graph visualization toolkit from AT&T, see the chapter on Graphviz in this book. It produces pleasing two dimensional layered graph layouts using a Sugiyama-style algorithm [20], see Section 4.2 in the Technical Foundations. The Wilma DOT layout engine runs DOT in a sub-process, pipes in the graph data converted into DOT file format and parses the DOT output to obtain the new layout. DOT also features æsthetically pleasing spline edges which Wilma is able to render as curved tubes.

Since the DOT layouts are strictly two-dimensional we are free to use the third dimension to capture additional information. For example Section 5.2 describes an application where the third dimension (the z-axis) is used to capture changes in the graph over time. That is, the nodes are rendered as tubes and the edges may appear at different levels in the z dimension.

4 Implementation

4.1 High Level Architecture

Conceived as a research project with open-ended goals Wilma was designed to be as flexible and extensible as possible. The intention was to allow different components such as new visual representations for graph elements, interfaces (either graphical user interfaces or remote programming interfaces)

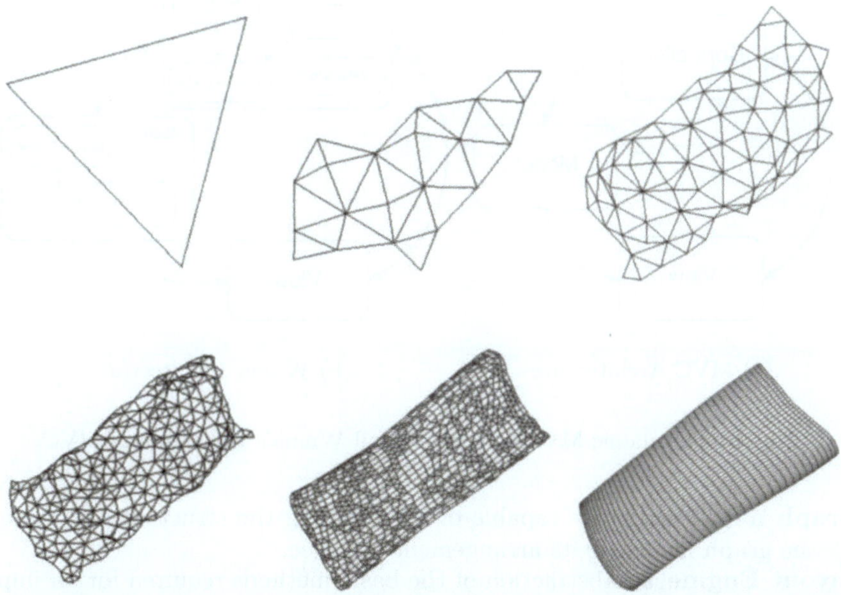

Fig. 4. Six screen shots showing the progress of the Wilma multi-scale layout engine as it finds an embedding for a regular mesh containing 900 nodes.

and different layout algorithm implementations to be added or removed easily. Therefore the design needed to decouple these components as much as possible so that altering one component would have minimal impact on the other components.

To achieve this we began by exploring the well known *Model-View-Controller* architecture (MVC) [9]. Briefly, the three primary components of the MVC architecture are as follows:

Model the core of the application, the data and algorithms that automatically modify the data.

View a user interface which displays information about the model to the user.

Controller a separate user interface that provides methods for the user to manipulate the application, i.e., to control the Model.

Each component's reference to the other components is via a carefully defined interface which should not require change when one of the components is modified in some way. The standard data flow diagram for the MVC architecture is shown in Figure 5(a).

In our system the Model component comprises two sub-components:

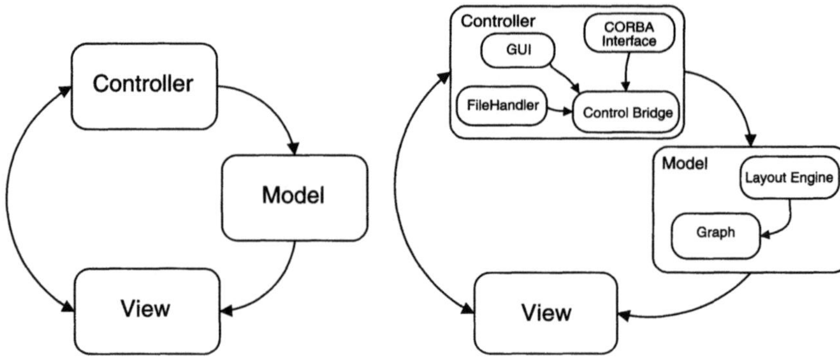

(a) MVC Architecture (b) Wilma Architecture

Fig. 5. The classic MVC framework and Wilma's utilization of MVC.

Graph a data structure capable of representing the structure and state of the graph including its arrangement in space.

Layout Engine an abstraction of the basic methods required for an implementation of any layout algorithm that will change the graph's arrangement in space.

A further requirement for our system is that the graph data model, the layout engine and the visual representation of the graph elements should be controllable from multiple sources, primarily:

Graphical User Interface a user can interactively construct or edit the graph structure. The user can also adjust the layout engine parameters and change the visual representation of the graph elements.

File Handler a previously constructed graph may be loaded from a file.

API Hooks supports remote control from a program running in another process or possibly on another machine.

The Controller component was therefore also broken down into several subcomponents. A "bridge" layer provides a common pro-grammatic interface to the Model. The methods provided by this bridge layer can then be called by either the GUI interface component, a component providing a CORBA interface for remote access or a component which can load and save files to an XML format.

Figure 5(b) depicts this expanded MVC architecture for graph visualization.

4.2 An Object-Oriented Graph Model

In designing the Graph Model, i.e., the data structures for storing the graph and the methods for manipulating them, some common elements were identified. From the definitions given in Section 2 of the Technical Foundations: a graph consists fundamentally of nodes and edges. These are the basic graph elements. A clustered graph has nodes which may themselves be graphs called clusters (see Section 2.5 of the Technical Foundations).

A clustered graph is modeled in a class hierarchy by defining an abstract class *GraphElement* which is implemented by both the *Node* and *Edge* classes. A Cluster will inherit all the properties of the *Node* class[2] and also contains an aggregation of *Nodes* and *Edges*. A Cluster also contains a reference to an abstract definition of a *LayoutEngine* which provides a common interface to an implementation of a layout algorithm for arranging the graph in two or three dimensional space. Since the details of the algorithm are kept separate it is easy to mix and match different layout styles to different graphs or even to clusters within the one graph. A similar class hierarchy was developed independently by Marshall *et al.* [12] around the same time. Figure 6(a) shows a UML diagram depicting this graph class hierarchy, and also shows how this relates to a force-directed *LayoutEngine* implementation, discussed further in Section 3.1. In Figure 6(b) we show a 3D interpretation of this UML diagram rendered by Wilma. This application of the system is described further in Section 5.1.

4.3 User Interface Design

A screen-shot of the main Wilma window, with labels describing the main features is shown in Figure 7. The majority of the space in this window is given over to the 3D canvas in which the graph structure is visualized. Users may "fly" through the virtual space rendered on this canvas by dragging with the various mouse buttons. The possible mouse navigation actions (rotate, zoom and translate) are shown in the reminder panel at the bottom of the window (which may be hidden to gain screen real-estate for the 3D canvas).

The user may also navigate through the cluster hierarchy through this window. Clusters are generally shown as transparent spheres or other convex shapes enveloping the nodes in the cluster. Right clicking on a cluster opens a pop-up menu in which the user may choose to expand or collapse that cluster. Collapsing the cluster removes its contents from the 3D scene, shrinks the cluster glyph to a size proportional to the sum of the mass of its child nodes and makes the (normally transparent) cluster glyph opaque.

For expanded spherical clusters calculating the radius such that all the cluster's children are enclosed is a simple matter. We set the radius of an expanded cluster $R_e(C)$ large enough to include the farthest child node v (of radius $R(v)$) from the cluster centroid c, i.e.,

$$R_e(C) = \max_{v \in C}(\|\overrightarrow{p_v} - \overrightarrow{p_c}\| + R(v))$$

[2] Whilst it is not strictly necessary that clusters should inherit all of the properties of nodes, in some domains it is rather useful to allow edges to be attached to clusters as a whole.

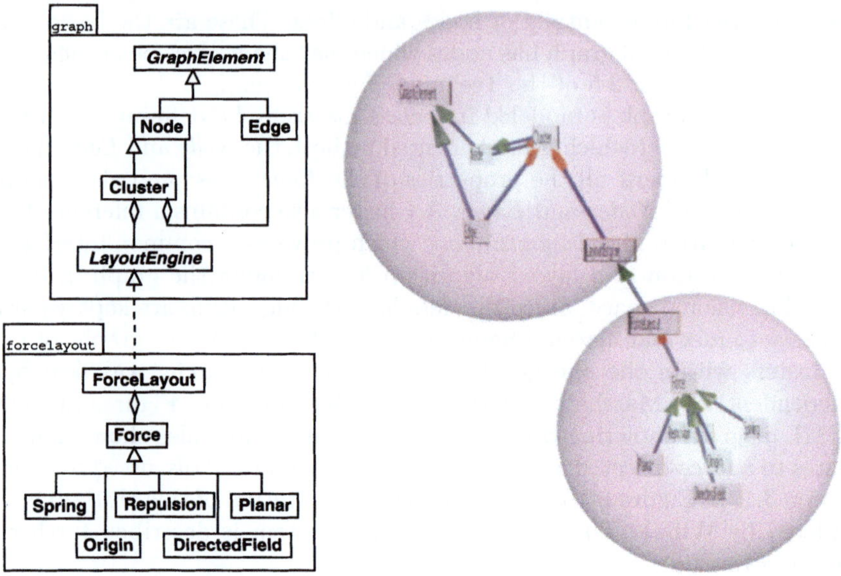

(a) UML Class diagram.

(b) A 3D interpretation of the class hierarchy.

Fig. 6. A class hierarchy for the graph model and the classes used in the Force-Directed Layout Engine implementation.

Thus the radius of expanded clusters depends on the layout algorithm used within the cluster and can be quite large.

We have found that a convenient way to determine the radius of a collapsed cluster $R_c(C)$ is to assume a volume for the cluster proportional to its total mass. The following is obtained from the formula for volume of a sphere:

$$R_c(C) = \sqrt[3]{\frac{3}{(4\rho\pi)} \sum_{v \in C} m_v}$$

We choose ρ to be a scale factor such that the size of a collapsed cluster of unit mass is slightly smaller than the expanded size. This method produces a collapsed cluster whose size gives the user a feeling for the number of children it contains. Yet, it is still compact enough to be useful in the elision of unnecessary detail from the collapsed parts of a clustered graph.

Note that a cluster's mass is the sum of its children so that a collapsed cluster's size will reflect the sum of all its descendents in the cluster tree. Section 3.1 describes how this mass is used to layout expanded clusters.

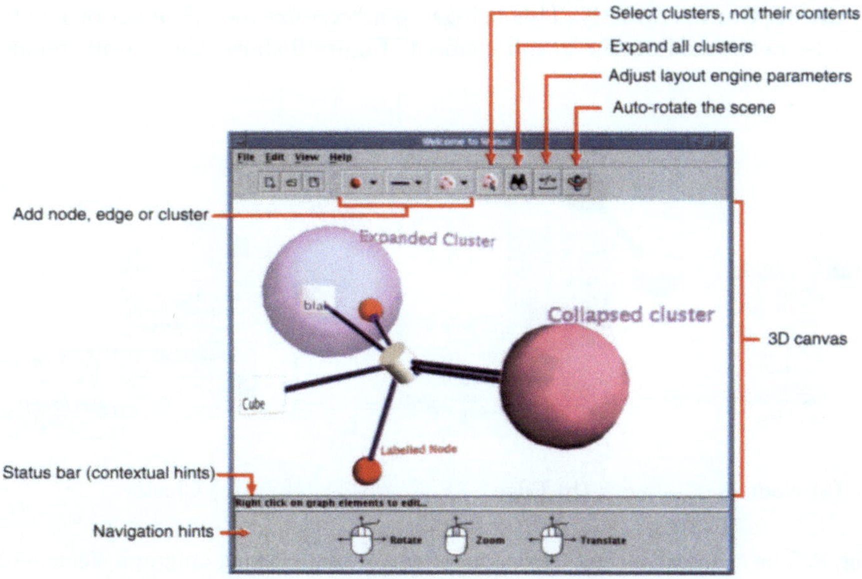

Fig. 7. The main WilmaScope window.

Wilma was conceived as an interactive graph editor and, therefore, there are a range of basic actions that a user may perform in editing the graph structure. A user may add nodes and edges or group nodes into clusters using the toolbar buttons. Clicking on the small arrow on a toolbar button produces a menu from which the default appearance for new graph elements may be selected, see Figure 8.

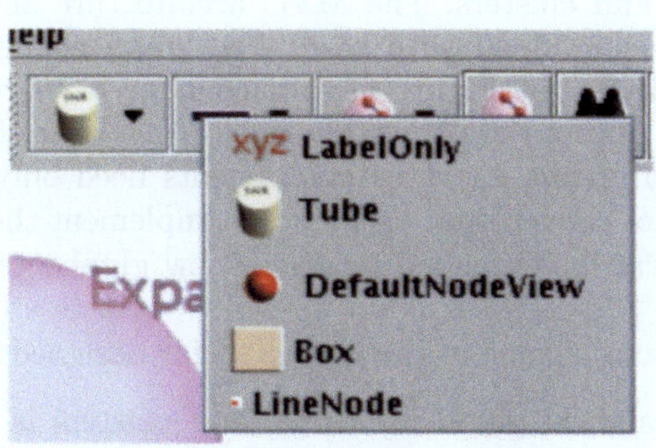

Fig. 8. Setting the default Node.

Alternately they can make changes to the graph or change the appearance of particular graph elements by right clicking on the nodes, edges or clusters on the 3D Canvas directly. This brings up a "context menu" of actions which may be performed on the graph element. Figure 9 shows the various menus.

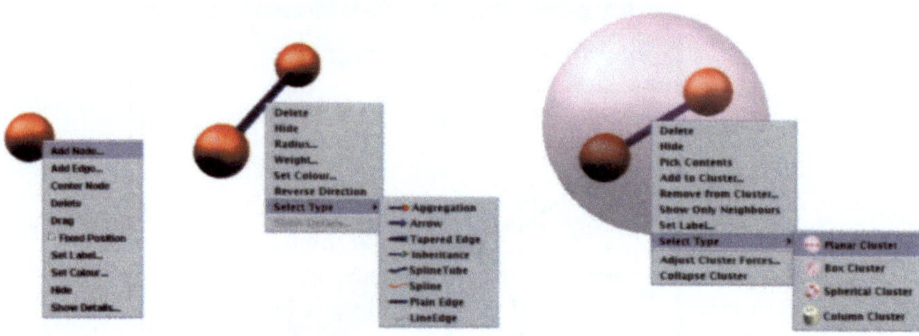

(a) Node (b) Edge (c) Cluster

Fig. 9. The "context menus" that appear when right-clicking on graph elements in Wilma.

Since Wilma is intended as a toolkit for exploring various layout algorithms an effort has been made to provide user controls for all parameters to these algorithms and to allow the user to change these parameters as layout proceeds. Figure 10 shows the various layout controls available to the user.

4.4 3D Graph Elements

Wilma provides a number of different 3D "widgets" or "glyphs"[3] representing nodes, edges and clusters. The MVC architecture allows other custom graph elements to be added with ease. The graph element classes defined in the *graph* package, see Figure 6(a), each have a reference to an object implementing the appropriate View interface (*NodeView*, *EdgeView* or *ClusterView*). Custom glyphs for these components need only implement these interfaces. Abstract convenience classes that implement these interfaces with default methods can be extended to define new glyphs with very little new code.

We briefly describe some of the glyphs so far designed for Wilma:

Defaults The standard glyph for nodes and clusters is a sphere and the default edge glyph is a simple cylinder. Such primitive shapes are useful

[3] "Glyph" refers to a graphical symbol, from the Greek word meaning carving. The term "Widget" usually implies a degree of interactivity, for example a button in a GUI. Our 3D graph elements are indeed interactive, so the latter might be more appropriate. In fact a Wilma graph could probably be used as a novel front end to an interactive application

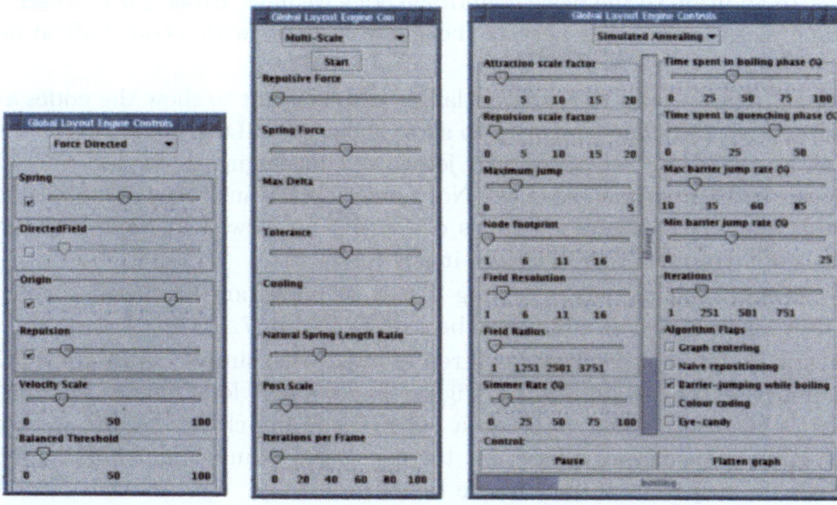

(a) Controls for the force-directed layout engine

(b) Controls for the multi-scale-force-directed layout engine

(c) Controls for the simulated-annealing layout engine

Fig. 10. The various layout engine control windows in Wilma.

because they look the same from all viewpoints. Level of Detail (LOD) scaling is used to improve rendering speed, thus maintaining high frame rates when the scene is rotated or zoomed. The underlying framework of all 3D shapes is a triangular mesh. LOD scaling reduces the total number of triangles that need to be displayed at any one time by drawing shapes distant from the view point in a courser fashion. This is, of course, at the expense of the additional video memory required to store both the detailed and course triangular meshes.

By default labels appear as banners hovering above the nodes and edges. These banners rotate to face the viewpoint so that they may be read even as the scene is being rotated.

Nodes Different applications require different node representations. For example, the 3D UML model shown in Figure 6(b) uses boxes to represent UML classes. The class name is texture mapped onto the surface of the box and in a similar fashion to the banner labels described above the boxes rotate to face the user. In order to enhance the 3D effect the edges of the boxes are beveled. An application that uses cylindrical nodes is described in Section 5.2. As can be seen in the example the top and bottom radii of these cylinders may be adjusted.

Edges In addition to the basic cylindrical edge we have arrows for representing directed edges. The head of the arrow is shown with a cone indicating direction.

A very efficient way to represent larger graphs is not to show the nodes at all and use only line segments to show the edges. 3D Graphics hardware can store a large set of vertices joined by line segments as a single 3D shape without surface normals. Not rendering the surfaces means graphs with tens of thousands of nodes can easily be viewed in their entirety. This style of rendering is shown in Figure 4.

In Wilma multiple edges joining a pair of nodes are displayed slightly offset, an example of which can be seen in Figure 7.

Clusters So far clusters have been represented with simple transparent 3D primitives: spheres and boxes. Figure 2 shows a style of cluster in which nodes are constrained to lie on a plane inside the cluster. Again we use a simple transparent sphere but the constraint plane is also highlighted with a transparent surface inside the cluster.

A more ambitious representation of a cluster might be a convex hull surrounding the cluster's children. Such a representation would probably be too computationally intensive to allow animated changes to the positions of the cluster's contents. However, it may be useful to show collapsed clusters in this way. Thus some of the cluster's internal structure would still be visible even when the individual nodes have been elided. Sprenger *et al.* [17] demonstrate such a visualization of clustered graphs without animation.

5 Examples

Wilma was designed to be as open and extensible as possible and evidence for the success of this design is shown in the array of domains to which Wilma has been applied.

5.1 3D UML Visualization

The first application of Wilma was an investigation into a 3D extension of the Unified Modeling Language [5]. UML diagram elements were translated into 3D glyphs and a simple class-diagram editor was constructed on top of the Wilma framework. A user study was then conducted to test the feasibility of such a paradigm for software design. Interesting anecdotal evidence was collected indicating that such 3D UML models, when coupled with a force-directed layout engine, could assist a software architect to understand structure within a reasonably complex system. An example of such a diagram is shown in Figure 6(b).

5.2 Fund Manager Flow Visualization

Most stock market visualizations involve a fairly straightforward mapping of share attributes into two- or three-dimensional space. The most obvious example is share price time series charts. In an experiment into graph based visualization techniques for stock market data, Dwyer [4] defined a graph model for Fund Manager movement within the stock market. The graph consists of nodes, which represent stocks, and edges, which represent a *movement* of a fund manager between a pair of stocks. Movement from one stock to another occurs when a fund manager reduces their holding in the first and increases their holding in the second.

The clients were particularly interested in seeing the changing behavior of fund managers over time. Effectively this means that we must find some way to visualize a changing graph. We showed these changes by arranging the graph for each time period on a plane and then stacking the time periods in the third dimension. Nodes representing stocks are extruded into columns whose width may be varied to indicate a stock attribute such as unit price. We call these 3D stacked graph visualizations *stratified graphs*, borrowing the geological term.

Various styles of layout were tried in arranging these stratified graphs in space. Force-directed layout was useful for showing clustering and centrality of highly active stocks while Sugiyama-style layout is useful for showing flow from source stocks to sinks. Figure 11 shows an example using the DOT layout engine in Wilma to produce 3D Sugiyama-style layout. A current research project is to tailor the heuristics used in these layout algorithms to suit such stratified graphs.

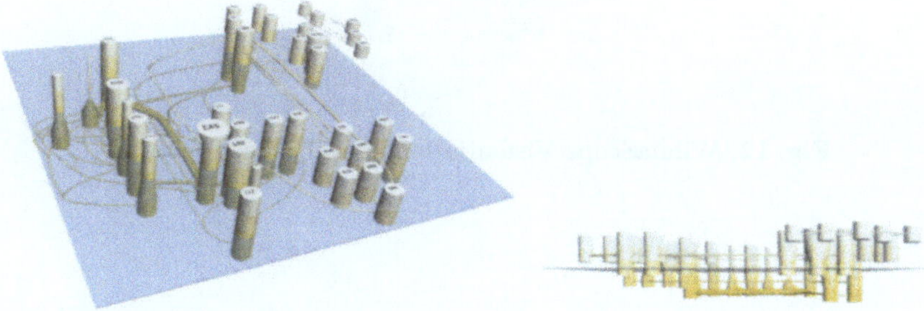

(a) Perspective view (b) Side view

Fig. 11. A visualization of fund manager movement within the UK Computer Services sector for five time periods over two weeks in December.

5.3 Web Structure Visualization

One early application of Wilma was in the representation of web structure, and to visualizing clustering algorithms for categorizing such structure [7].

An example of web structure visualization is shown in Figure 12. This is a dataset collected in 2000 from the web-site `www.linuxlinks.com`. Each node is a page and edges indicate links between pages. The clusters are defined over similarity[4] between pages. Note that the density of edges in the visualization is due to 17 pages (linked to every other page) which form the site's navigation bar.

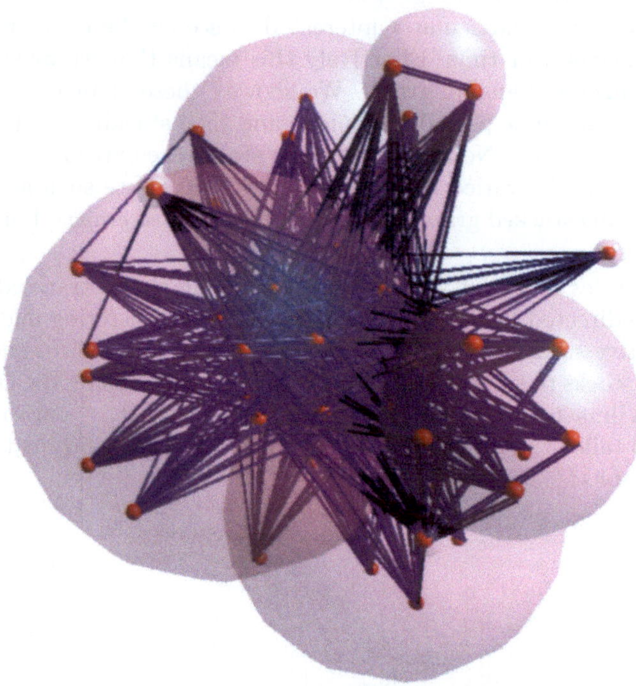

Fig. 12. WilmaScope Visualization of Web Site Structure.

5.4 Concept Maps

A common application of automated graph drawing systems is to visualize "concept map" graphs or "semantic webs" in which nodes represent ideas and edges, the connections between them. These visualizations can be useful

[4] This similarity measure is described in detail in [7].

for recognizing the important concepts which lie at the heart of expansive ontological frameworks.

Wilma's extensive range of features allows it to produce concept maps effortlessly and with a number of visual enhancements over simple embeddings. One example of this is shown in Figure 13.

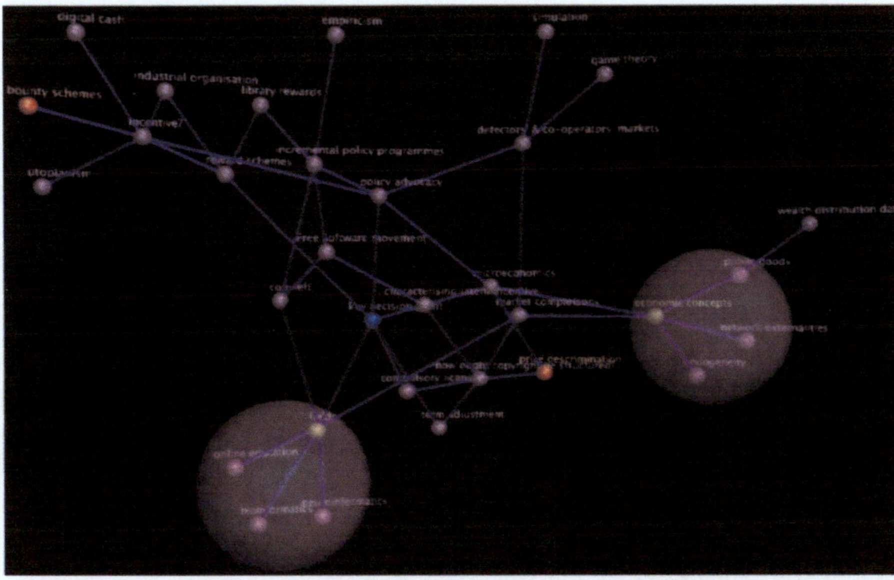

Fig. 13. Example of a WilmaScope Concept Map.

6 Software

6.1 Tools and Libraries Used By Wilma

WilmaScope has been implemented in Java, using the Java3D graphics library. Java provides a good tradeoff between high level language constructs, portability and performance. Java3D provides access to 3D graphics accelerator hardware through a high-level Java API and useful features such as a scene graph structure and methods for coupling animation into the render cycle.

As mentioned in Section 3.4 the GraphViz toolkit is also used by one of the layout engines. It should be noted that this functionality is optional and the GraphViz toolkit is not distributed with WilmaScope.

6.2 The WilmaScope System

WilmaScope is released under a free software license – the Lesser GNU General Public License (`http://www.gnu.org/copyleft/lesser.html`), which maximizes benefits for the user community, guarantees an open development ecology and thus encourages creative input all round. The software and source-code is freely down-loadable from `http://wilma.sourceforge.net` and may be used subject to the conditions of the above license in creating other applications.

References

1. Brandes, U., Kääb, V., Löh, A., Wagner, D., Willhalm, T. (2000) Dynamic www structures in 3d. Journal of Graph Algorithms and Applications **4** (3), 183–191
2. Cowling, J. (2002) Wilmascope fast layout engine product development report. Technical report, School of Information Technologies, The University of Sydney `http://www.wilmascope.org/FastlayoutReport.pdf`.
3. Davidson, G. S., Wylie, B. N., Boyack, K. W. (2001) Cluster stability and the use of noise in interpretation of clustering. In: Proceedings of the IEEE Symposium on Information Visualization
4. Dwyer, T., Eades, P. (2002) Visualising a fund manager flow graph using columns and worms. In: Proceedings of IEEE IV'02, London, IEEE Computer Society, 147–158
5. Dwyer, T. (2001) 3D UML Using Force Directed Layout. In: Proceedings of the Australian Symposium on Information Visualisation, `http://www.wilmascope.org/3DUML-dwyer.pdf`
6. Eades, P., Feng, Q. (1996) Multilevel visualization of clustered graphs. In: S. North (ed.) Graph Drawing '96, Lecture Notes in Computer Science 1190, Springer-Verlag, 101–112
7. Eckersley, P. (2000) Classiscope: Building better magnets for the web haystack. Honours Thesis, Department of Computer Science & Software Engineering, University of Melbourne, `http://www.cs.mu.oz.au/\textasciitildepde/hons/thesis.pdf`
8. Fruchtermann, T., Reingold, E. (1990) Graph drawing by force-directed placement. Technical report, Department of Computer Science, University of Illinois at Urbana-Champagne
9. Gamma, E., Helm, R., Johnson, R., Vlissides, J. (1994) Design Patterns, Elements of Reusable Object-Oriented Software. Addison-Wesley Publishing Company, Reading, Massachusetts
10. Hendley, R., Drew, N., Wood, A., Beale, R. (1995) Narcissus: Visualising information. In: Proceedings of the IEEE Symposium on Information Visualisation (InfoVis 1995), 90–96
11. Hendrickson, B., Leland, R. (1995) A multilevel algorithm for partitioning graphs. In: Proceedings of Supercomputing 1995, ACM Press
12. Herman, I., Marshall, M. S., Melançon, G. (2000) An object-oriented design for graph visualization. Technical report, Centrum voor Wiskunde en Informatica: CWI, The Netherlands

13. Huang, M., Eades, P. (1995) A fully animated interactive system for clustering and navigating huge graphs. In: S. H. Whitesides (ed.) Graph Drawing '98, Lecture Notes in Computer Science 1547, Springer-Verlag, 374–383
14. Misue, K., Eades, P., Lai, W., Sugiyama, K. (1995) Layout adjustment and the mental map. Journal of Visual Languages and Computing **6** (2), 183–210
15. Parker, G., Franck, G., Ware, C. (1998) Visualization of large nested graphs in 3d: Navigation and interaction. Journal of Visual Languages and Computing **9** (3), 299–317
16. Risden, K., Czerwinski, M., Munzner, T., Cook, D. (2000) An initial examination of ease of use for 2d and 3d information visualizations of web content. International Journal of Human Computer Studies **53** (5), 695–714
17. Sprenger, T., Gross, M., Bielser, D., Strasser, T. (1998) Ivory – an object-oriented framework for physics-based information visualization in java. In: Proceedings of the IEEE Symposium on Information Visualisation (InfoVis 1998), 79–86
18. Stallman, R. M. (1992) Why software should be free. Free Software Foundation `http://www.gnu.org/philosophy/shouldbefree.html`.
19. Sugiyama, K., Misue, K. (1995) Graph drawing by the magnetic spring model. Journal of Visual Languages and Computing **6** (3), 217–231
20. Sugiyama, K., Tagawa, S., Toda, M. (1981) Methods for visual understanding of hierarchical system structures. *IEEE Transactions on Systems, Man, and Cybernetics* **11**, pp. 109–125
21. Walshaw, C. (2000) A multilevel algorithm for force-directed graph drawing. In: J. Marks (ed.) Graph Drawing '00, Lecture Notes in Computer Science 1984, Springer-Verlag, 171–182
22. Ware, C., Franck, G. (1996) Evaluating stereo and motion cues for visualizing information nets in three dimensions. ACM Transactions on Graphics **15** (2), pp. 121–139

Pajek – Analysis and Visualization of Large Networks*

Vladimir Batagelj[1] and Andrej Mrvar[2]

[1] Department of Mathematics, Faculty of Mathematics and Physics, University of Ljubljana, Slovenia
[2] Faculty of Social Sciences, University of Ljubljana, Slovenia

1 Introduction

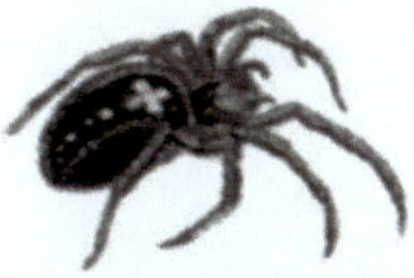

Pajek is a program, for Windows, for analysis and visualization of *large networks* having some ten or hundred of thousands of vertices. In Slovenian language *pajek* means spider.

The design of Pajek is based on experience gained in the development of the graph data structure and algorithm libraries Graph [2] and X-graph [15], the collection of network analysis and visualization programs STRAN, RelCalc, Draw, Energ [9], and the SGML-based graph description markup language NetML [8]. We started the development of Pajek in November 1996.

The main goals in the design of Pajek are [10,13]:

- to support abstraction by (recursive) decomposition of a large network into several smaller networks that can be treated further using more sophisticated methods;
- to provide the user with some powerful visualization tools;
- to implement a selection of efficient (*sub-quadratic*) algorithms for the analysis of large networks.

With Pajek we can (see Figure 1): *find* clusters (components, neighborhoods of 'important' vertices, cores, etc.) in a network, *extract* vertices that belong to the same clusters and *show* them separately, possibly with the parts of the context (detailed local view), *shrink* vertices in clusters and show relations among clusters (global view).

Besides ordinary (directed, undirected, mixed) networks Pajek supports also:

- 2-mode networks, bipartite (valued) graphs – networks between two disjoint sets of vertices. Examples of such networks are: (authors, papers, *cites the paper*), (authors, papers, *is the (co)author of the paper*), (people, events, *was present at*), (people, institutions, *is member of*), (articles, shopping lists, *is on the list*).

* This work was partially supported by the Ministry of Education, Science and Sport of Slovenia, Projects J1-8532 and Z5-3350.

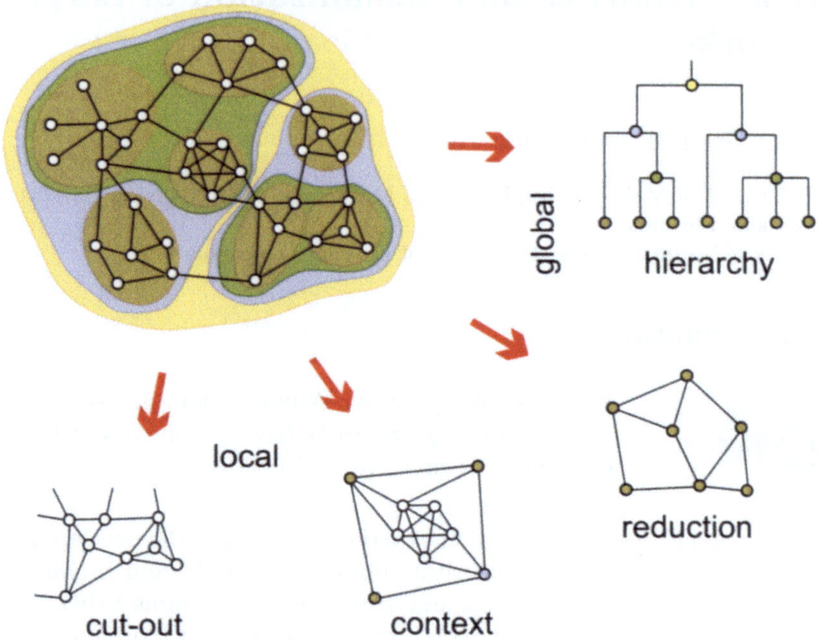

Fig. 1. Approaches to deal with large networks.

- temporal networks, dynamic graphs – networks changing over time.

In this chapter we present the main characteristics of `Pajek`. Since large networks can't be visualized in detail in a single view we first have to identify interesting substructures in such a network and then visualize them as separate views. The central, algorithmic section of this chapter deals mainly with different efficient approaches to this problem.

2 Applications

There exist several sources of large networks that are already in machine-readable form. `Pajek` provides tools for analysis and visualization of such networks and is applied by researchers in different areas: social network analysis [11], chemistry (organic molecules), biomedical/genomics research (protein-receptor interaction networks) [50], genealogies [49,28], internet networks [22], citation networks [38], diffusion networks (AIDS, news), analysis of texts [17], data-mining (2-mode networks) [14], etc. Although it was developed primarily for analysis of large networks it is often used also for, especially visualization of, small networks.

In the last months of 2002 we had over 500 downloads of `Pajek` per month.

Pajek is also used at several universities: Ljubljana, Rotterdam, Stanford, Irvine, The Ohio State University, Penn State, Wisconsin/Madison, Vienna, Freiburg, Madrid, and some others as a support in courses on network analysis. Together with Wouter de Nooy of the University of Rotterdam we wrote a course book *Exploratory Social Network Analysis With* Pajek [25].

3 Algorithms

To support the design goals we implemented several algorithms known from the literature (see Section 4.2), but for some tasks new, efficient algorithms, suitable to deal with large networks, had to be developed. They mainly provide different ways of identifying interesting substructures in a given network.

3.1 Citation Weights

In a given set of units/vertices U (articles, books, works, etc.) we introduce a *citing relation*/set of arcs $R \subseteq U \times U$

$$uRv \equiv v \text{ cites } u$$

which determines a *citation network* $N = (U, R)$.

The citation network analysis started in 1964 with the paper of Garfield *et al.* [29]. In 1989 Hummon and Doreian [35] proposed three indices – weights of arcs that provide us with an automatic way to identify the (most) important part of the citation network. For two of these indices we developed algorithms to efficiently compute them [4].

A citing relation is usually *irreflexive* (no loops) and (almost) *acyclic.* In the following we shall assume that it has these two properties. Since in real-life citation networks the strong components are small (usually 2 or 3 vertices) we can transform such a network into an acyclic network by shrinking strong components and deleting loops. For other approaches see [4]. It is also useful to transform a citation network to its *standardized* form by adding a common *source* vertex $s \notin U$ and a common *sink* vertex $t \notin U$. The source s is linked by an arc to all minimal elements of R; and all maximal elements of R are linked to the sink t. Thus we get an st-digraph (see Section 2.2 in the Technical Foundations). Finally, to make the theory smoother, we also add the 'feedback' arc (t, s).

The *search path count* (SPC) method is based on counters $n(u, v)$ that count the number of different paths from s to t through the arc (u, v). To compute $n(u, v)$ we introduce two auxiliary quantities: $n^-(v)$ counts the number of different paths from s to v, and $n^+(v)$ counts the number of different paths from v to t.

It follows by basic principles of combinatorics that

$$n(u, v) = n^-(u) \cdot n^+(v), \qquad (u, v) \in R$$

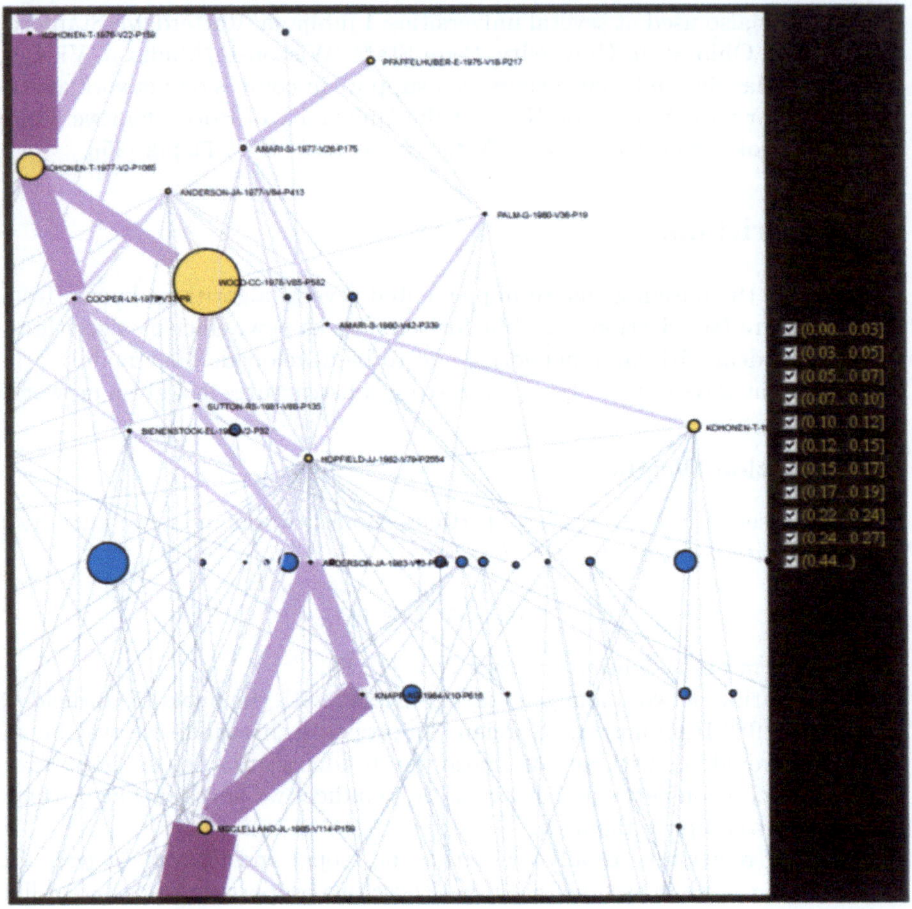

Fig. 2. Part of SOM main subnetwork at level 0.001.

where

$$n^-(u) = \begin{cases} 1 & \text{if } u = s, \\ \sum_{v:vRu} n^-(v) & \text{otherwise,} \end{cases}$$

and

$$n^+(u) = \begin{cases} 1 & \text{if } u = t, \\ \sum_{v:uRv} n^+(v) & \text{otherwise.} \end{cases}$$

This is the basis of an efficient algorithm for computing $n(u, v)$ – after a topological sorting (see Section 2.2 in the Technical Foundations) of the *st*-digraph we can compute, using the above relations in topological order, the weights in $O(|R|)$ time. The topological ordering ensures that all the quantities in the right hand sides of the above equalities are already computed when needed.

The Hummon and Doreian indices are defined as follows:

- *search path link count* (SPLC) method: $w_l(u,v)$ equals the number of "*all possible search paths through the network emanating from an origin node*" through the arc $(u,v) \in R$,
- *search path node pair* (SPNP) method: $w_p(u,v)$ accounts for "*all connected vertex pairs along the paths*" through the arc $(u,v) \in R$.

We get the SPLC weights by applying the SPC method on the network obtained from a given standardized network by linking the source s by an arc to each non-minimal vertex from U; and the SPNP weights by applying the SPC method on the network obtained from the SPLC network by additionally linking by an arc each non-maximal vertex from U to the sink t.

The values of the counters $n(u,v)$ form a flow in the citation network and *Kirchoff's vertex law* holds: For every vertex u in a standardized citation network *incoming flow = outgoing flow*:

$$\sum_{v:vRu} n(v,u) = \sum_{v:uRv} n(u,v) = n^-(u) \cdot n^+(u)$$

The weight $n(t,s)$ is equal to the total flow through network and provides a natural normalization of the weights

$$w(u,v) = \frac{n(u,v)}{n(t,s)} \quad \Longrightarrow \quad 0 \le w(u,v) \le 1$$

and, if C is a minimal arc-cut-set, we have

$$\sum_{(u,v)\in C} w(u,v) = 1.$$

In large networks the values of weights can grow very large. This should be considered in the implementation of the algorithms.

From a given network we can obtain subnetworks by using *cuts* as follows: If we *edge-cut* a network $N = (V,E,w)$ where $w : E \to \mathbb{R}$ at a selected level t we get a subnetwork $N_w(t) = (V[E'],E',w)$, where $E' = \{e \in E \mid w(e) \ge t\}$ and $V[E']$ is the set of all end-vertices of the edges from E'. The *vertex-cut* of network $N = (V,E,p)$ where $p : V \to \mathbb{R}$ at a selected level t is the subnetwork $N_p(t) = (V',E[V'],p)$ determined by the set $V' = \{v \in V \mid p(v) \ge t\}$ and $E[V']$ is the set of edges from E that have both end-vertices in V'.

In Figure 2 the main subnetwork obtained as an edge-cut at level 0.001 of the citation network ($|U| = 4470$, $|R| = 12731$) in the SOM (*self-organizing maps*) literature is presented. The picture is exported in SVG with additional JavaScript support that provides the user with options to inspect the subnetwork at different predetermined levels.

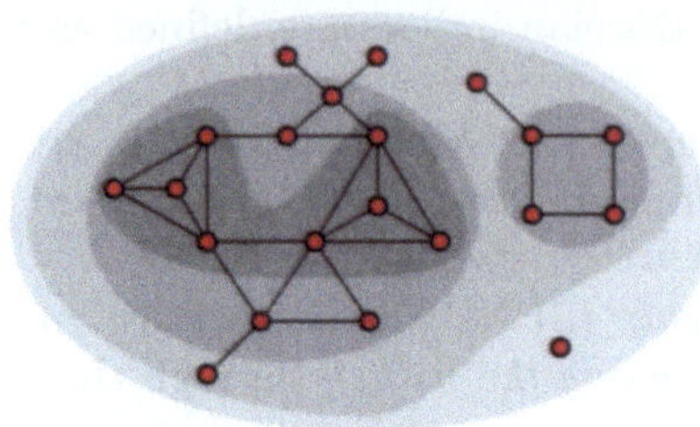

Fig. 3. 0, 1, 2 and 3 core.

3.2 Cores and Generalized Cores

The notion of core was introduced by Seidman in 1983 [44]. Let $G = (V, E)$ be a graph. A subgraph $H = (W, E[W])$ induced by the vertex set W is a *k-core* or a *core of order k* iff $\deg_H(v) \geq k$ for all $v \in W$ and H is a maximal subgraph with this property. The core of maximum order is also called the *main* core. The *core number* core[v] of vertex v is the highest order of a core that contains this vertex. The degree deg(v) can be: in-degree, out-degree, in-degree + out-degree, etc., determining different types of cores.

In Figure 3 an example for a core decomposition of a given graph is presented. From this figure we can see the following properties of cores:

- The cores are nested: $i < j \implies H_j \subseteq H_i$
- Cores are not necessarily connected subgraphs.

Our algorithm for determining the cores hierarchy is based on the following property [16]:

> If from a given graph $G = (V, E)$ we recursively delete all vertices, and edges incident with them, of degree less than k, the remaining graph is the k-core.

Its outline is given in Algorithm 1.

In the refinements of the algorithm we have to provide efficient implementations of sorting the *degrees* and their reordering. Since the values of degrees are in the range $0 \ldots n-1$ we can order them in $O(|V|)$ time using a variant of bucket sort, the update of the ordering can be done in a constant time. For details see [18].

The cores, because they can be determined very efficiently, are one among few concepts that provide us with meaningful decompositions of large networks. We expect that different approaches to the analysis of large networks can be built on this basis. For example, we get the following bound on the chromatic number of a given graph G

$$\chi(G) \leq 1 + \mathrm{core}(G)$$

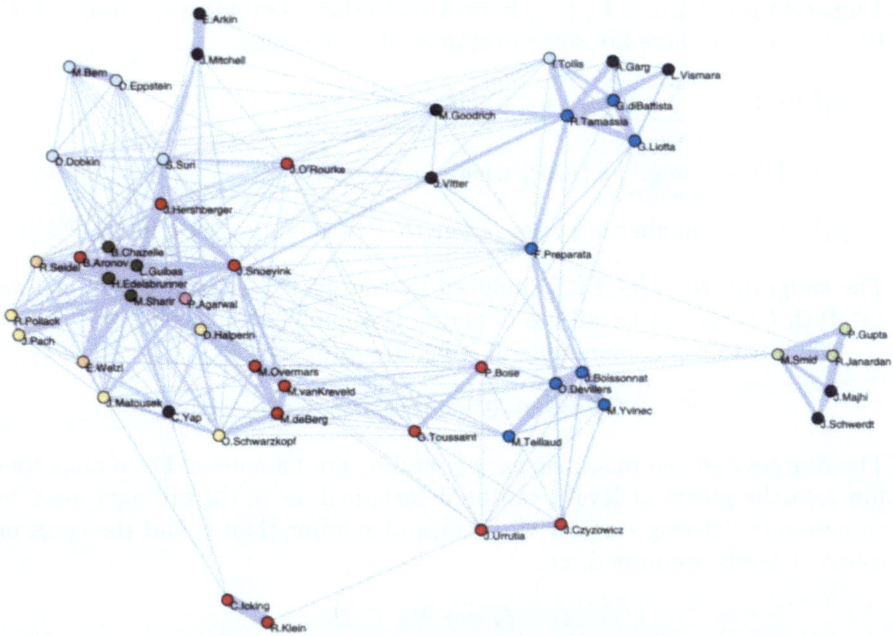

Fig. 4. p_S-core at level 46 of Geomlib network.

Algorithm 1: Core numbers algorithm

Input : Graph $G = (V, E)$ represented by adjacency lists
Output: Table *core*$[V]$ with the core number for each vertex
Compute the *degrees* of vertices
Order the set of vertices V by increasing degrees
for *each* $v \in V$ *in this order* **do**
  Set *core*$[v]$ = *degree*$[v]$
  for *each* $u \in \text{adj}(v)$ **do**
    if *degree*$[u]$ > *degree*$[v]$ **then**
      Set *degree*$[u]$ = *degree*$[u] - 1$
      Reorder V accordingly
    end
  end
end

---

where $\text{core}(G) = \max_{v \in V} \text{core}[v]$. Cores can also be used to localize the search for interesting subnetworks in large networks: If it exists, a k-component is contained in a k-core; and a k-clique is contained in a k-core.

The notion of core can be generalized to networks. Let $N = (V, E, w)$ be a network, where $G = (V, E)$ is a graph and $w : E \rightarrow \mathbb{R}$ is a function assigning values to edges. A *vertex property function* on N, or a *p-function* for short, is a function $p(v,U)$, $v \in V$, $U \subseteq V$ with real values. Let $\mathrm{adj}_U(v) = \mathrm{adj}(v) \cap U$. Besides degrees, here are some examples of p-functions:

$$\begin{aligned} p_S(v,U) &= \sum_{u \in \mathrm{adj}_U(v)} w(v,u), \text{ where } w : E \to \mathbb{R}_0^+ \\ p_M(v,U) &= \max_{u \in \mathrm{adj}_U(v)} w(v,u), \text{ where } w : E \to \mathbb{R} \\ p_k(v,U) &= \text{number of cycles of length } k \text{ through vertex } v \text{ in } (U, E[U]) \end{aligned}$$

The subgraph $H = (C, E[C])$ induced by the set $C \subseteq V$ is a *p-core at level* $t \in \mathbb{R}$ iff $t \leq p(v,C)$ for all $v \in C$ and C is a maximal such set.

The function p is *monotone* iff it has the property

$$C_1 \subset C_2 \Longrightarrow \forall v \in V : (p(v,C_1) \leq p(v,C_2)).$$

The degrees and the functions p_S, p_M and p_k are monotone. For a monotone function the p-core at level t can be determined, as in the ordinary case, by successively deleting vertices with value of p lower than t; and the cores on different levels are nested, i.e.,

$$t_1 < t_2 \Longrightarrow H_{t_2} \subseteq H_{t_1}.$$

The p-function is *local* iff

$$p(v,U) = p(v, \mathrm{adj}_U(v)).$$

The degrees p_S and p_M are local, but p_k is **not** local for $k \geq 4$. For a local p-function an $O(|E| \max(\mathrm{maxdeg}(G), \log |V|))$ algorithm for determining the p-core levels exists, assuming that $p(v, \mathrm{adj}_C(v))$ can be computed in $O(\deg_C(v))$ time [19].

In Figure 4 a p_S-core at level 46 of the *collaboration network* in the field of computational geometry [36] is presented.

3.3 Pattern Searching

If a selected *pattern* determined by a given graph does not occur frequently in a sparse network, the straightforward backtracking algorithm applied for pattern searching finds all appearances of the pattern very fast even in the case of very large networks.

To speed up the search or to consider some additional properties of the pattern, a user can set some additional options:

- the vertices in the network should match with the vertices in the pattern in some nominal, ordinal or numerical property (for example, type of atom in a molecule);
- the values of the edges must match (for example, edges representing male/female links in the case of p-graphs [49]);

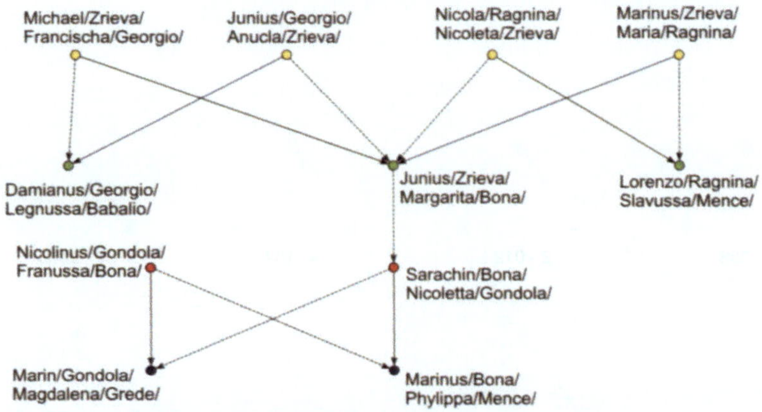

Fig. 5. Marriages among relatives in Ragusa.

- the first vertex in the pattern can be selected only from a given subset of vertices in the network.

Pattern searching was successfully applied to searching for patterns of atoms in molecules (carbon rings) and searching for relinking marriages in genealogies. Figure 5 presents three connected relinking marriages which are non-blood marriages found in the genealogy of ragusan noble families [28]. The genealogy is represented as a p-graph. A solid arc indicates the _ *is a son of* _ relation, and a dotted arc indicates the _ *is a daughter of* _ relation. In all three patterns a brother and a sister from one family found their partners in the same other family.

3.4 Triads

Let $G = (V, R)$ be a simple directed graph without loops. A *triad* is a subgraph induced by a given set of three vertices. There are 16 non-isomorphic (types of) triads [47, page 244]. They can be partitioned into three basic types (see Figure 6):

- the *null* triad 003;
- *dyadic* triads 012 and 102; and
- *connected* triads: 111D, 201, 210, 300, 021D, 111U, 120D, 021U, 030T, 120U, 021C, 030C and 120C.

Several properties of a graph can be expressed in terms of its *triadic spectrum*, i.e., the distribution of all its triads. It also provides ingredients for p^* network models [48]. A direct approach to determine the triadic spectrum is of order $O(|V|^3)$; but in most large graphs it can be determined much faster [12]. The algorithm is based on the following observation: *In a large and sparse graph most triads are null triads.* Let T_1, T_2, T_3 be the number of null, dyadic and

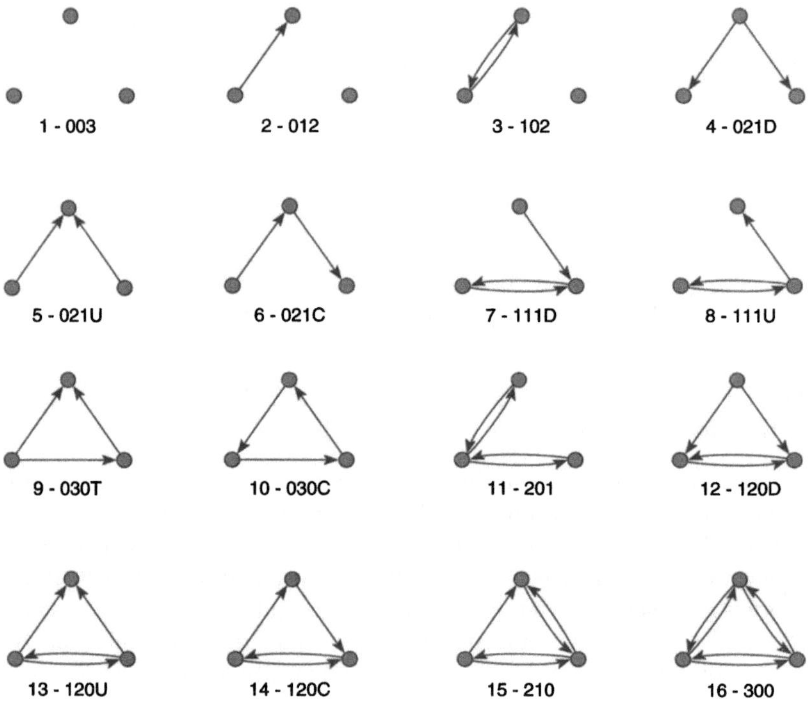

Fig. 6. Triads.

connected triads, respectively. Since the total number of triads is $T = \binom{n}{3}$ and the above types partition the set of all triads, the idea of the algorithm is as follows:

- count all dyadic T_2 and all connected T_3 triads with their subtypes;
- compute the number of null triads $T_1 = T - T_2 - T_3$.

In the algorithm we have to assure that every non-null triad is counted exactly once while scanning the set of arcs. A set of three vertices $\{v, u, w\}$ can generally be selected in 6 different ways: (v, u, w), (v, w, u), (u, v, w), (u, w, v), (w, v, u), (w, u, v). We solve the isomorphism problem by introducing the *canonical* selection that contributes to the triadic count; the other, non-canonical selections need not to be considered in the counting process.

Every connected dyad forms a dyadic triad with every vertex both members of the dyad are not adjacent to. Let $\hat{R} = R \cup R^{-1}$. Each pair of vertices (v, u), $v < u$ connected by an arc contributes

$$n - |\hat{R}(u) \cup \hat{R}(v) \setminus \{u, v\}| - 2$$

triads of type 3-102, if u and v are connected in both directions; and of type 2-012 otherwise. The condition $v < u$ determines the canonical selection for dyadic triads. A selection (v, u, w) of connected triad is canonical iff $v < u < w$.

The triads isomorphism problem can be efficiently solved by assigning to each triad a code consisting of an integer number between 0 to 63 obtained by treating the out-diagonal entries of the triad adjacency matrix as a binary number. Each triad code corresponds to a unique triad type that can be determined from a precomputed table.

For a connected triad we can always assume that v is the smallest of its vertices. So we have to determine the canonical selection from the remaining two selections (v, u, w) and (v, w, u). If $v < w < u$ and $v\hat{R}w$, then the selection (v, w, u) was already counted before. Therefore we have to consider it as canonical only if it is not $v\hat{R}w$.

In an implementation of the algorithm we must also take care of the range overflow in the case of T and T_1.

The total running time of the algorithm is $O(\text{maxdeg}(G)|E|)$ and thus, for graphs with small maximum degree $\text{maxdeg}(G) \ll |V|$, since $2|E| \leq |V| \,\text{maxdeg}(G)$, of order $O(|V|)$.

3.5 Triangular Connectivities

In this subsection we present an extension of the notion of connectivity to connectivity by chains of triangles.

Undirected Graphs

We call a subgraph isomorphic to K_3 a *triangle*. A subgraph $H = (V', E')$ of $G = (V, E)$ is *triangular* if each vertex in V' and each edge in E' belongs to at least one triangle in H.

A sequence $(T_1, T_2, \ldots, T_s)$ of triangles of G *(vertex) triangularly connects* the vertices $u, v \in V$ iff $u \in T_1$ and $v \in T_s$ or $u \in T_s$ and $v \in T_1$ and $V(T_{i-1}) \cap V(T_i) \neq \emptyset$, $i = 2, \ldots s$. Such sequence is called a *triangular chain*. It *edge triangularly connects* the vertices $u, v \in V$ iff a stronger version of the second condition holds, namely $E(T_{i-1}) \cap E(T_i) \neq \emptyset$, $i = 2, \ldots s$.

A pair of vertices $u, v \in V$ is *(vertex) triangularly connected* iff $u = v$ or there exists a chain that triangularly connects u and v. Triangular connectivity is an equivalence relation on the set of vertices V; and the nontrivial triangular connectivity components are exactly the maximal connected triangular subgraphs.

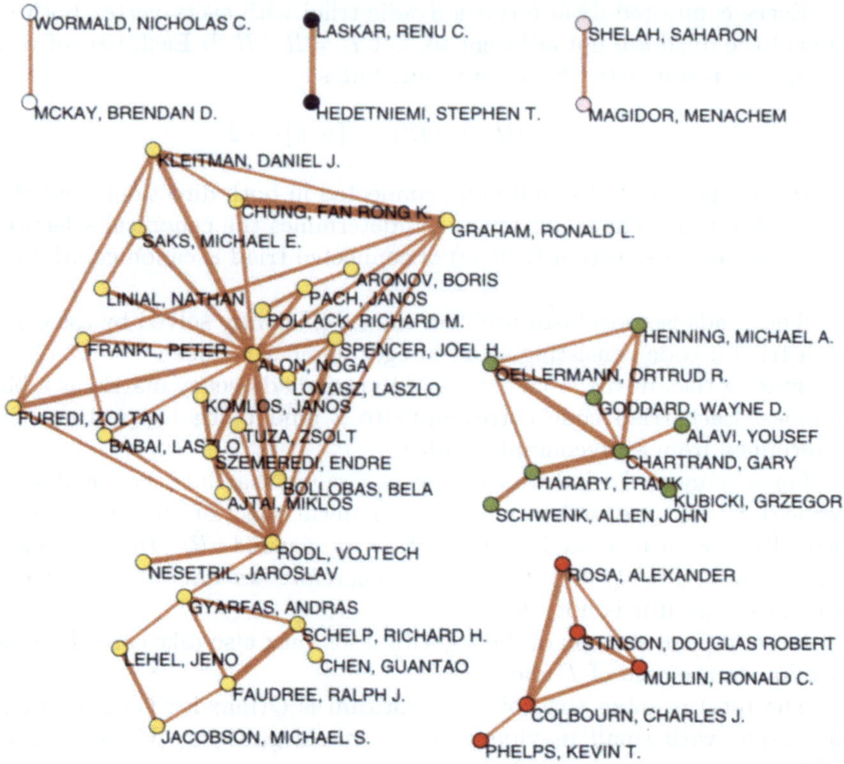

Fig. 7. Edge-cut at level 16 of triangular network of Erdős collaboration graph.

A pair of vertices $u, v \in V$ is *edge triangularly connected* iff $u = v$ or there exists a chain that edge triangularly connects u and v. Edge triangular connectivity components determine an equivalence relation on the set of edges E. Each non-triangular edge is in its own component.

Let G be a simple undirected graph. A *triangular network* $N_T(G) = (V, E_T, w)$ determined by G is a subgraph $G_T = (V, E_T)$ of G whose set of edges E_T consists of all triangular edges of $E(G)$. For $e \in E_T$ the weight $w(e)$ is equal to the number of different triangles in G to which e belongs.

A procedure for determining E_T and $w(e)$, $e \in E_T$ simply collects all edges with $w(e) = |\text{adj}(u) \cap \text{adj}(v)| > 0$, $e = \{u, v\} \in E$. If the sets of neighbors $\text{adj}(v)$ are ordered we can use merging to compute $w(e)$ faster. Nontrivial triangular connectivity components are exactly the components of G_T.

Triangular networks can be used to efficiently identify dense clique-like parts of a graph. If an edge e belongs to a k-clique in G then $w(e) \geq k - 2$.

In Figure 7 the edge-cut at level 16 of a triangular network of the *Erdős collaboration graph* [33,11] (without Erdős, $|V| = 6926$, $|E| = 11343$) is presented.

Directed Graphs

If the graph G is mixed, we replace edges with pairs of opposite arcs. In the following let $G = (V, A)$ be a simple directed graph without loops. For a selected arc $(u, v) \in A$ there are four different types of directed triangles: **cyc**lic, **tra**nsitive, **in**put and **out**put.

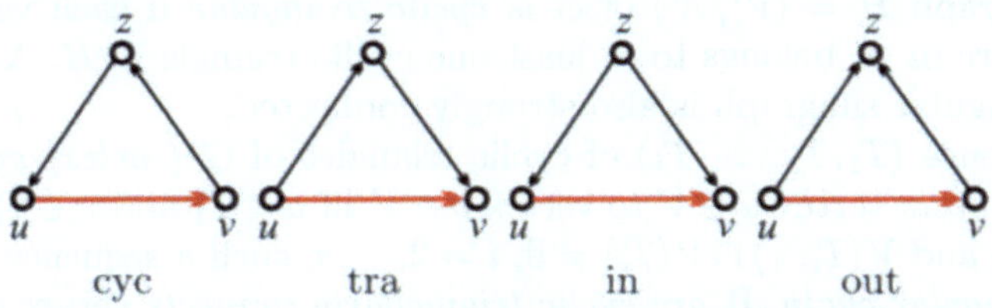

For each type we get the corresponding triangular network N_{cyc}, N_{tra}, N_{in} and N_{out}. Also procedures for determining the networks are similar to the undirected case. For example, for the cyclic network $N_{cyc} = (V, A_{cyc}, w_{cyc})$ we have for $(u, v) \in A_{cyc}$

$$w_{cyc}(u, v) = |\,\text{outadj}(v) \cap \text{inadj}(u)|.$$

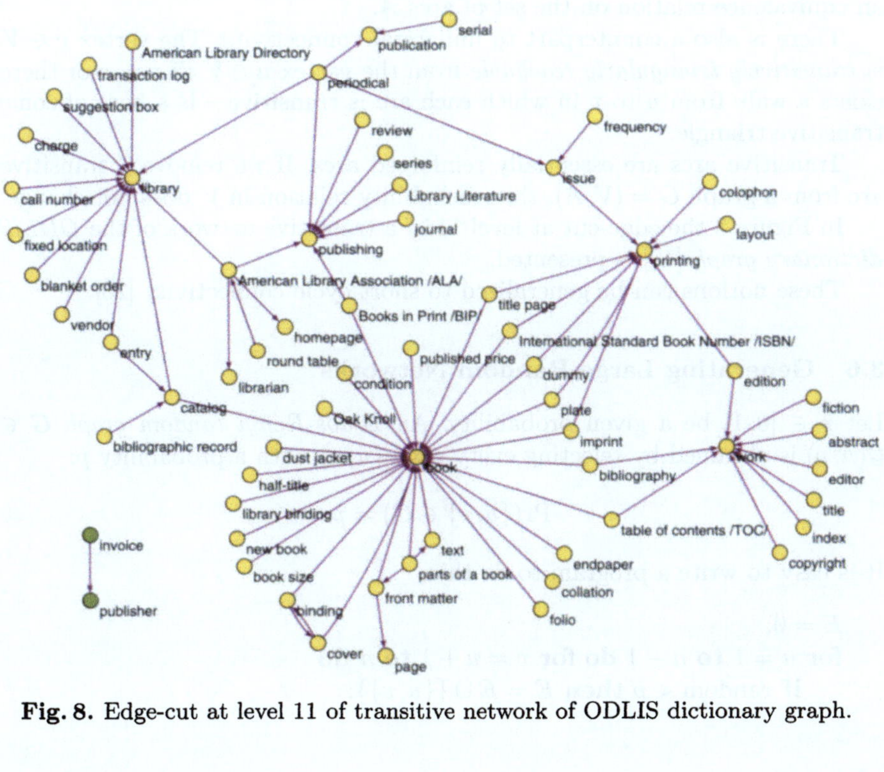

Fig. 8. Edge-cut at level 11 of transitive network of ODLIS dictionary graph.

In directed graphs we distinguish weak and strong connectivity. The weak connectivity can be reduced to the undirected concepts in the skeleton $S = (V, E_S)$ of the given graph G where

$$E_S = \{\{u, v\} : u \neq v \wedge (u, v) \in A\}.$$

A subgraph $H = (V', A')$ of G is *cyclic triangular* if each vertex in V' and each arc in A' belongs to at least one cyclic triangle in H. A connected cyclic triangular subgraph is also strongly connected.

A sequence $(T_1, T_2, \ldots, T_s)$ of cyclic triangles of G *(vertex) cyclic triangularly connects* vertex $u \in V$ to vertex $v \in V$ iff $u \in T_1$ and $v \in T_s$ or $u \in T_s$ and $v \in T_1$ and $V(T_{i-1}) \cap V(T_i) \neq \emptyset$, $i = 2, \ldots s$; such a sequence is called a *cyclic triangular chain*. It *arc cyclic triangularly connects* vertex u to vertex v iff $A(T_{i-1}) \cap A(T_i) \neq \emptyset$, $i = 2, \ldots s$ holds; such a sequence is called an *arc cyclic triangular chain.*

Again, we can introduce two types of cyclic triangular connectivity:

A pair of vertices $u, v \in V$ is *(vertex) cyclic triangularly connected* iff $u = v$ or there exists a cyclic triangular chain that connects u to v.

A pair of vertices $u, v \in V$ is *arc cyclic triangularly connected* iff $u = v$, or there exists an arc cyclic triangular chain that connects u to v.

Cyclic triangular connectivity is an equivalence relation on the set of vertices V; and the arc cyclic triangular connectivity components determine an equivalence relation on the set of arcs A.

There is also a counterpart to unilateral connectivity. The vertex $v \in V$ is *transitively triangularly reachable* from the vertex $u \in V$ iff $u = v$ or there exists a walk from u to v in which each arc is transitive – is a base of some transitive triangle.

Transitive arcs are essentially reinforced arcs. If we remove a transitive arc from a graph $G = (V, A)$, the reachability relation in V does not change.

In Figure 8 the edge-cut at level 11 of a transitive network of the *ODLIS dictionary graph* [40] is presented.

These notions can be generalized to short cycle connectivity [20].

3.6 Generating Large Random Networks

Let $p \in [0, 1]$ be a given probability. An *Erdős-Rényi random graph* $G \in \mathcal{G}(n, p)$ is obtained by selecting every edge $\{u, v\}$ with a probability p:

$$\Pr(\{u, v\} \in G) = p$$

It is easy to write a program to do this:

$E = \emptyset$;
for $u = 1$ **to** $n - 1$ **do for** $v = u + 1$ **to** n **do**
  if random $< p$ **then** $E = E \cup \{\{u, v\}\}$;

But for large and very sparse networks this is too slow. A faster procedure can be built on the following idea: move by random steps over the $M = \binom{n}{2}$ cells and mark the touched cells.

How to select the length of the random step? For our Bernoulli model we have $\Pr(\text{step} = s) = q^{s-1}p,\ s = 1, 2, 3, \ldots$ and $F(s) = \Pr(\text{step} < s) = \sum_{t=1}^{s-1} q^{t-1}p = 1 - q^{s-1}$. Therefore we get the random step s from the equation $F(s) = \text{random}$:

$$s = F^{-1}(\text{random}) = 1 + \left\lfloor \frac{\log(1 - \text{random})}{\log q} \right\rfloor$$

This is the basis of the fast random graph generation procedure presented in Algorithm 2. The expected number of steps of this procedure is Mp.

Algorithm 2: Sparse Erdős-Rényi random graph generator

Input : Probability p, number of vertices n
Output: Random graph $G = (1 \ldots n, E)$
Set $q = 1 - p$; $f = 1$; $u = 2$; $k = 0$; $E = \emptyset$; $M = n(n-1)/2$; *again* = *true*
while *again* **do**
    Set $k = k + 1 + \left\lfloor \frac{\ln(1 - \text{random})}{\ln q} \right\rfloor$
    if $k > M$ **then** set *again* = *false* **else**
        while $f < k$ **do** set $f = f + u$; $u = u + 1$
        Set $v = k + u - f - 1$; $E = E \cup \{\{u, v\}\}$
    end
od

The same approach is easy to adapt to generate different types of random graphs: undirected, directed, acyclic, undirected bipartite, directed bipartite, acyclic bipartite, 2-mode, and others [5].

`Pajek` contains also a refinement of the model for generating *scale free networks*, proposed in [41]. At each step of the growth a new vertex and k edges are added to the network N. The endpoints of the edges are randomly selected among all vertices according to the probability

$$\Pr(v) = \alpha \frac{\text{indeg}(v)}{|E|} + \beta \frac{\text{outdeg}(v)}{|E|} + \gamma \frac{1}{|V|}$$

where $\alpha + \beta + \gamma = 1$. It is easy to check that $\sum_{v \in V} \Pr(v) = 1$. The running time of this procedure is $O(|E|)$.

3.7 2-Mode Networks

A 2-*mode network* is a structure $N = (U, V, A, w)$, where U and V are disjoint sets of vertices, A is the set of arcs with the initial vertex in the set U and the terminal vertex in the set V, and $w : A \to \mathrm{I\!R}$ is a *weight*. If no weight is defined we can assume a constant weight $w(u,v) = 1$ for all arcs $(u,v) \in A$. The set A can also be viewed as a relation $A \subseteq U \times V$. A 2-mode network can be formally represented by a rectangular matrix $\mathbf{A} = [a_{uv}]_{U \times V}$ where

$$a_{uv} = \begin{cases} w(u,v) & \text{if } (u,v) \in A, \\ 0 & \text{otherwise.} \end{cases}$$

For a direct analysis of 2-mode networks we can use the eigenvector approach, clustering and blockmodeling. But most often we transform a 2-mode network into an ordinary (1-mode) network $N_1 = (U, E_1, w_1)$ or/and $N_2 = (V, E_2, w_2)$, where E_1 and w_1 are determined by the matrix $\mathbf{A}^{(1)} = \mathbf{A}\mathbf{A}^T$, $a_{uv}^{(1)} = \sum_{z \in V} a_{uz} \cdot a_{zv}^T$. Evidently $a_{uv}^{(1)} = a_{vu}^{(1)}$. There is an edge $\{u,v\} \in E_1$ in N_1 iff $\mathrm{adj}(u) \cap \mathrm{adj}(v) \neq \emptyset$. Its weight is $w_1(u,v) = a_{uv}^{(1)}$. The network N_2 is determined in a similar way by the matrix $\mathbf{A}^{(2)} = \mathbf{A}^T\mathbf{A}$. The networks N_1 and N_2 are analyzed using standard methods.

3.8 Normalizations

The *normalization* approach was developed for quick inspection of (1-mode) networks obtained from 2-mode networks [14,51] – a kind of network based data-mining. In networks obtained from large 2-mode networks there are often huge differences in weights. Therefore it is not possible to compare the vertices according to the raw data. First we have to normalize the network to make the weights comparable. There exist several ways how to do this. Some of them are presented in Table 1. They can also be used on other networks.

$$\mathrm{Geo}_{uv} = \frac{w_{uv}}{\sqrt{w_{uu} w_{vv}}} \qquad \mathrm{GeoDeg}_{uv} = \frac{w_{uv}}{\sqrt{\deg(u)\deg(v)}}$$

$$\mathrm{Input}_{uv} = \frac{w_{uv}}{w_{vv}} \qquad \mathrm{Output}_{uv} = \frac{w_{uv}}{w_{uu}}$$

$$\mathrm{Min}_{uv} = \frac{w_{uv}}{\min(w_{uu}, w_{vv})} \qquad \mathrm{Max}_{uv} = \frac{w_{uv}}{\max(w_{uu}, w_{vv})}$$

$$\mathrm{MinDir}_{uv} = \begin{cases} \frac{w_{uv}}{w_{uu}} & \text{if } w_{uu} \leq w_{vv} \\ 0 & \text{otherwise} \end{cases} \qquad \mathrm{MaxDir}_{uv} = \begin{cases} \frac{w_{uv}}{w_{vv}} & \text{if } w_{uu} \leq w_{vv} \\ 0 & \text{otherwise} \end{cases}$$

Table 1. Weight normalizations.

In the case of networks without loops we define the diagonal weights for undirected networks as the sum of out-diagonal elements in the row (or column)

$$w_{vv} = \sum_u w_{vu}$$

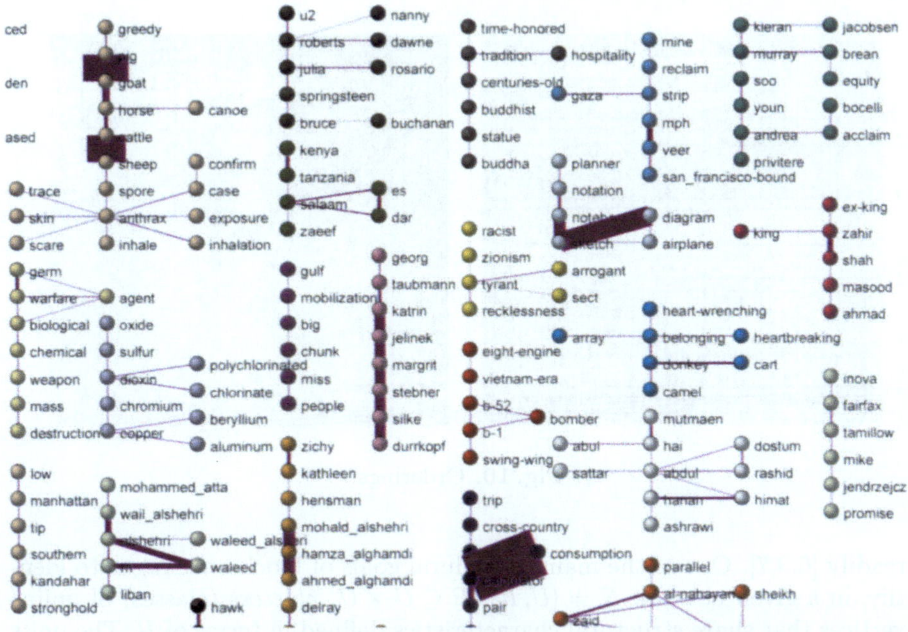

Fig. 9. GeoDeg normalization of Reuters terror news network.

and for directed networks as some mean value of the row and column sum, for example

$$w_{vv} = \frac{1}{2}\left(\sum_u w_{vu} + \sum_u w_{uv}\right).$$

Usually we assume that the network does not contain any isolated vertex.

After a selected normalization, the important parts of a network are obtained by edge-cutting the normalized network at a selected level t and preserving components with at least k vertices.

In Figure 9 a part of 'themes' from *Reuters terror news network* [14] determined by a cut of its GeoDeg normalization is presented.

3.9 Blockmodeling

In Figure 10 the *Snyder and Kick's world trade network* is represented by its matrix: on the left side the units (states) are ordered in the alphabetic order of their names; on the right side they are ordered on the basis of clustering results. It is evident that a 'proper' ordering can reveal structure in the network. Such orderings can be produced in different ways [39]. For networks of moderate size (up to some hundreds of units) we can also use the blockmodeling methods.

The goal of *blockmodeling* is to reduce a large, potentially incoherent network to a smaller comprehensible structure that can be interpreted more

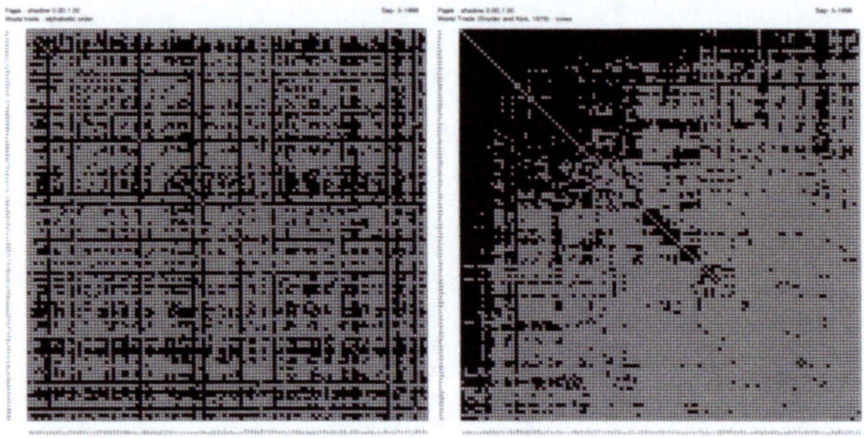

Fig. 10. Orderings.

readily [6,3,7]. One of the main procedural goals of blockmodeling is to identify, in a given network $N = (U, R)$, $R \subseteq U \times U$, *clusters* (classes) of units/vertices that share structural characteristics defined in terms of R. The units within a cluster have the same or similar connection patterns to other units.

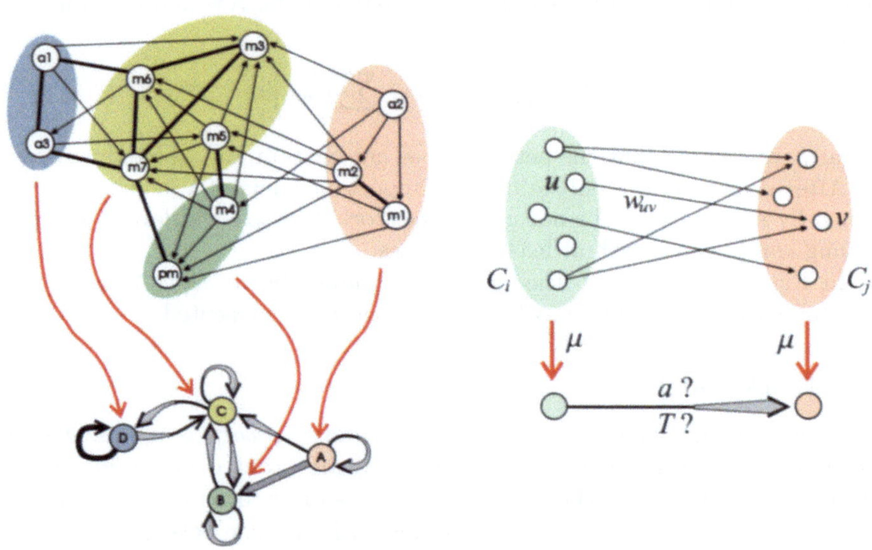

Fig. 11. Blockmodeling.

They form a *clustering* $\mathbf{C} = \{C_1, C_2, \ldots, C_k\}$ which is a *partition* of the set U. Each partition determines an equivalence relation (and vice versa).

A clustering $\mathbf{C}$ also partitions the relation R into *blocks*

$$R(C_i, C_j) = R \cap C_i \times C_j.$$

Each such block consists of units belonging to the clusters C_i and C_j and all arcs leading from cluster C_i to cluster C_j. If $i = j$, a block $R(C_i, C_i)$ is called a *diagonal* block.

A *block-model* consists of structures obtained by identifying all units from the same cluster in the clustering $\mathbf{C}$, see the left side of Figure 11. For an exact definition of a blockmodel, see the right side of Figure 11, we must also be precise about which blocks produce an arc in the *reduced graph* and which do not, and of what *type*. Some types of connections are presented in Figure 12. The reduced graph can be represented by a relational matrix, also called *image matrix*.

Furthermore, by *reordering* a network matrix so that the units from each cluster of the optimal clustering are located together, we obtain a matrix representation of the network with visible structure.

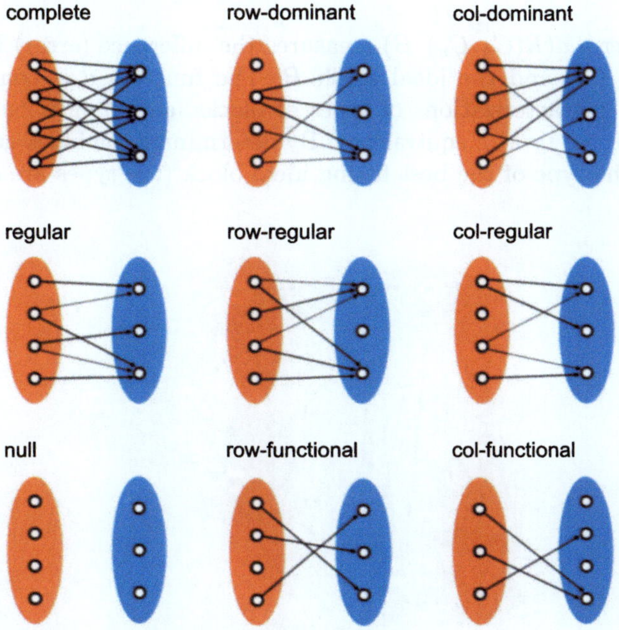

Fig. 12. Block types.

How to determine an appropriate block-model? The blockmodeling can be formulated as a *clustering problem* (Φ, P) as follows:

Determine the clustering $\mathbf{C}^\star \in \Phi$ for which

$$P(\mathbf{C}^\star) = \min_{\mathbf{C} \in \Phi} P(\mathbf{C}).$$

Since the set of units U is finite, the set of feasible clusterings Φ is also finite. Therefore the set $\text{Min}(\Phi, P)$ of all solutions of the problem (optimal clusterings) is not empty. In theory, the set $\text{Min}(\Phi, P)$ can be determined by exhaustive search, but it turns out that most cases of the clustering problem are $\mathcal{NP}$-hard. The blockmodeling problems are usually solved by using local optimization methods based on moving a unit from one cluster to another or interchanging two units between two clusters.

One of the possible ways of constructing a criterion function that directly reflects the considered equivalence is to measure the fit of a clustering to an ideal one with perfect relations within each cluster and between clusters according to the considered equivalence.

Given a clustering $\mathbf{C} = \{C_1, C_2, \ldots, C_k\}$, let $\mathcal{B}(C_u, C_v)$ denote the set of all ideal blocks corresponding to block $R(C_u, C_v)$. Then the global error of clustering $\mathbf{C}$ can be expressed as

$$P(\mathbf{C}) = \sum_{C_u, C_v \in \mathbf{C}} \min_{B \in \mathcal{B}(C_u, C_v)} d(R(C_u, C_v), B)$$

where the term $d(R(C_u, C_v), B)$ measures the difference (error) between the block $R(C_u, C_v)$ and the ideal block B. The function d is constructed on the basis of characterizations of types of blocks, and it must be compatible with the selected type of equivalence. By determining the block error, we also determine the type of the best fitting ideal block (the types are ordered).

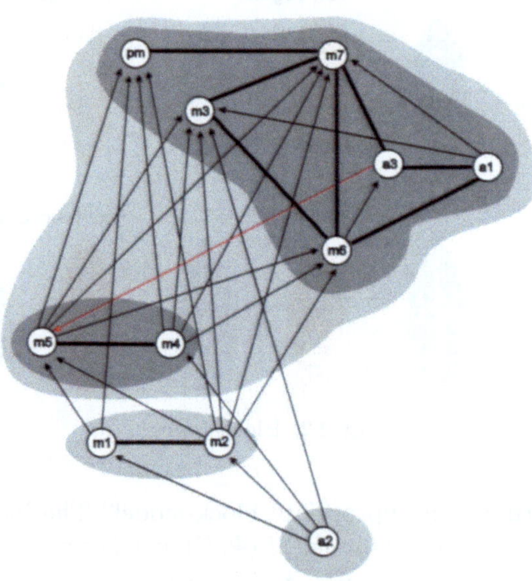

Fig. 13. A symmetric acyclic block-model of Student Government.

The criterion function $P(\mathbf{C})$ is *sensitive* iff $P(\mathbf{C}) = 0 \iff \mathbf{C}$ determines an exact blockmodeling. For all presented block types, sensitive criterion functions can be constructed. Once a clustering $\mathbf{C}$ and the types of blocks are determined, we can also compute the values of connections by using averaging rules.

In Figure 13 a symmetric acyclic (edge connected inside clusters, acyclic reduced graph) block-model [27] of *Student Government* at the University of Ljubljana [34] is presented. The obtained clustering in 4 clusters is almost exact. The only error is produced by the arc $(a3, m5)$.

4 Implementation

4.1 Data Structures

In Pajek analysis and visualization are performed using 6 data types:

- *network* (graph),
- *partition* (nominal or ordinal properties of vertices),
- *vector* (numerical properties of vertices),
- *cluster* (subset of vertices),
- *permutation* (reordering of vertices, ordinal properties), and
- *hierarchy* (general tree structure on vertices).

In the near future we intend to extend this list with a support of multiple networks and partitions of edges.

The power of Pajek is based on several transformations that support different transitions among these data structures. Also the menu structure (see Figure 14) of the main Pajek window is based on them. Pajek's main window uses a 'calculator' paradigm with list-accumulator for each data type. The operations are performed on the currently active (selected) data and are also returning the results through accumulators.

The values of vectors can be used to determine several elements of network display such as X, Y, Z coordinates and the size of the vertex shape. The partition can be graphically represented by the color and the shape of the vertices. The values of edges can be represented by their thickness and/or color.

4.2 Implemented Algorithms

In Pajek, besides the algorithms described in Section 3, several known efficient algorithms are implemented, like:

- *simplifications and transformations*: deleting loops, multiple edges, transforming arcs to edges etc.;
- *components*: strong, weak, biconnected, symmetric;
- *decompositions*: symmetric-acyclic, hierarchical clustering;

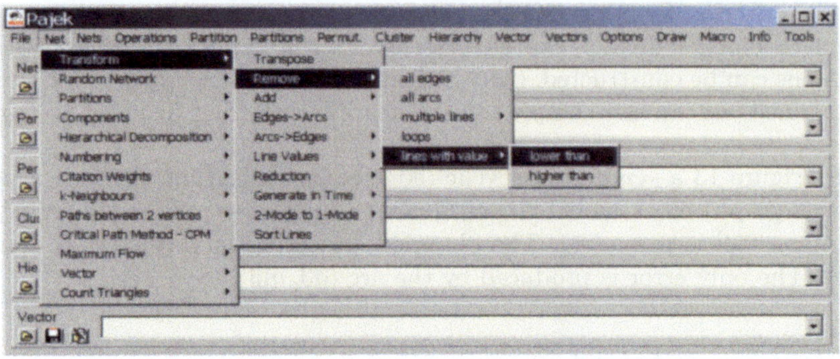

Fig. 14. `Pajek`'s main window.

- *paths*: shortest path(s), all paths between two vertices;
- *flows*: maximum flow between two vertices;
- *neighborhood*: k-neighbors;
- *CPM* – critical paths;
- *social networks algorithms*: centrality measures, hubs and authorities, measures of prestige, brokerage roles, structural holes, diffusion partitions;
- *measures of dependencies among partitions / vectors*: Cramer's V, Spearman rank correlation coefficient, Pearson correlation coefficient, Rajski coefficient;
- *extracting* subnetwork;
- *shrinking* clusters in network (generalized blockmodeling);
- *reordering*: topological ordering, Richards's numbering, Murtagh's seriation and clumping algorithms, depth/breadth first search.

`Pajek` contains also some data analysis procedures which have higher order running times and can therefore be used only on smaller networks or selected parts of large networks: hierarchical clustering, generalized blockmodeling, partitioning signed graphs [26], TSP (Traveling Salesman Problem), computing geodesics matrices, etc.

The procedures are available through the main window menus. Frequently used sequences of operations can be defined as *macros*. This allows the adaptations of `Pajek` to groups of users from different areas (social networks, chemistry, genealogy, computer science, mathematics, ...) for specific tasks.

4.3 Layout Algorithms and Layout Features

Special emphasis is given in `Pajek` to the automatic generation of network layouts. Several standard algorithms for automatic graph drawing are implemented: spring embedders (Kamada-Kawai and Fruchterman-Reingold), layouts determined by eigenvectors (Lanczos algorithm), drawing in layers (genealogies and other acyclic structures), fish-eye views and block (matrix) representation.

These algorithms were modified and extended to enable additional options: drawing with constraints (optimization of the selected part of the network, fixing some vertices to predefined positions, using values of edges as similarities or dissimilarities), drawing in 3D space. Pajek also provides tools for the manual editing of graph layouts.

Properties of vertices/edges (given as data or computed) can be represented by using colors, sizes and/or shapes of vertices/edges.

Pajek also supports drawing sequences of networks in its Draw window, and exports sequences of networks in suitable formats that can be examined with special 2D or 3D viewers (e.g., SVG and Mage). Pictures in SVG can be further controlled by using support written in JavaScript.

4.4 Interfaces

Pajek supports also some non-native input formats: UCINET DL files [45]; Vega graph files [46]; chemical MDLMOL [37] and BS; and genealogical GEDCOM [30].

The layouts can be exported in the following output graphic formats that can be examined by special 2D and 3D viewers: Encapsulated PostScript (EPS) [31], Scalable Vector Graphics (SVG) [1], VRML [24], MDLMOL/chime [37], and Kinemages (Mage) [43].

The main window menu *Tools* provides the export of Pajek's data to the statistical program R [42,21]. In the *Tools* menu, the user can prepare calls to her/his favorite viewers and other tools. It is also possible to run Pajek (+macros) from other programs (R, Ucinet, and others).

5 Examples

Several examples of applications of Pajek were already presented as illustrations while describing selected algorithms.

In Figure 15 a 3D layout of a graph obtained using *eigenvectors* is presented.

Figure 16 presents a snapshot of our 3D layout of graph A from the Graph drawing contest 1997, displayed in a VRML viewer [32].

6 Software

6.1 Architecture

Pajek is implemented in Delphi and runs on Windows operating systems. On the *things to do* list we have: support for GraphML format, implementing Pajek on Unix, and replacing macros by a JavaScript based network scripting language.

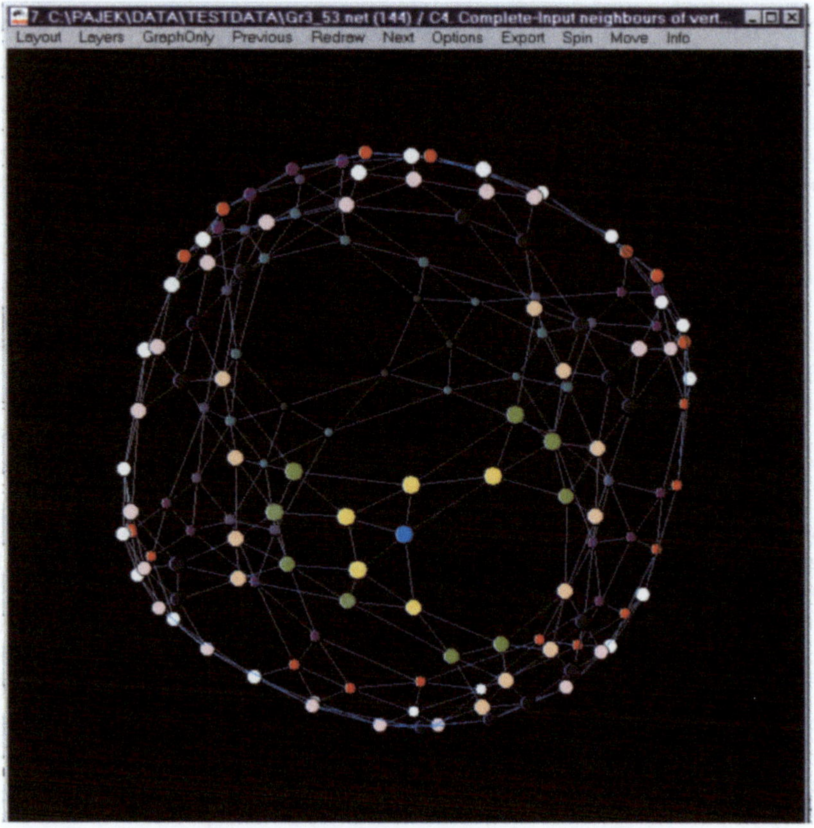

Fig. 15. 3D layout obtained using eigenvectors.

6.2 Availability

`Pajek` is still under development. The latest version is freely available, for noncommercial use, at its home page:
`http://vlado.fmf.uni-lj.si/pub/networks/pajek/`

References

1. Adobe SVG Viewer (2002) `http://www.adobe.com/svg/viewer/install/`
2. Batagelj, V. (1986) Graph – data structure and algorithms in pascal. Research report
3. Batagelj, V. (1997) Notes on blockmodeling. Social Networks **19**, 143–155
4. Batagelj, V. (2002) Efficient Algorithms for Citation Network Analysis, in preparation
5. Batagelj, V., Brandes, U. (2002) Fast generation of large sparse random graphs. in preparation

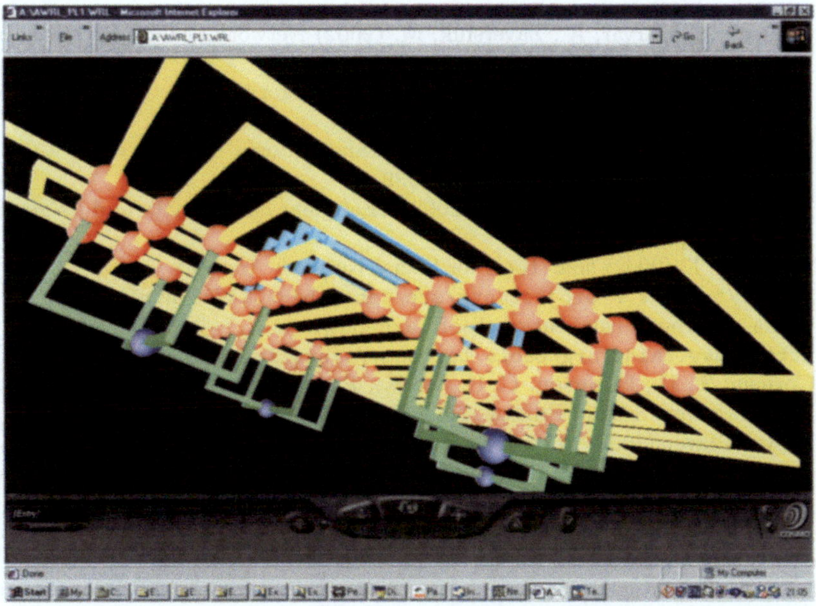

Fig. 16. GD '97 contest graph A in VRML.

6. Batagelj, V., Doreian, P., Ferligoj, A. (1992) An Optimizational Approach to Regular Equivalence. Social Networks **14**, 121–135
7. Batagelj, V., Ferligoj, A. (2000) Clustering relational data. In: W. Gaul, O. Opitz, M. Schader (eds.) Data Analysis, Springer-Verlag, Berlin, 3–15
8. Batagelj, V., Mrvar, A. (1995) Towards NetML Networks Markup Language. Presented at International Social Network Conference, London, July 6-10, 1995. `http://www.ijp.si/ftp/pub/preprints/ps/95/trp9515.ps`
9. Batagelj, V., Mrvar, A. (1991-94) Programs for Network Analysis. `http://vlado.fmf.uni-lj.si/pub/networks/`
10. Batagelj, V., Mrvar, A. (1998) `Pajek` – A Program for Large Network Analysis. Connections **21** (2), 47–57
11. Batagelj, V., Mrvar, A. (2000) Some Analyses of Erdős Collaboration Graph. Social Networks **22**, 173–186
12. Batagelj, V., Mrvar, A. (2001) A Subquadratic Triad Census Algorithm for Large Sparse Networks with Small Maximum Degree. Social Networks **23**, 237–243
13. Batagelj, V., Mrvar, A. (2002) `Pajek` - Analysis and Visualization of Large Networks. In: P. Mutzel, M. Jünger, S. Leipert (eds.) Graph Drawing '01, Lecture Notes in Computer Science 2265, Springer-Verlag, 477–478
14. Batagelj, V., Mrvar, A. (2002) Density based approaches to Reuters terror news network analysis. submitted
15. Batagelj, V., Pisanski, T. (1989) Xgraph project documentation
16. Batagelj, V., Mrvar, A., Zaveršnik, M. (1999) Partitioning Approach to Visualization of Large Graphs. In: J. Kratochvíl (ed.) Graph Drawing '99, Štiřin Castle, Czech Republic. Lecture Notes in Computer Science 1731, Springer-Verlag, 90–97

17. Batagelj, V., Mrvar, A., Zaveršnik, M. (2002) Network analysis of texts. Language Technologies, Ljubljana, 143–148
18. Batagelj, V., Zaveršnik, M. (2001) An $O(m)$ Algorithm for Cores Decomposition of Networks. submitted
19. Batagelj, V., Zaveršnik, M. (2002) Generalized Cores. submitted `http://arxiv.org/abs/cs.DS/0202039`
20. Batagelj, V. and Zaveršnik, M. (2002) Triangular connectivity and its generalizations, in preparation
21. Butts, C. T. (2002) sna: Tools for Social Network Analysis. `http://cran.at.r-project.org/src/contrib/PACKAGES.html\#sna`
22. Caida: Internet Visualization Tool Taxonomy. `http://www.caida.org/tools/taxonomy/visualization/`
23. Cormen, T. H., Leiserson, C. E., Rivest, R. L., Stein, C. (2001) Introduction to Algorithms, Second Edition, MIT Press
24. Cosmo Player (2002) `http://ca.com/cosmo/`
25. de Nooy, W., Mrvar, A., Batagelj, V. (2002) Exploratory Social Network Analysis With **Pajek**. to be published by the Cambridge University Press
26. Doreian, P., Mrvar, A. (1996) A Partitioning Approach to Structural Balance. Social Networks **18**, 149–168
27. Doreian, P., Batagelj, V., Ferligoj, A. (2000) Symmetric-acyclic decompositions of networks. J. classif. **17** (1), 3–28
28. Dremelj, P., Mrvar, A., Batagelj, V. (2002) Analiza rodoslova dubrovačkog vlasteoskog kruga pomoću programa **Pajek**. Anali Dubrovnik XL, HAZU, Zagreb, Dubrovnik, 105–126 (in Croatian)
29. Garfield, E., Sher, I. H., Torpie, R. J. (1964) The Use of Citation Data in Writing the History of Science. Philadelphia: The Institute for Scientific Information `http://www.garfield.library.upenn.edu/papers/useofcitdatawritinghistofsci.pdf`
30. GEDCOM 5.5. `http://homepages.rootsweb.com/~pmcbride/gedcom/55gctoc.htm`
31. Ghostscript, Ghostview and GSview, `http://www.cs.wisc.edu/~ghost/`
32. Graph Drawing Contest 1997. `http://vlado.fmf.uni-lj.si/pub/gd/gd97.htm`
33. Grossman, J. (2002) The Erdős Number Project. `http://www.oakland.edu/~grossman/erdoshp.html`
34. Hlebec, V. (1993) Recall versus recognition: Comparison of two alternative procedures for collecting social network data. Metodološki zvezki **9**, Ljubljana: FDV, 121–128
35. Hummon, N. P., Doreian, P. (1989) Connectivity in a citation network: The development of DNA theory. Social Networks **11**, 39–63
36. Jones B. (2002). Computational geometry database. `http://compgeom.cs.uiuc.edu/~jeffe/compgeom/biblios.html`
37. MDL Information Systems, Inc. (2002) `http://www.mdli.com/`
38. James Moody home page (2002) `http://www.soc.sbs.ohio-state.edu/jwm/`
39. Murtagh, F. (1985) Multidimensional Clustering Algorithms, *Compstat lectures* **4**, Vienna: Physica-Verlag
40. ODLIS (2002) Online dictionary of library and information science. `http://vax.wcsu.edu/library/odlis.html`

41. Pennock, D.M. et al. (2002) Winners don't take all, PNAS **99** (8), 5207–5211
42. The R Project for Statistical Computing. `http://www.r-project.org/`
43. Richardson, D. C., Richardson, J. S. (2002) The Mage Page. `http://kinemage.biochem.duke.edu/index.html`
44. Seidman, S. B. (1983) Network structure and minimum degree, Social Networks **5**, 269–287
45. UCINET (2002) `http://www.analytictech.com/`
46. Project Vega (2002) `http://vega.ijp.si/`
47. Wasserman, S., Faust, K. (1994) Social Network Analysis: Methods and Applications. Cambridge University Press, Cambridge
48. Wasserman, S., and Pattison, P. (1996) Logit models and logistic regressions for social networks: I. An introduction to Markov graphs and p^*. Psychometrika **60**, 401–42, `http://kentucky.psych.uiuc.edu/pstar/index.html`
49. White, D. R., Batagelj, V., Mrvar, A. (1999) Analyzing Large Kinship and Marriage Networks with Pgraph and `Pajek`. Social Science Computer Review **17** (3), 245–274
50. Yuen Ho et al. (2002) Systematic identification of protein complexes in Saccharomyces cerevisiae by mass spectrometry. Nature **415**, 180–183, `http://www.mshri.on.ca/tyers/pdfs/proteome.pdf`
51. Zaveršnik, M., Batagelj, V., Mrvar, A. (2002) Analysis and visualization of 2-mode networks. In: Proceedings of Sixth Austrian, Hungarian, Italian and Slovenian Meeting of Young Statisticians, October 5–7, 2001, Ossiach, Austria. University of Klagenfurt, 113–123

Tulip – A Huge Graph Visualization Framework*

David Auber

LaBRI-Université Bordeaux 1, 351 Cours de la Libération, 33405 Talence, France

1 Introduction

The research by the *information visualization* community ("*InfoViz*") shows clearly that using a visual representation of data-sets enables faster analysis by the end users. Several scientific reasons explain these results. First of all, the visual perception system is the most powerful of all the human perception systems. In the human brain, 70% of the receptors and 40% of the cortex are used for the vision process [27,34]. Furthermore, human beings are better at "recognition" tasks than at "memorization" tasks [10]. This implies that textual representations are less efficient than visual metaphors when one wants to analyze huge data-sets. This comes from the fact that reading is both a memorization task and a recognition task.

The research by Bertin [5], Fairchild [12] and Ware [34] shows that two types of information exist: entities and relations. Thus, all kinds of data-sets can be represented by a graph with attributes. In this graph, the nodes are the entities and the edges are the relations. The graph visualization framework that we present in this chapter has been set-up in order to devise, experiment and use, for the information-visualization purpose, new tools based on the results coming from graph theory. For instance, one of our results [4] consists of using the statistical properties of random trees having a fixed maximum-degree or/and a fixed maximum segment-length in order to detect automatically the irregularities in the visualized data-set.

Even if the Tulip framework enables the visualization, the drawing and the edition of small graphs, all parts of the framework have been built in order to be able to visualize graphs having up to 1,000,000 elements. When one wants to visualize such structures, interaction is necessary. Ideally, the human perception system requires an interactive system to respond to an operation in less than fifty milliseconds [34]. Such time constraints imply that special emphasis should be layed on the running time of the algorithms. Furthermore, when the size of graphs becomes huge, both due to the limits and the architecture of existing memories, reducing the memory consumption is one of the most important requirements.

Moreover, if we follow the information retrieval method introduced by Shneiderman [26]:

* I gratefully acknowledge the constructive remarks on earlier drafts by Marie Cornu, Michael Jünger and Petra Mutzel.

"Overview first, zoom and filters, then details on demand",

a visualization system must draw and display huge graphs, enable to navigate through geometric operations as well as extract subgraphs of the data and allow to change the representation of the results obtained by filtering [20]. Thus, a graph visualization system must allow three things: graph drawing, graph clustering and interaction. The Tulip framework is especially designed to support such a visualization method on huge graphs.

This chapter presents some of the direct applications of the Tulip framework in research and bioinformatics. Then, it introduces different kinds of algorithms implemented in Tulip such as graph drawing, graph parameters and graph clustering. Subsequently, we will describe the general functioning of the Tulip data structure that enables the management of a graph hierarchy and the manipulation of algorithms; we will also give a short description of the Tulip [1] software functioning. Finally, after giving several examples of graph drawing results obtained on real graphs, which come from file-systems, web sites and program analysis, we will conclude with general information about the terms of use of the framework.

2 Applications

2.1 Research

The first application of the Tulip graph visualization framework is to provide an environment in which tools can be experimentally evaluated for the purpose of information visualization research. In particular, our team and others are using it in order to devise new kinds of human computer interfaces and new tools. Huge data-sets can consequently be manipulated. Using graphs for information visualization is a complex task in which graph drawing algorithms have an important place. The most important pieces of research currently supported by the Tulip framework are: using graph parameters in order to show information in data [3,4], using graphs in order to make a visual analysis of semantic networks [6], and studying general new concepts of data exploration. These different pieces of research take place in the University of Bath (UK), the University of Chicoutimi (Canada), Virginia Tech (USA), the University of Montpellier (France) and the University of Bordeaux (France).

2.2 Biochemistry

One of the direct applications of the Tulip framework occurs in a European project that consists of giving access to information about some protein-protein interactions to biologists. The protein-protein interaction (PPI) data are developing into increasingly important resources for the analysis of metabolic pathways, signal transduction chains and other cellular mechanisms.

This allows, for instance, to find specific drug treatments to inhibit or activate a precise and selected metabolic pathway. Therefore, it decreases side effects. One reason for this current increase in the utilization of technologies which yield the PPI data is the fact that these technologies, in particular the yeast two-hybrid technology, are relatively well-studied for the development of high throughput experiments conducted by different groups. However, the comparisons of results obtained by different groups is currently very labor-intensive. Thus, one of the applications of the Tulip framework is to use the graph visualization method in order to simplify the comparisons of results through an intuitive human computer interface that uses graph visualization methods and interaction with the data.

2.3 Others

The architecture of the software has been split into different parts that can be reused in order to build new graph visualization applications easily. Thus, the use of this framework into direct applications is growing quickly. For instance, it is used in order to display the results of an automatic analysis of videos in the MEPGS format in which the generated data are graphs and trees. Another application is the visualization and the comparison of sequences and secondary structures of DNA, in which graph drawing algorithms are used for an automatic display of the data and the combinatoric properties of the trees are used to simplify the comparisons.

3 Algorithms

Since the Tulip software is dedicated to graph visualization, several kinds of algorithms are available. The most important are: graph drawing algorithms, clustering algorithms, metrics algorithms and visual attribute mapping algorithms. Afterwards, we will present some of the algorithms available through the Tulip framework.

3.1 Graph Drawing

A large variety of graph drawing algorithms dedicated to graphs, directed acyclic graphs and trees is presented in the Technical Foundations chapter. Here we will focus on some algorithms that can be applied for the visualization of huge "real" graphs. When we consider huge graphs, running time is very important and special emphasis should be layed on the minimization of the quantity of memory used in all algorithms. This necessity comes from the fact that, in most cases, even if an algorithm is linear, the access to the memory on the hard disk drive (swap) makes the algorithm unusable. One of the reasons is that a graph structure is not linear by definition, thus, the memory management algorithms (like cache, or prefetch) are inefficient most of the time.

Afterwards, we will introduce a version of the Reingold and Tilford algorithm [24] that reduces the memory consumption and which permits to include nodes of arbitrary individual size and edges of arbitrary individual length. Then we will introduce the Cone Tree algorithm originally designed by Robertson *et al.* [25] for file-system visualization. This algorithm is of general interest for the purpose of information visualization. We will discuss in detail one of the improvements by Carriere and Kazman [9] and then we will present a heuristic that produces a better drawing if the tree has a non-constant node degree. To finish, we will present a graph drawing algorithm for Sugiyama-style layout that is especially designed to handle huge graphs. This algorithm draws graphs with at the most two bends per edge, it runs in $O([V| \cdot |E|)$ time and $O([V| + |E|)$ space. Other algorithms such as the so-called GEM algorithm of Frick *et al.* [14], the well-known Tutte algorithm [31] and the Tree map algorithm [7] are also available in Tulip.

Reingold and Tilford. As described in Section 4.1 of the Technical Foundations, the original algorithm of Reingold and Tilford [24] is a recursive algorithm that consists of drawing separately each subtree of a node and then move each subtree until the distance between the subtrees is minimal. The algorithm described by Reingold and Tilford needs to store data inside nodes in order to make all the operations.

In order to obtain a usable drawing in terms of information visualization, one must produce a layout in which the individual size of a node and the individual length of an edge are taken into account. Our tree drawing algorithm manages the node height by fixing the height of a layer L to be the maximum height of a node in L. The node width is taken into account by managing the left and right contours for each node. This can be done with slight modifications of the original Reingold and Tilford algorithm. The method used to manage the edge length consists in an augmentation step that adds nodes and edges to the tree. Figure 1 summarizes the augmentation method. In the following, let T denote the tree obtained after augmentation.

Let $h : E \rightarrow \mathbb{N}^+$ be a function that represents edge lengths. If one uses the standard Reingold and Tilford algorithm, the running time of the algorithm is $O(\sum_{e \in E} h(e))$ and the space requirement is $O(\sum_{e \in E} h(e))$ because one must build a tree of $1 + \sum_{e \in E} h(e)$ nodes and $\sum_{e \in E} h(e)$ edges.

When one wants to draw huge trees, the memory requirement of the algorithm presented above makes it unusable if the edge lengths are important. However, if we look carefully at the Reingold and Tilford algorithm, we can notice that in order to compute the layout, we only need to store two contours at the same time and not two values inside each node like proposed in the original version by Reingold and Tilford. Figure 2 illustrates this. Another important property of the Reingold and Tilford algorithm is that each node

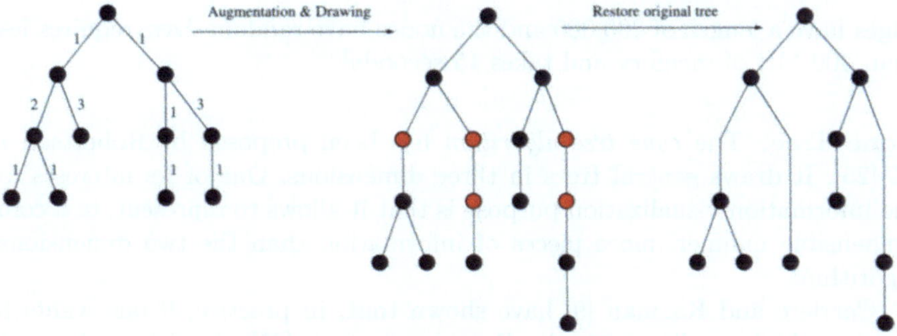

Fig. 1. Edge length management.

(different from the root) of degree equal to two is lined up with its neighbors. Therefore, it is not necessary to store the coordinates of each virtual node added during the augmentation step. Furthermore, the contours induced by an edge with length greater than one can be stored efficiently. This enables us to preserve the memory usage when having a lot of different edge lengths. If we take these two considerations into account, it is possible to add dynamically, and efficiently, the virtual nodes during the contour building of each subtree and then, when the contour is not used anymore, to free all the unused virtual nodes. This results in an algorithm with $O(\sum_{e \in E} h(e))$ running time and $O(|V|)$ memory consumption.

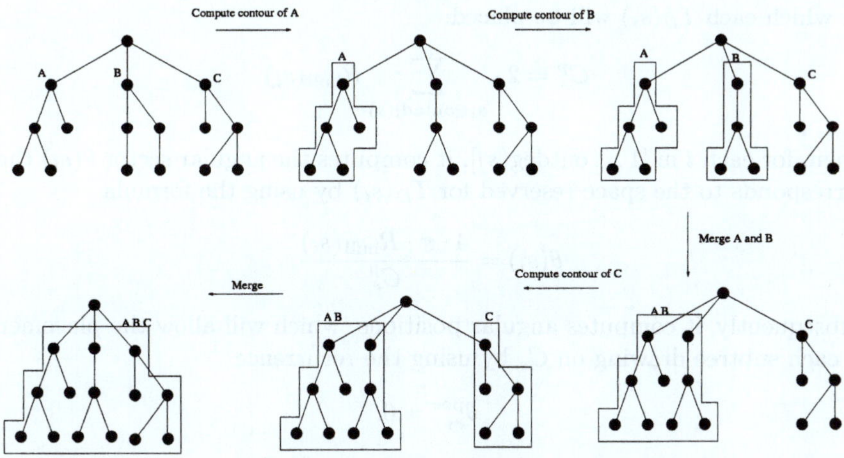

Fig. 2. Tree contours.

The hierarchical tree drawing algorithm proposed in Tulip is the one presented above. For instance, the storing, the drawing and the displaying of a complete binary tree of depth 20 (2^{20} nodes and $2^{20} - 1$ edges) in which all edges have a length of 200.000 and the nodes have random sizes, requires less than 400 MB of memory and takes 15 seconds[1].

Cone Tree. The *cone tree algorithm* has been proposed by Robertson *et al.* [25]. It draws general trees in three dimensions. One of its interests for the information visualization purpose is that it allows to represent, in a comprehensible manner, more pieces of information than the two dimensional algorithms.

Carriere and Kazman [9] have shown that, in practice, if one wants to obtain a high quality with the Robertson *et al.* [25] algorithm, the node degrees must be constant. This comes from the fact that the Robertson *et al.* algorithm assigns the same amount of space to each subtree without taking their sizes into account. Thus, when two subtrees have a different size (a different number of nodes), they have the same size in the final drawing. The solution proposed by Carriere and Kazman consists of using a divide and conquer algorithm. Similar in concept to the one of Reingold and Tilford, the algorithm draws each subtree inside an enclosing circle and then places each enclosing circle at a minimum distance on a circle. The third coordinate of the nodes is obtained by using their depths in the tree. The principle of the recursive algorithm is the following:

Let $T_D(x)$ be the drawing of the subtree induced by node x, and let $R_{\text{hull}}(x)$ be the radius of an enclosing circle of $T_D(x)$. Let s be a node. For simplification, we denote the ith element of $\text{outadj}(s)$ by s_i. In order to compute $T_D(s)$, the algorithm first computes the perimeter C_s^p of the circle C_s on which each $T_D(s_i)$ will be placed:

$$C_s^p = 2 \cdot \sum_{s_i \in \text{outadj}(s)} R_{\text{hull}}(s_i)$$

Then, for each i in $[1 \dots \text{outdeg}(s)]$, it computes the angular sector $\theta(s_i)$ that corresponds to the space reserved for $T_D(s_i)$ by using the formula

$$\theta(s_i) = \frac{4 \cdot \pi \cdot R_{\text{hull}}(s_i)}{C_s^p}.$$

Subsequently, it computes angular positions, which will allow the placement of each subtree drawing on C_s by using the recurrence

$$\theta_{s_1}^{\text{pos}} = 0,$$

$$\theta_{s_i}^{\text{pos}} = \theta_{s_{i-1}}^{\text{pos}} + \frac{\theta(s_{i-1}) + \theta(s_i)}{2}.$$

Finally, the algorithm computes the enclosing circle of the new drawing by using the formula

$$R_{\text{hull}}(s) = \max(\{R_{\text{hull}}(s_i) \mid s_i \in \text{outadj}(s)\}) + \frac{C_s^p}{2 \cdot \pi}.$$

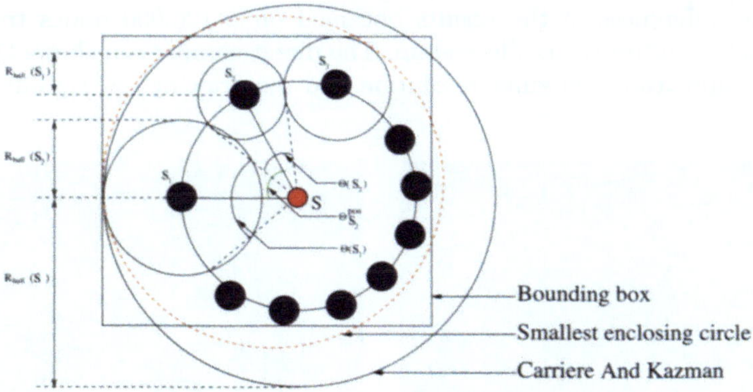

Fig. 3. Carriere and Kazman algorithm.

Figure 3 summarizes the algorithm. It shows that the enclosing circle used by the Carriere and Kazman algorithm is far from being optimal (i.e., the smallest enclosing circle). It is straightforward that minimizing the size of the enclosing circle has the effect of reducing the drawing size and of providing a better angular resolution in the final layout. Therefore, the algorithmic set-up in Tulip is different from the one by Carriere and Kazman. The most important difference is that the center of the enclosing circle can be different from a node position. This change is necessary if one wants to find a better enclosing circle. Finding the optimal enclosing circle is a special case of a more general problem, called the "Smallest enclosing ball problem". This problem can be formulated as a convex optimization problem. For more information on this subject see [16,22,35].

In our algorithm, we have set up a fast approximation. It uses the fact that one can directly compute the optimal enclosing circle of two circles. Thus, it is possible to compute an enclosing circle incrementally by successively merging two circles. This enables us to obtain an enclosing circle of $T_D(s)$ in $O(\text{outdeg}(s))$ time. The fact that all circles are placed on a circle at a defined angular position is taken into account by choosing the order in which the merging operations are done. In the current version of our heuristic we use the internal circle of the bounding box of all subtrees as a starting circle. The Carriere and Kazman heuristic is optimal if the enclosing-circle size of each subtree is identical. This is why we compute the enclosing circle obtained by both methods and then choose one that has minimum size.

Experiments have shown that the results obtained on trees having a non-constant degree are better than those obtained by using the method suggested by Carriere and Kazman. E.g., we have measured that when the degrees are chosen randomly, the average area of an enclosing circle is 40% smaller than the area obtained by the Carriere and Kazman algorithm. Figures 4 and 5

[1] On an x86 computer running at 1.5 GHz.

show the differences of the results obtained on a 120.000 nodes tree that represents an entire Linux file-system. The direct comparison shows that our method improves the angular resolution and the drawing size significantly.

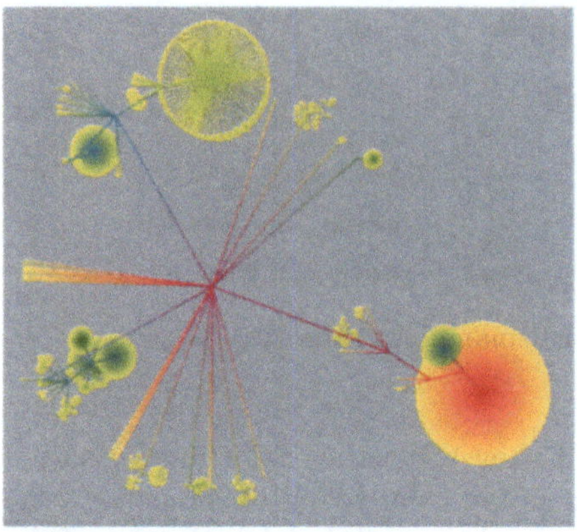

Fig. 4. Carriere and Kazman file-system drawing.

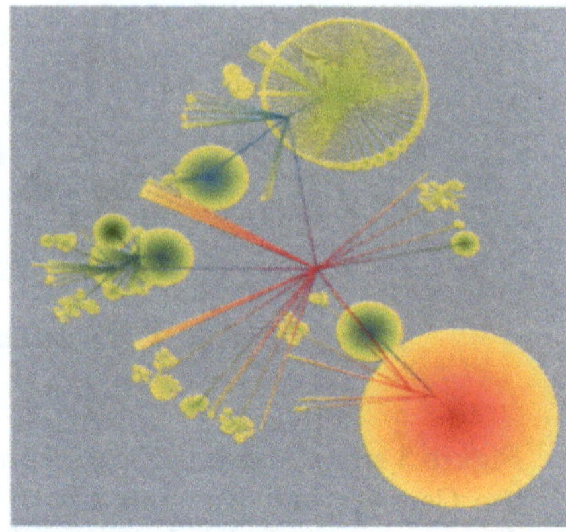

Fig. 5. Improvement of the Carriere and Kazman algorithm.

Like in the Reingold and Tilford algorithm, the linear running time is achieved by delaying all the placements of the subtrees to a second phase. The implemented version in Tulip can draw and display trees such as those of Figures 4 and 5 in less than one second[2].

Hierarchical Drawing. The advantages of the Sugiyama approach [29] described in Section 4.2 of the Technical Foundations are numerous and its usefulness for information visualization is well-known. However, the memory consumption of the existing algorithms makes them unusable for drawing of huge graphs. The problem comes from the artificial node insertion step that can add $O(|V| \cdot |E|)$ nodes in the worst case. Even when using fast Sugiyama algorithms, such as the one proposed by Buchheim *et al.* [8], the problem is still the memory usage. For instance, a drawing of a complete dag (directed acyclic graph) with 200 nodes and 19.900 edges requires 900 MB. Figure 6 shows a typical graph in which the augmentation step requires a quadratic number of insertions. In order to allow the layered layout of a huge graph that prevents edge superposition, reduces the crossings and uses at most two bends per edge, we have set up an algorithm that uses only $O(|V| + |E|)$ memory in the worst case [2]. For ease of exposition, we consider directed acyclic graphs with one source. Using a well-known preprocessing step for

[2] On an x86 computer running at 1.5 GHz.

the Sugiyama algorithm, one can always transform a general graph into such a graph (see Section 4.2 in the Technical Foundations).

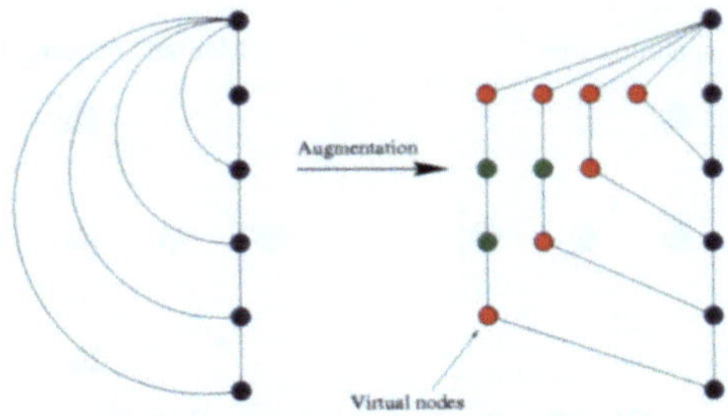

Fig. 6. Quadratic augmentation.

In the layer assignment step of our algorithm we use *longest path layering* as described in Section 4.2 of the Technical Foundations. This method amounts to a standard topological walk in a dag. Let k be the number of layers and $L(x)$ be the layer number of the node x. The algorithm ensures that there is a path P in the graph between layer 1 and layer k, in which for each edge (u, v) we have $L(u) = L(v) - 1$. Thus, the depth of a spanning tree after the artificial node insertion is equal to the depth of a spanning tree in the original dag.

The augmentation step is performed by replacing the edges of the original graph and by building a function $E_h : E \rightarrow \mathbb{N}$. Let $\lambda(s, d) = |L(s) - L(d)|$. The transformation method of an edge $e(s, d)$ is the following:

$$e(s,d) \rightarrow \begin{cases} \text{If } \lambda = 2, & \text{then we add one node } u_1 \text{ and two edges } e_1 = (s, u_1), \\ & e_2 = (u_1, d) \text{ and we set } E_h(e_1) = E_h(e_2) = 1. \\ \text{If } \lambda > 2, & \text{then we add two nodes } u_1, u_2 \text{ and three edges} \\ & e_1 = (s, u_1),\ e_2 = (u_1, u_2),\ e_3 = (u_2, d) \text{ and we set} \\ & E_h(e_1) = E_h(e_3) = 1 \text{ and } E_h(e_2) = \lambda. \end{cases}$$

Furthermore, we assign the following layer numbers to the added nodes: $L(u_1) = L(s) + 1$ and $L(u_2) = L(v) - 1$. This method avoids a quadratic augmentation and ensures the insertion of at most $O(2 \cdot |E|)$ artificial nodes into the graph (i.e., we do not insert the green nodes in Figure 6). Then, in order to reduce the number of crossings, we use the barycenter heuristic described in Section 4.2 of the Technical Foundations. By default, the number of up and down sweeps is fixed to 4.

For the coordinate assignment step, we first extract a spanning tree. For each node v, the building of a spanning tree consists of removing all the edges in instar(v) but one. In order to obtain a drawing in which v is placed in the center of its ancestors, this edge is chosen so that the barycenter value (obtained during the crossing minimization step) of its source s is the median of the barycenter values of the elements in $\mathrm{inadj}(v)$. Figure 7 shows the effect of this choice on a simple layout.

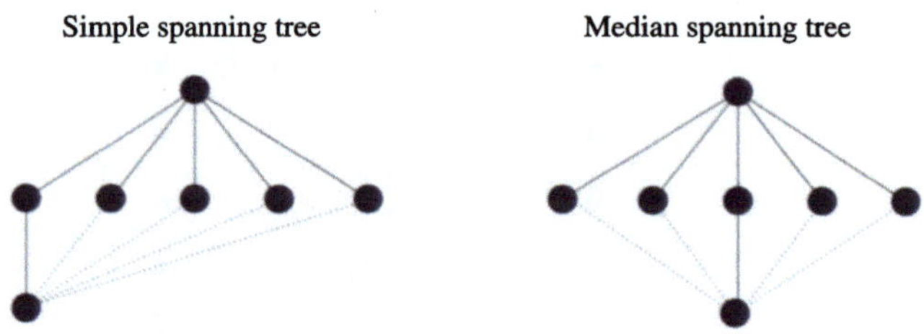

Fig. 7. Spanning tree building.

The final layout is obtained by drawing the spanning tree with the variant of the Reingold and Tilford algorithm introduced above, in which we use E_h for the edge lengths and user-defined sizes of the nodes. The result of the algorithm is an upward forward drawing with at the most two bends per edge that needs $O(|V| + |E|)$ space and $O(|V| \cdot |E|)$ time. The proof of the space consumption uses the properties of the longest path layering [2]. For example, with the implemented version of this algorithm in Tulip, it takes 9 seconds and 24 MB for a complete dag with 200 nodes and 19.900 edges, or 65 seconds and 100 MB for a complete dag with 500 nodes and 124.750 edges[3]. Even if this algorithm was designed to be usable for huge graphs, when we use it on small graphs we observe that the layouts obtained are very similar to those obtained by the existing "Sugiyama style layout" algorithms. Figures 8 and 9 show the results of the Buchheim *et al.* [8] algorithm and of our algorithm on a little graph.

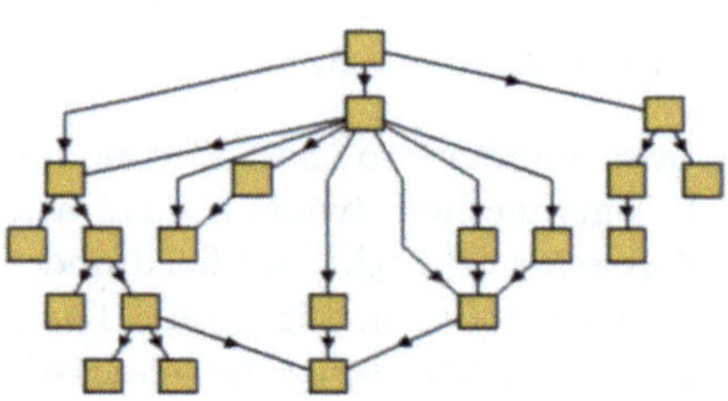

Fig. 8. Our algorithm.

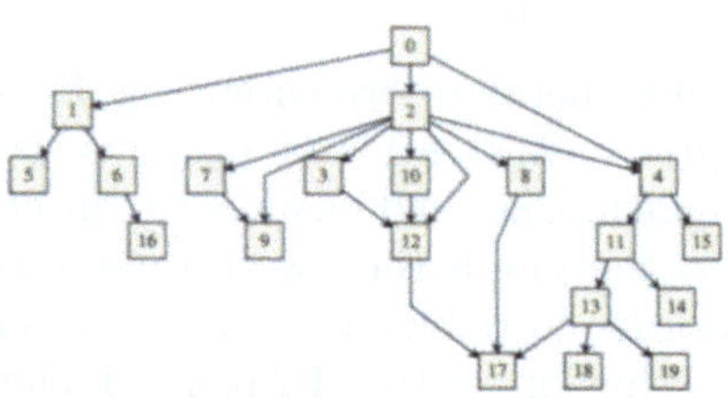

Fig. 9. Buchheim *et al.* algorithm.

[3] On an x86 computer running at 1.5 GHz.

3.2 Graph Measure

When working with huge graphs, representing them by using graph drawing algorithms is not sufficient to produce a usable view of the data for the end-users. Therefore, we use intrinsic measures in order to show the relevant information in graphs. Displaying automatically such pieces of information enables the users to detect them easily, even on huge data-sets [20,34].

One of the most important parameters that we use is the Strahler parameter. The *Strahler number* of binary trees has been introduced in the context of the morphological structure of river networks [28]. It consists of associating an integer value to each of the nodes of a binary tree. These values give quantitative information about the complexity of each subtree of the original tree [33]. Furthermore, if we consider an arithmetical expression A and its evaluation binary tree T, Ershov [11] has proved that the Strahler number of T increased by one is exactly the minimal number of registers needed to compute A. The Strahler number can be computed by Algorithm 1; Figure 10 shows an example of the result.

Algorithm 1: Strahler algorithm.

```
binaryStrahler(node η of a binary tree T)
begin
  if η is a leaf of T return 1
  let η_left and η_right be the left and the right child of η, respectively
  if binaryStrahler(η_left) = binaryStrahler(η_right)
    return binaryStrahler(η_left) + 1
  else
    return max(binaryStrahler(η_left),binaryStrahler(η_right))
end binaryStrahler
```

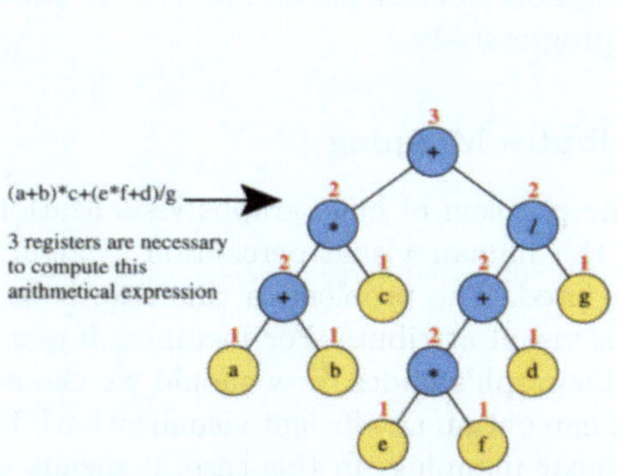

Fig. 10. Arithmetical expression tree.

The algorithmic set-up in Tulip [3] is an extension of the Strahler algorithm that can be performed on graphs. The idea is to use the extension of the Strahler number parameter introduced by Fédou [13] and to extend it to graphs. To summarize the algorithm, in the original Strahler version, trees are seen as arithmetical expressions on which we count the number of registers they need to be evaluated on a computer. When we treat graphs, we consider that a graph can be seen as a program. In this case, to evaluate a program, we need registers and nested calls to a stack. Thus, the parameter is in two dimensions: the first counts the number of registers and the second counts the number of stacks. Such a parameter can be used for different tasks. In Tulip we use it to automatically build the ordering of elements needed in the incremental rendering method (implemented in Tulip) introduced by Wills [36]. The results [3] enable to obtain a good abstraction of the graph drawing during the visual exploration in $O(|V|)$ for dags and in $O(|V| \log |V|)$ for general graphs.

3.3 Graph Clustering

To enable the visual exploration of a large data-set one must propose automatic clustering algorithms to end-users. These algorithms can be divided into two groups: the intrinsic clustering algorithms and the extrinsic clustering algorithms [19]. In Tulip, different kinds of clustering algorithms, based on the density functions of attributes, enable users to manage both cases.

One important graph clustering algorithm available in Tulip is dedicated to trees. The idea is to use the well-known intrinsic parameters on trees in order to cluster them. This algorithm [4] uses node-degree and segment-length (a path in which each node has a degree equal to 2) in trees. Using the combinatoric results on the distributions of these two parameters on random trees with fixed degree or/and fixed segment length, we have extracted statistical tables that enable us to test in constant time whether or not a subtree is closed to the distribution. The final algorithm [4] enables pruning a tree in order to reduce its number of elements and to detect "abnormal" phenomena automatically and progressively.

3.4 Visual Attributes Mapping

In order to treat the problem of huge graphs visualization one must use all the capabilities of the human visual perception system. Thus, size, shape and colors must be used. The problem in this case is to map a parameter (of any kind) into a visual attribute. For instance, if one wants to visualize the outdegrees of the graph's nodes, how should we choose the colors of the elements so that we can obtain an efficient visualization? The straightforward solution is to use linear mapping. In this case, it means using a gradient of colors and then choosing a color proportional to the element's value. Such a method works very well when the distribution of the values is uniform.

However, when the distribution is not uniform, in most of the cases this solution allows detection of only few different values.

To solve this problem in Tulip, we are using the *color mapping algorithm* proposed by Herman *et al.* [17]. This algorithm consists of building an approximation of the probability distribution by computing the frequency histogram of an attribute. Once normalized, this histogram gives a discrete form of the attribute distribution. By accumulating the frequencies along the range of values, it produces a discrete density function that can be used to map an attribute to colors. Figures 11 and 12 give an example of the differences between a linear mapping and a "distribution mapping". In these figures the colors represent values of the "fission" parameter described by Marshall in [20]. It is clear that in this case, using the "distribution mapping" enables users to detect both the existence of several different values and which values are higher than the others.

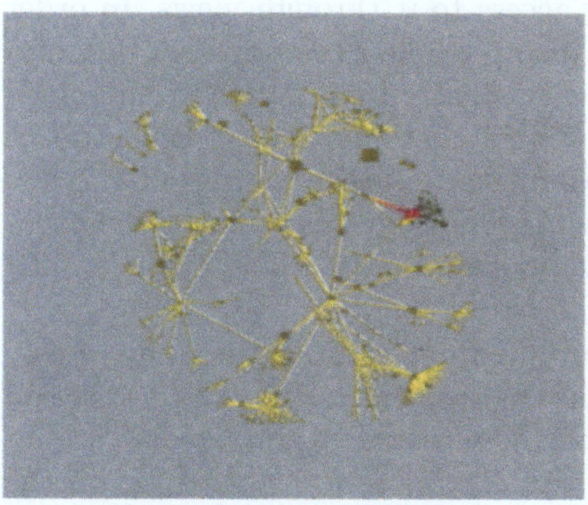

Fig. 11. Linear mapping.

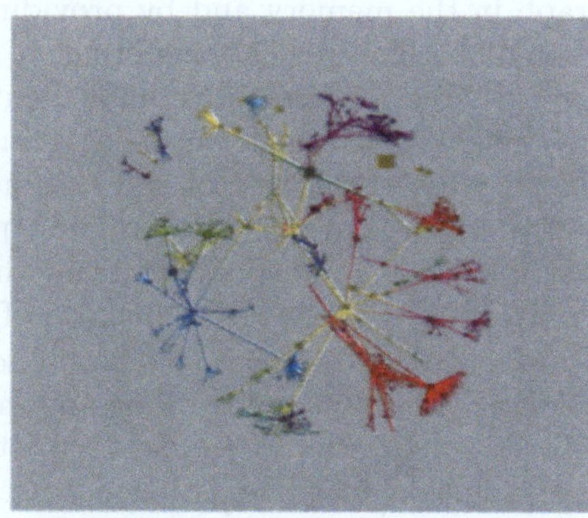

Fig. 12. Herman *et al.* mapping.

4 Implementation

In this section we will describe the data structure used in the Tulip framework. To manage huge graphs, we have put a special emphasis on it. It allows all the operations needed by the Shneiderman exploration process [26] and includes mechanisms that make it possible to minimize the memory usage. The whole Tulip framework has been written in C++. It is based on the standard template library [18] and on a free implementation of the OpenGl library [23]. Then, we will describe the Tulip software [1] that uses the QT [30] library for its dynamic human-computer interface. We will also present briefly the TlpRender software that provides usage of graphs through a web service. We will conclude by an overview of all the possible extensions of the framework.

4.1 Data Structure

Tulip has been built in order to handle graphs having up to 1,000,000 elements (nodes and edges). In this case, the memory management is a crucial factor for building an efficient framework. In order to limit the memory swapping and the processor cache faults, one must put a special emphasis on the trade-off between the memory space and the processor time used. In most of the cases, minimizing the necessary memory implies the need for a global knowledge of all the stored data. Furthermore, in order to provide a framework for the purpose of information visualization, one must treat the problem of attributes storing. Afterwards, we will present the general concepts of the Tulip data structure that are the base of the whole Tulip framework.

Graph Hierarchy. In Tulip, cluster management is done by using only one graph in the memory and by providing access to it through views. In order to enable a hierarchical clustering, it is also possible to obtain the view of a view. Such a model can be implemented efficiently by using the well-known "fly-weight" pattern (for elements) and "chain of responsibility" pattern (for cluster trees) [15]. One of the best advantages is a real sharing of the elements between graphs with a good memory management. This implementation solves the memory problem that appears in the Marshall *et al.* [21] architecture without any reduction of the functionalities.

It is easy to obtain very efficient solutions when using a hierarchy of partitions. However, when working on graphs that represent data, the restriction to partitions does not enable us to store the clusters of graphs that are already defined in the existing data-set. For instance, when working on the human metabolism data-set, the data are composed of links (edges) between enzymes and compounds (nodes) that form a graph. The set of metabolic pathways is a set of subgraphs of this graph. In many cases, compounds and enzymes can be found in different pathways (for instance, water), thus, this set of subgraphs cannot be stored if one uses the standard cluster tree definition (see Section 2.5 in the Technical Foundations).

The Tulip solution can be considered as graph filtering. In Figure 13, one can see a graph G and a set of clusters $\{G_1, G_2, G_3, G_4, G_5\}$. In this example, the clusters are subgraphs induced by the nodes inside the colored boxes. Figure 14 is the cluster tree that represents the hierarchy of graphs of Figure 13. On the tree-edges of Figure 14, the boxes represent adjustable filters. The idea of adjustable filters is to store in memory a minimum amount of information that allows dynamical cluster reconstruction. For instance, for filter $F2$ it is better to store the difference between G_2 and G if one wants to minimize the memory usage. On the contrary, for filter $F3$, it is better to store all the nodes and edges of G_3. For a study describing how adjustable filters can be chosen in order to minimize the memory consumption, and to preserve efficient access to the graph structure, we refer to [2].

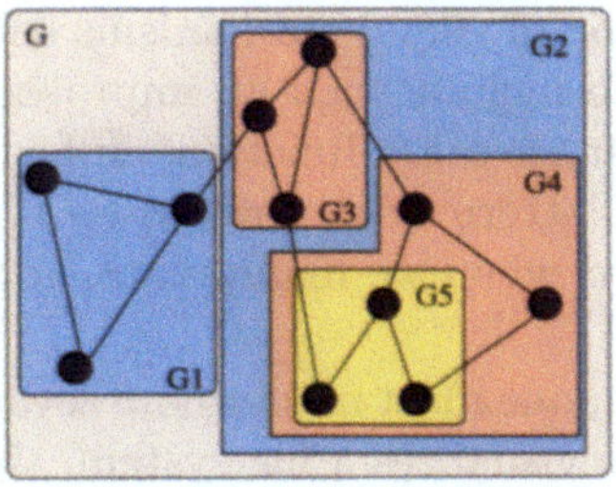

Fig. 13. A clustered graph.

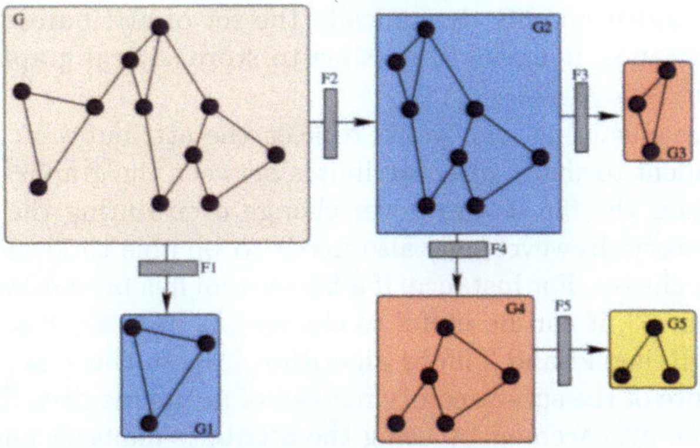

Fig. 14. A cluster hierarchy.

In order to maintain the coherence of the data structure, one must state the modification operations precisely. When one wants to add a node or edge to a cluster, this node or edge must be inserted into all the upper-graphs of the cluster. When one wants to delete a node or an edge in a cluster, this node or this edge must be deleted from all the subgraphs of the cluster. In practical cases of graph visualization, the processor time-cost due to the management of the hierarchy coherence is offset by the reduction in the memory usage and by the improvements in important operations such as graphs cloning or elements sharing.

Graph Attributes. An *attribute* is a value attached to a node or an edge. In a graph visualization framework we can divide the attributes in two types: those predefined in the data or set by the user, and those computed by the algorithms provided by the framework. For instance, when we load a labeled graph, the nodes' labels are predefined attributes, and when we compute a graph layout, the nodes' coordinates are computed attributes. It is easy to see that in both cases, we can abstract the attributes with a set of two functions that return a value for an element. In Tulip, this abstraction allows the optimization of the memory consumption. For instance, setting to zero all elements of a graph $G(V, E)$ is equivalent to building a function $F_V : V \rightarrow \{0\}$.

It also allows the inclusion of useful mechanisms such as buffered evaluation of recursive functions. To include such an improvement we have built functions called proxies which use other functions. Information about proxies can be found in the Design Pattern book written by Gamma *et al.* [15]. Such a mechanism is widely used when we manipulate combinatoric parameters on graphs.

In graph visualization, one must manipulate several attributes at the same time. For example, if one visualizes a file-system, the names, sizes and types of the files are attributes of the graph nodes. In Tulip, an attribute manager is used to manage a set of functions. It allows us to store an unbounded number of attributes and to modify dynamically the set of attributes attached to a graph. For instance, it makes it possible to store several graph drawings at the same time.

During the clustering, one wants to keep the attributes on the elements. This is equivalent to sharing the attributes between the graphs. For example, in a file-system, the file names never change even during the visualization of a sub-directory. However, one also needs to be able to locally change the attribute of a cluster. For instance, if a file-system has been drawn with a tree map algorithm [7], it can be useful to change the drawing of a sub-directory by using the Reingold and Tilford algorithm [24]. In this case, one can look at the structure of the sub-directory instead of at the file sizes. In Tulip, both cases are taken into account by using the attribute manager and the Cluster tree. The mechanism set-up is analogous to those included in object oriented languages that permit the inheritance, redefinition and dynamic change of the object structure [32]. The difference in Tulip is that we allow the inheritance of data. A complete example is presented below.

In Figure 15 we can see a set of graphs with attributes. G is a loaded graph that contains two attributes: a layout and labels. G_1 is a spanning directed acyclic graph (dag) of G. Due to the inheritance of the attributes we have directly the layout and the labels of its elements without any cloning of data. G_2 is also a spanning dag of G that has been redrawn using a dag dedicated algorithm. In this case, we redefine the layout attribute locally in G_2. Thus, labels are still inherited from G and the layout is contained in G_2. In the graph G_3, we can see that to define the set of inherited attributes, we choose those closest in the cluster tree. Therefore, the layout of G_3 is the one of G_2 and not the one of G.

Extension Mechanism. In order to include new features easily, a plug-in mechanism has been built inside Tulip. It works as follows. During the initialization of the Tulip data structure, Tulip's configuration directories are scanned to find new functions (plug-ins). Those found are added to a function factory. Now, when one asks for a graph attribute (or function) named A, if it doesn't exist (locally or inherited) the attribute manager queries the function factory for a function that has the same name. If it exists, after initialization

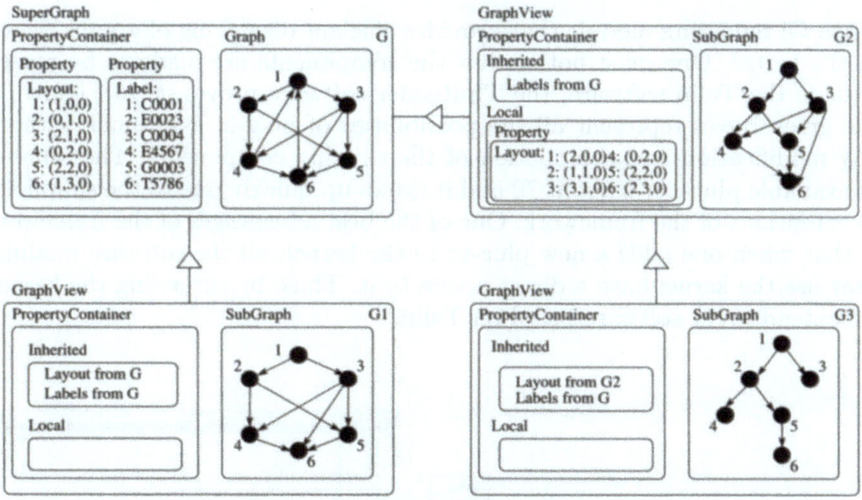

Fig. 15. Inheritance of attributes.

and calculability checks, the function (or attribute) is added to the graph. If such a function does not exist, then a data function is created. Tulip includes other plug-in mechanisms in order to support the addition of algorithms that do not return attributes. The existing ones are the import/export of graphs, the clustering of graphs, and glyphs used for the 3D representation of elements.

4.2 Tulip and TlpRender

The first implementation made with the Tulip graph visualization framework is the Tulip software. This software enables the manipulation of all the existing plug-ins and attributes available in the framework. The human-computer interface of the software is dynamically built according to the plug-ins available in the framework. Thus, it can be seen as a generic software for graphs visualization.

Another software called TlpRender enables to input a graph and then, after applying a graph drawing algorithm (available in the framework) allows to produce an html file in which image maps are used to enable interaction with the drawn graph. This software is used to make web services that use graphs.

4.3 Overview

Figure 16 presents an overview of the available components in the Tulip package. The first one is the kernel itself that accepts all the plug-ins and that manages the data structure introduced above. The second one is an

Open Gl rendering module that provides efficient displaying of graphs stored in the kernel. One must notice that the components are made to be reused outside the Tulip software, the TlpRender software proves it. In Figure 16, the green boxes represent all the possibilities of plug-in extensions without any modification and compilation of the existing components. The number of available plug-ins is about 70 and it grows up quickly due to the simplicity of extensions of the framework. One of the best advantages of the framework is that when one adds a new plug-in to the kernel, all the software modules that use the kernel have a direct access to it. Thus, by extending the kernel, we extend every software based on Tulip.

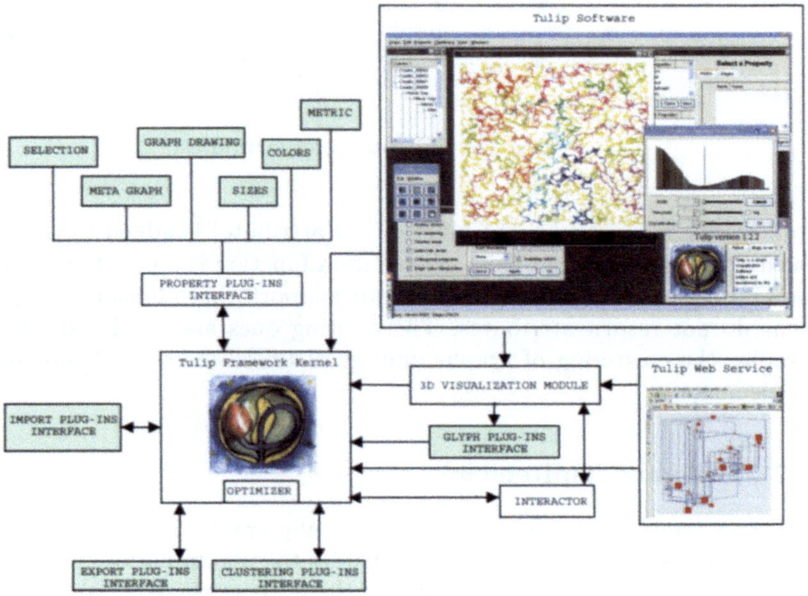

Fig. 16. Tulip Framework overview.

5 Examples

We will give here several examples obtained with the graph drawing algorithms available in the Tulip framework. Figures 17, 18, 19, 20, and 21 show different automatic drawings of a file-system with 110.000 files that can be used in order to detect problems, as for instance, duplications or hidden files. Figures 23, 24, 25, and 26 are different automatic drawings of the LaBRI's web site ($|V| = 800$, $|E| = 1400$). Figure 22 is a meta-graph that has been built by using the results of Tulip's clustering algorithm on the graph of the inclusions of the Tulip source code. The final graph is the quotient graph (automatically built) of the subgraphs obtained by the clustering algorithm. In this figure one can see that Tulip can manage Meta-Graph rendering.

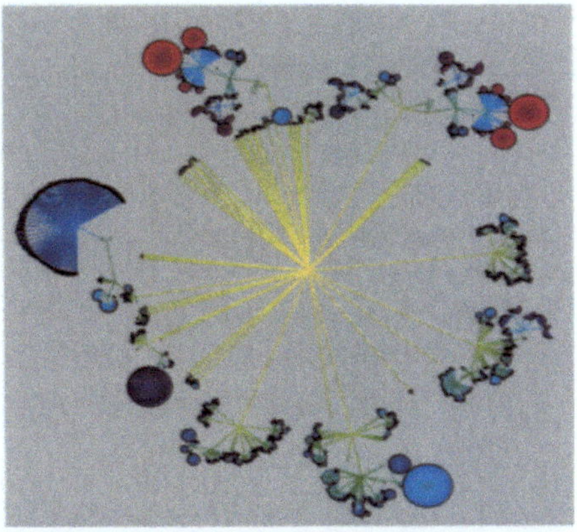

Fig. 17. Balloon drawing (< 10s).

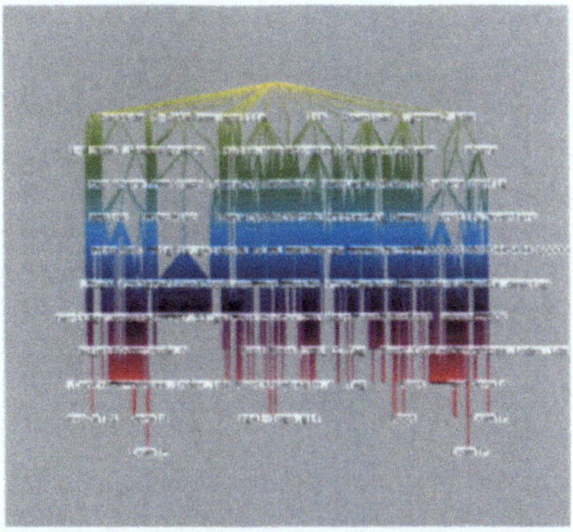

Fig. 18. Hierarchical drawing (< 1s).

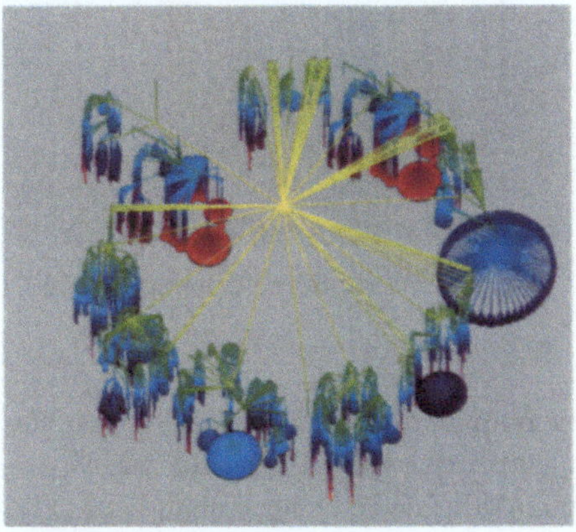

Fig. 19. Cone tree drawing (< 1s).

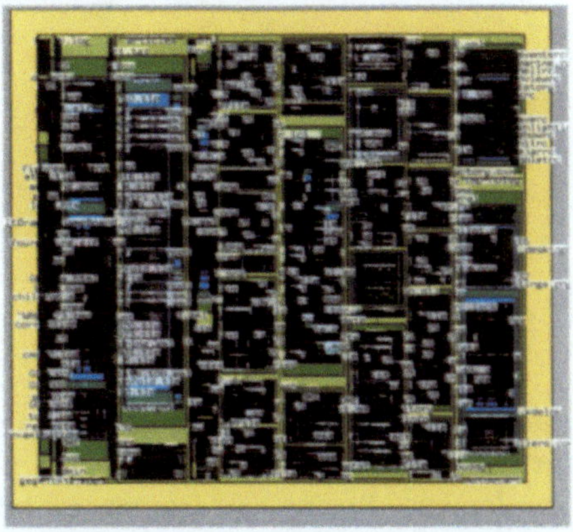

Fig. 20. Tree Map drawing (< 1s).

6 Software

The Tulip framework can be downloaded from `www.tulip-software.org`. The whole software is under the general public license (GPL), thus, it can be downloaded and used freely. One of the GPL license restrictions is that each

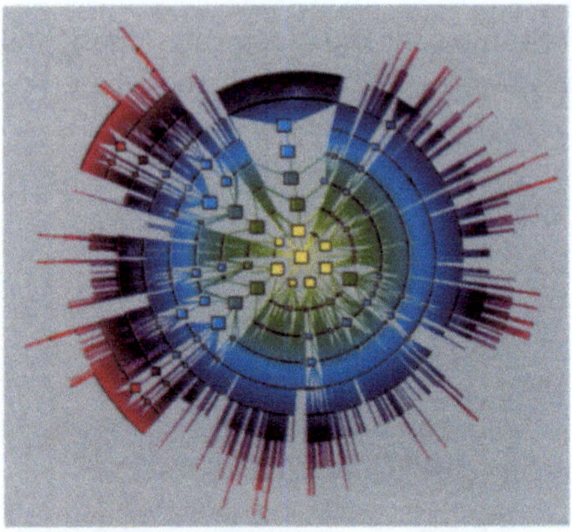

Fig. 21. Radial drawing ($< 1s$).

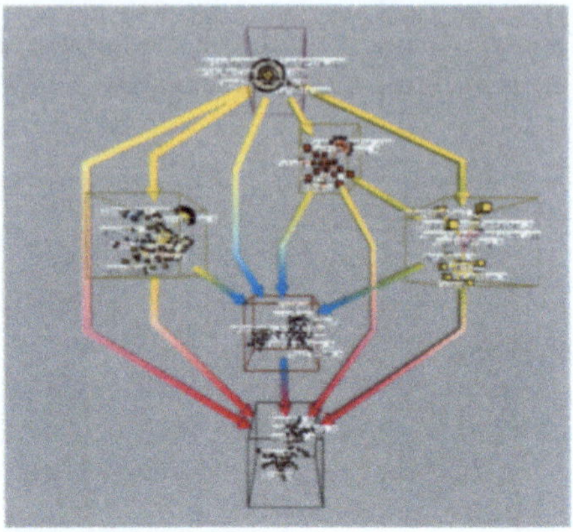

Fig. 22. Meta graph drawing ($< 1s$).

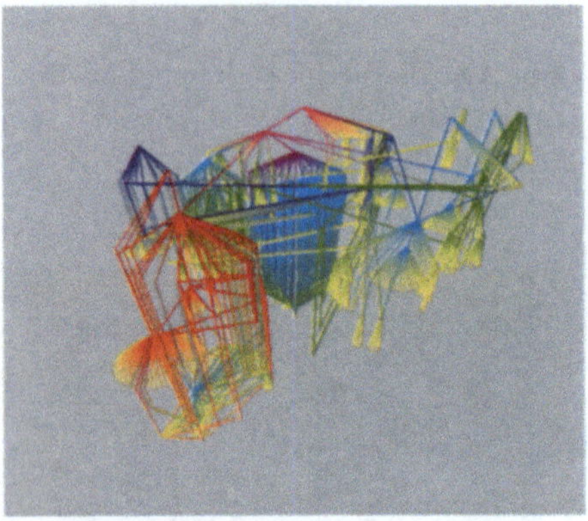

Fig. 23. 3D drawing ($< 1s$).

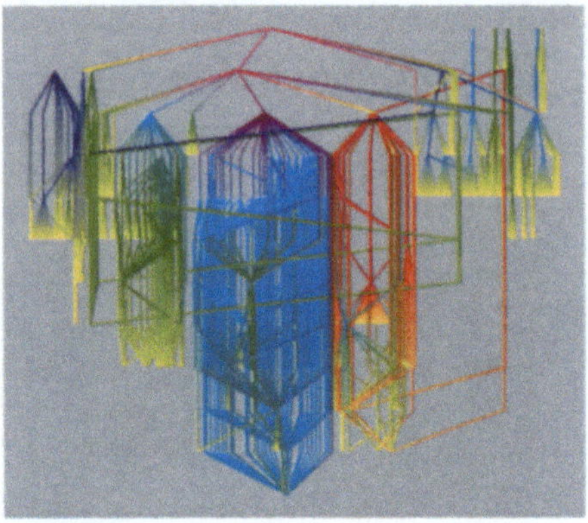

Fig. 24. Hierarchical drawing ($< 1s$).

program using the Tulip framework must respect the GPL license. Thus, the project is growing up quickly and new graph drawing algorithm which are implemented using this framework become available to other researchers. The advantage is that it enables us to compare easily graph drawing algorithms, and consequently, to study efficiently with the end-users the efficiency of each algorithm for solving a visualization task.

References

1. Auber, D. (2001) Tulip. In: S. Leipert, P. Mutzel, M. Jünger (eds.) Graph Drawing '01, Lecture Notes in Computer Science 2265, Springer-Verlag, 335–337
2. Auber, D. (2002) Outils de visualisation de larges structures de données. PhD thesis, University Bordeaux I

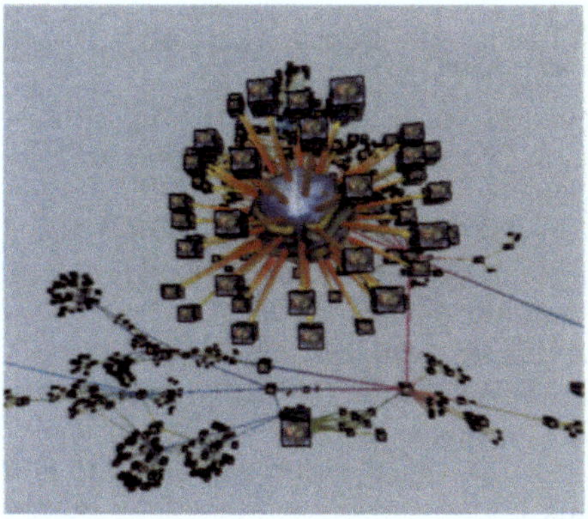

Fig. 25. Spring 3D drawing (< 90s).

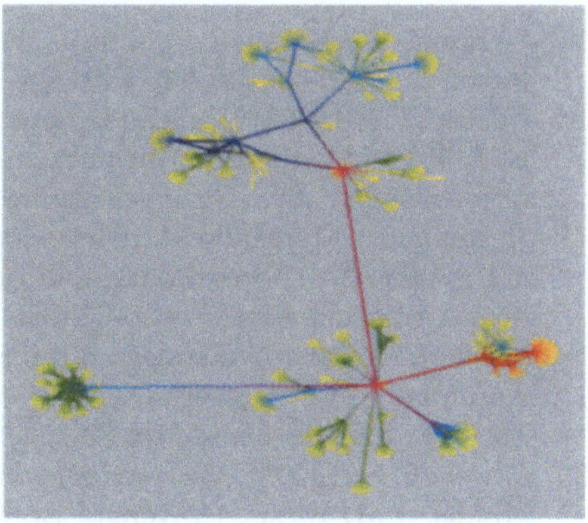

Fig. 26. GEM drawing (< 12s).

3. Auber, D. (2002) Using Strahler numbers for real time visual exploration of huge graphs. International Conference on Computer Vision and Graphics, 56–69
4. Auber, D., Delest, M. (to appear) A clustering algorithm for huge trees. Advances in Applied Mathematics
5. Bertin, J. (1977) La graphique et le traitement graphique de l'information. Flammarion
6. Le Blanc, B., Dion, D., Auber, D., Melançon, G. (2001) Constitution et visualisation de deux réseaux d'associations verbales. Colloque Agents Logiciels, Coopération, Apprentissage et Activité Humaine (ALCAA), 37–43
7. Bruls, D. M., Huizing, C., VanWijk, J. J. (2000) Squarified treemaps. In: Data Visualization 2000, Proceedings of the joint Eurographics and IEEE TCVG Symposium on Visualization, Springer-Verlag, 33–42
8. Buchheim, C., Jünger, M., Leipert, S. (2000) A fast layout algorithm for k-level graphs. In: J. Marks (ed.) Graph Drawing '00, Lecture Notes in Computer Science 1984, Springer-Verlag, 229–240
9. Carriere, J., Kazman, R. (1995) Interacting with huge hierarchies: Beyond cone trees. In: G. and S. Eick (eds.) IEEE Symposium on Information Visualization, Atlanta, Georgia Institute for Electrical and Electronics Engineers, 74–78
10. Dix, A., Finlay, J. (1998) Human-Computer Interaction. Prentice-Hall
11. Ershov, A. P. (1958) On programming of arithmetic operations. Communication of the ACM **1** (8), 3–6
12. Fairchild, K. M., Poltrock, S. E., Furnas, G. W. (1998) Semnet: Three-dimensional graphic representation of large knowledge bases. In: R. Guindon and L. Erlbaum (eds.) Cognitive Science and its Applications for Human-Computer Interaction, 201–233
13. Fédou, J. M. (1999) Nombre de Strahler sur les arbres généraux. In: GDR ALP (ed.) Ecole jeunes chercheurs en algorithmique et calcul formel
14. Frick, A. K., Mehldau, H., Ludwig, A. (1994) A fast adaptive layout algorithm for undirected graphs. In: I. G. Tollis and R. Tamassia (eds.) Graph Drawing '94, Lecture Notes in Computer Science 894, Springer-Verlag, 388–403

15. Gamma, E., Helm, R., Johnson, R., Vlissides, J., Booch, G. (1995) Design Patterns. Addison-Wesley Pub Co
16. Gärtner, B. (1999) Fast and robust smallest enclosing balls. In: Algorithms-ESA'99: 7th Annual European Symposium Proceedings, Lecture Notes in Computer Science 1643, Springer-Verlag, 325–338
17. Herman, I., Marshall, M., Melançon, G. (2000) Density functions for visual attributes and effective partitioning in graph visualization. IEEE Symposium on Information Visualization, IEEE Computer Society, 49–56
18. Hewlett-Packard. Stl standard template library. `www.sgi.com/tech/stl/`
19. Kauffman, M., Wagner, D. (2001) Drawing Graphs: Methods and Models. Lecture Notes in Computer Science 2025, Springer-Verlag
20. Marshall, S. (2001) Methods and tools for the visualization and navigation of graphs. PhD thesis, University Bordeaux I
21. Marshall, S., Herman, I., Melançon, G. (2001) An object-oriented design for graph visualization. Software - Practice and Experience **31** (8), 739–756
22. Megiddo, N. (1983) Linear-time algorithms for linear programming in R^3 and related problems. SIAM Journal on Computing **12**, 759–776
23. Paul, B. The mesa 3-d graphics library. `www.mesa3d.org`
24. Reingold, E. M., Tilford, J. S. (1981) Tidier drawings of trees. IEEE Transactions on Software Engineering **7** (2), 223–228
25. Robertson, G. G., Mackinlay, J. D., Card, S. K. (1991) Cone trees: Animated 3d visualizations of hierarchical information. SIGCHI, Conference on Human Factors in Computing Systems, ACM, 189–194
26. Shneiderman, B. (1996) The eyes have it: A task by data type taxonomy for information visualization. In: Boulder (ed.) IEEE Conference on Visual Languages, 336–343
27. Spence, R. (2001) Information Visualization. Addison-Wesley
28. Strahler, A. N. (1952) Hypsomic analysis of erosional topography. Bulletin Geological Society of America **63**, 1117-1142
29. Sugiyama, K., Tagawa, S., Toda, M. (1981) Methods for visual understanding of hierarchical system structures. IEEE Transactions on Systems, Man, and Cybernetics **SMC-11** (2), 109–125
30. Trolltech. Qt the crossplatform C++ gui framework. `www.trolltech.com`
31. Tutte, W. T. (1963) How to draw a graph. In: Proceedings of the London Mathematical Society **3** (13), 743–768
32. Ungar, D., Chambers, C., Chang, B. W., Hölzle, U. (July 1991) Organizing programs without classes. Lisp and Symbolic Computation **4** (3), 223–242
33. Viennot, G. (1990) Trees everywhere. In: A. Arnold (ed.) Colloquium on Trees in Algebra and Programming, Lecture Notes in Computer Science 431, Springer-Verlag, 18–41
34. Ware, C. (2000) Information Visualization: Perception for design. Interactive Technologies, Moragn Kaufmann
35. Welzl, E. (1991) Smallest enclosing disks (balls and ellipsoids). In: H. A. Maurer (ed.) New Results and New Trends in Computer Science, Lecture Notes in Computer Science 555, Springer-Verlag
36. Wills, G. J. (1997) NicheWorks : Interactive visualization of very large graphs. In: G. Di Battista (ed.) Graph Drawing '97, Lecture Notes in Computer Science 1353, Springer-Verlag, 403–414

Graphviz and Dynagraph – Static and Dynamic Graph Drawing Tools

John Ellson, Emden R. Gansner, Eleftherios Koutsofios, Stephen C. North, and Gordon Woodhull

AT&T Labs - Research, Florham Park NJ 07932, USA

1 Introduction

Graphviz is a collection of software for viewing and manipulating abstract graphs. It provides graph visualization for tools and web sites in domains such as software engineering, networking, databases, knowledge representation, and bioinformatics. Hundreds of thousands of copies have been distributed under an open source license.

The core of Graphviz consists of implementations of various common types of graph layout. These layouts can be used via a C library interface, stream-based command line tools, graphical user interfaces and web browsers. Aspects which distinguish the software include a retention of stream-based interfaces in conjunction with a variety of tools for graph manipulation, and support for a wide assortment of graphical features and output formats. The former makes it possible to write high-level programs for querying, modifying and displaying graphs. The latter allows Graphviz to be useful in a wide range of areas, with applications far removed from academic exercises.

The algorithms of Graphviz concentrate on static layouts. Dynagraph is a sibling of Graphviz, with algorithms and interactive programs for incremental layout. At the library level, it provides an object-oriented interface for graphs and graph algorithms.

2 Applications

Many applications employ Graphviz to produce graph layouts in order to assist their users to better understand domain information or to perform some task visually. In particular, the stream model supported by Graphviz lends itself to applications that need an external graph visualization service with a graphical or web interface. It is simple to emit graph models in the DOT language [15] and then load them into a customized version of one of the Graphviz viewers, or to generate server-side web content as clickable images, Adobe PDF or SVG meta-files.

We will briefly survey some successful application areas.

2.1 Software Engineering

The complexity of large software modules, programs and protocols is a serious impediment to understanding and changing them, and thus is a problem with great economic significance. Software visualization is one attack on this problem. The idea is to model some aspect of software as a graph, and present the graph as a drawing to make it easier to understand the model. Graphs are convenient for describing the data types, functions, variables, control structures, files and even bugs in source code programs, or the structure of finite state machines and grammars. They can be created from static analysis, dynamic traces, or other sources. Some practical systems that rely on Graphviz for software visualization are the Acacia [4], Doxygen [38], and Mono [10] static analysis systems, the Syntacs toolkit for Java compiler generation [24], the Spin concurrent protocol analyzer [21] and the Bugzilla bug tracking system [1] originally created for the Mozilla (Netscape) open source project.

Graphviz has also been applied to digital logic design, database schema design, knowledge representation, Bayesian networks and decision diagrams, to name a few other areas in related branches of engineering and technology.

2.2 Bioinformatics

Graphs arise naturally in metabolic network models, gene and protein sequences and in studies of other biological structures. Graphs are often generated from experimental data, or extracted by cross-referencing the literature. For example, PubGene [23] is a biological database application that employs Graphviz as a web visualization service. The database describes the co-citation of mouse, rat and human gene symbols in an archive of over 10 million articles from PubMed. Interactive queries allow exploring the neighborhood around a set of genes given by standard names.

The Protein Interaction Extraction System (PIES) [42] is a platform for exploring biomedical abstracts using Graphviz. With it, the user can call up research abstracts from online sources, extract relevant information from the texts and manipulate interaction pathways. The system uses Graphviz to display interactions graphically.

The Bioconductor Graph Project, based on the R statistics language, incorporates Graphviz as a rendering module, along with other graph libraries. The integration of statistical and graph models is a promising area for data mining and visualization research.

2.3 Internet and Web Structures

Many Internet and web mapping and analysis tools are based on graphs. In the area of web structure, a central effort of the World Wide Web (W3C) consortium is to define a "semantic web" in XML. One of its contributions is the RDF Resource Description Framework (RDF) dialect of XML which formally describes web site contents. RDF models naturally give rise to graphs. IsaViz and FRODO RDFSViz are translators which map aspects of RDF into Graphviz diagrams. Other examples in the realm of web and Internet engineering are Webdiff [5] (for tracking changes in web site contents), the Apache2Dot translator (for viewing links followed by clients within a web site), Gnucleus [7] (a visualizer for Gnutella peer-to-peer networks), DNS Bajaj [22] (for viewing and debugging domain name server delegation graphs) and net-map [36] (for traceroute visualization).

A common technique used in web pages for creating interactive content based on graphs is to rely on a *webdot* HTTP server. It is invoked by a URL which specifies a remote graph file to be retrieved, the Graphviz layout program to run, and the MIME type of the image to be created. For example, the line

```
<img src=/cgi-bin/webdot/tut1.dot.neato.png>
```

in a web page indicates that the graph described in `tut1.dot` should be drawn using *neato* and the output should be in PNG format. In addition to providing inline images, if a node or edge in the graph specifies a URL attribute, the corresponding image will act as a link to that URL. This type of web service followed naturally from the basic stream orientation of the Graphviz software.

Histograph is an application of Dynagraph that displays a nonlinear web click history graph for Microsoft Internet Explorer. In the conventional linear history view of most browsers, it is difficult or even impossible to understand branching URL visit structures. Histograph instead makes a map of the pages visited by the browser using nodes in a graph. As the user follows links in the browser, Histograph dynamically adjusts the map, and the user can easily jump to any previously explored page by clicking on its node in the map. Histograph is a concise C++ program that passes events between the Internet Explorer and Dynagraph components of the application.

Histograph was created with Montage, a generic OLE client-server module for integrating Dynagraph (or other applications) with Microsoft OLE-aware Windows programs. Montage supports user interface modes (collections of behaviors), event management and persistence of non-hierarchical collections of objects to enable state file saving and loading and cut-and-paste operations. Its generic features enable the creation of sophisticated applications. Beyond the Histograph demonstration, it supports general embeddable diagrams, and Visual Basic programming with graph diagrams.

2.4 Dynamic Distributed Communication Services

Distributed Feature Composition (DFC) is an architecture for specifying the structured composition of modular communication service features. DFC appears to solve many of the difficulties that have been encountered in specifying telecommunication services. Of principal concern here, it models the invocation and interaction of communication services as an evolving graph of feature boxes. Building Box [2] is a platform for applying DFC to Internet Protocol services. An extension of Graphviz was created to monitor and validate service protocols and feature setups in real time. In particular, DFC models are naturally represented as a set of boundary nodes surrounding a cloud of internal feature nodes, and drawn using a modified spring embedder.

3 Algorithms

The algorithms forming the fabric of the Graphviz software range from standard graph and graph drawing algorithms, implemented for robustness and flexibility, to novel variations of standard algorithms or standard algorithms used in novel ways. It seems most natural to describe these techniques in the context of the graph drawing model where each is used, saving those serving multiple models to the end.

3.1 Static Layered Drawings

For layered drawings, Graphviz relies on an implementation of the Sugiyama-style approach as described in Section 4.2 of the Technical Foundations. As with all Graphviz drawing tools, the design goal is to make æsthetically pleasing drawings of modest-sized graphs approaching the quality of handmade diagrams. We concentrate here on the aspects where the Graphviz implementation differs significantly from the description in the Technical Foundations Chapter.

Ranking. The first major pass in creating a Sugiyama-type layout is to place nodes on discrete ranks, honoring the direction of the edges. There are many ways of doing this, depending on which aspects of the ranking are deemed most important. Graphviz models node ranking as the following linear integer program:

$$\text{minimize} \sum_{(u,v)\in E} \omega(u,v)(y_u - y_v) \tag{1}$$

$$\text{subject to } y_u - y_v \geq \delta(u,v) \text{ for all } (u,v) \in E \tag{2}$$

where y_u denotes the rank of node u and hence is a nonnegative integer, and $\delta(u,v)$ is the minimum length of the edge. By default, δ is taken as 1, but the general case supports flat edges, when the nodes are placed on the same rank ($\delta = 0$), or the times when it is important to enforce a greater separation

($\delta > 1$). The weight factor $\omega(u, v)$ allows one to specify the importance of having the rank separation of two nodes be as close to minimum as possible.

Using this criterion for placing nodes on ranks has the effect of reducing the total length of all the edges where, in this context, the length of an edge is the difference in ranks of its endpoints. This is important from an æsthetic and cognitive sense, since it is generally agreed that having short edges in the drawing of a graph is important. This approach also has the practical effect of reducing the number of artificial nodes introduced for the remainder of the layout. As the time to finish the later phases is strongly influenced by the number of nodes, real and artificial, anything that reduces the number of artificial nodes needed can have a beneficial effect on performance. On the other hand, for shallow but wide hierarchies, minimizing the total edge length, or the number of ranks, can lead to a layout with a very poor aspect ratio. This can be overcome by the use of additional constraints, such as adding invisible edges between nodes which would normally be placed on the same rank.

Despite the proposed advantages of using the integer program (1)–(2) to determine ranks, if one could not solve it efficiently, it would not be worthwhile. Fortunately, the problem allows many polynomial-time solutions. Since its corresponding constraint matrix is totally unimodular, a rational solution obtained from a network flow formulation or the basic linear program is equivalent to the desired integer solution.

Here, we describe the network simplex algorithm used in Graphviz. We expand the notion of ranking to be any assignment of y coordinates to the nodes. A *feasible* ranking is one satisfying the length constraints (2). Given any ranking, not necessarily feasible, the *slack* of an edge is the difference of its length and its minimum length. Thus, a ranking is feasible if the slack of every edge is nonnegative. An edge is *tight* if its slack is zero.

A spanning tree of a graph induces a ranking, or rather, a family of equivalent rankings. (Note that the spanning tree is on the underlying unrooted undirected graph, and is not necessarily a directed tree.) This ranking is generated by picking an initial node and assigning it a rank. Then, for each node adjacent in the spanning tree to a ranked node, assign it the rank of the adjacent node, incremented or decremented by the minimum length of the connecting edge, depending on whether it is the head or tail of the connecting edge. This process is continued until all nodes are ranked. A spanning tree is *feasible* if it induces a feasible ranking. By construction, all edges in a feasible tree are tight.

Given a feasible spanning tree, we can associate an integer *cut value* with each tree edge as follows. If the tree edge is deleted, the tree breaks into two connected components, the tail component containing the tail node of the edge, and the head component containing the head node. The cut value is defined as the sum of the weights of all edges from the tail component to the head component, including the tree edge, minus the sum of the weights of all edges from the head component to the tail component.

Typically (but not always, because of degeneracy) a negative cut value indicates that the weighted edge length sum could be reduced by lengthening the tree edge as much as possible, until one of the head component-to-tail component edges becomes tight. This corresponds to replacing the tree edge in the spanning tree with the newly tight edge, obtaining a new feasible spanning tree. An example of this interchange is given in Figure 1. The graph has 8 nodes and 9 edges, the minimum edge length is 1, and non-tree edges are dotted. The numbers attached to tree edges are the cut values of the edge. In (a), the tree edge (g, h) has cut value -1. In (b), it is removed from the tree and replaced by edge (a, e), strictly decreasing the total edge length.

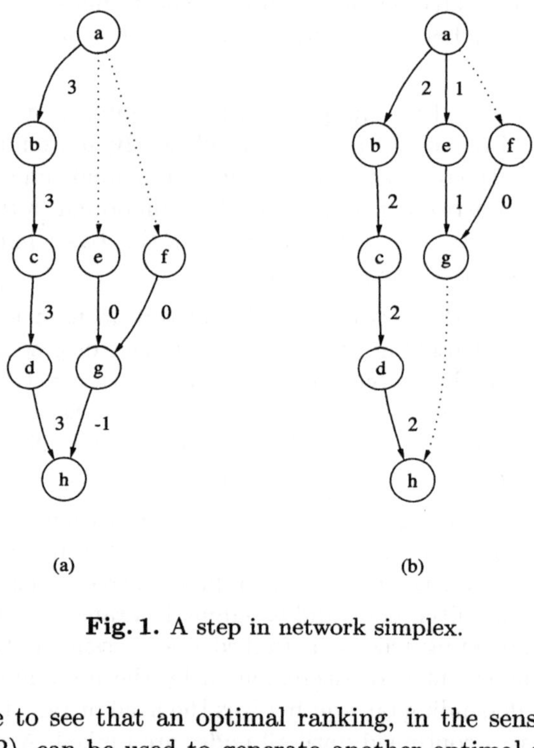

Fig. 1. A step in network simplex.

It is simple to see that an optimal ranking, in the sense of the integer program (1)–(2), can be used to generate another optimal ranking induced by a feasible spanning tree. These observations are the key to solving the ranking problem in a graphical rather than algebraic context, as described in Algorithm 1. Tree edges with negative cut values are replaced by appropriate non-tree edges, until all tree edges have nonnegative cut values. The resulting spanning tree corresponds to an optimal ranking.

For further discussion of the termination of the network simplex algorithm and optimality of the result, as well as implementation tricks, the

Algorithm 1: Network simplex

Input : Directed acyclic graph $G = (V, E)$
Output: Optimal ranking of V
Create initial feasible spanning tree T
while *edge* $e \in T$ *has negative cut value* **do**
    Pick edge $f \in E \setminus T$ with minimum slack
    Set $T = T \cup \{f\} \setminus \{e\}$
end

interested reader is referred to the literature, e.g., Cook *et al.* [9], Chvátal [6] or Gansner *et al.* [16].

Coordinate Assignment. As noted in Section 4.2 of the Technical Foundations, the assignment of y coordinates for top-down drawings is basically trivial. On the other hand, picking good x coordinates in order to minimize edge bends and obtain a compact, neat layout takes some work. We attempted to use heuristics similar to those used for crossing reduction, but the heuristics became increasingly complex and started to interfere with each other. It was then recognized that we could again model node placement as a nonlinear integer program:

$$\text{minimize} \sum_{(u,v)\in E} \Omega(u,v)\,\omega(u,v)\,|x_u - x_v| \tag{3}$$

$$\text{subject to } x_a - x_b \geq \rho(a,b) \text{ for all } a \text{ and } b \text{ where } a \text{ is the left neighbor of } b \text{ on the same rank.}$$

In this program, $\rho(a, b)$ gives the minimum horizontal separation of a and b, which is usually taken as the sum of half their respective widths, plus some constant internode spacing. Ω is an additional weight function favoring the straightening of long edges. Specifically, Ω is greatest where both vertices are artificial, less when only one vertex is, and least when both vertices are real.

A standard transformation in linear programming introduces additional variables to remove the absolute value. Graphically, this corresponds to creating a new graph G' as illustrated in Figure 2. (For this presentation, we are ignoring flat edges in G.) The new graph has the same vertex set as G plus a new vertex n_e for each edge. There are two kinds of edges in G'. The first class is defined by creating two edges $e_u = (n_e, u)$ and $e_v = (n_e, v)$ for every edge $e = (u, v)$ in G. These edges have $\delta = 0$ and $\omega = \omega(e)\Omega(e)$, and thereby encode the cost of the original edge. The other type of edges separates adjacent nodes on the same rank. If v is immediately to the left of w

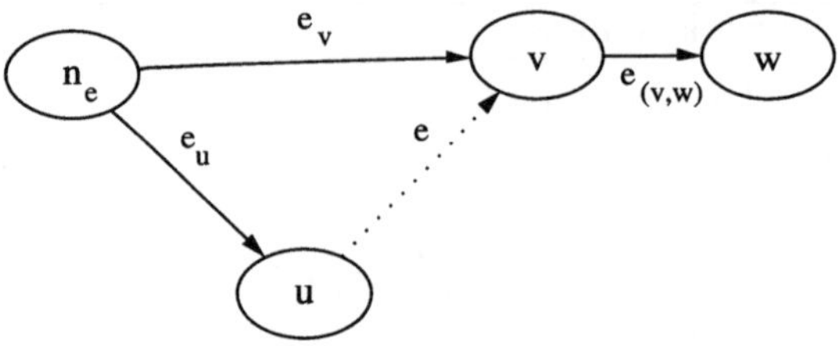

Fig. 2. Constructing G'.

on its rank, we add an edge $f = e_{(v,w)}$ to G' with $\delta(f) = \rho(v,w)$ and $\omega = 0$. Note that this edge will not effect the cost of the layout.

With this construction, solving the original optimization problem becomes equivalent to finding an optimal ranking in the derived graph G', and we can just reuse the network simplex algorithm.

This formulation has an additional advantage. By appropriately setting the minimum edge lengths, rather than using the default of 0, the derived graph can encode horizontal shifts in edge endpoints to allow node ports. This enables the drawing of arrows between fields in records, as shown in Figure 3.

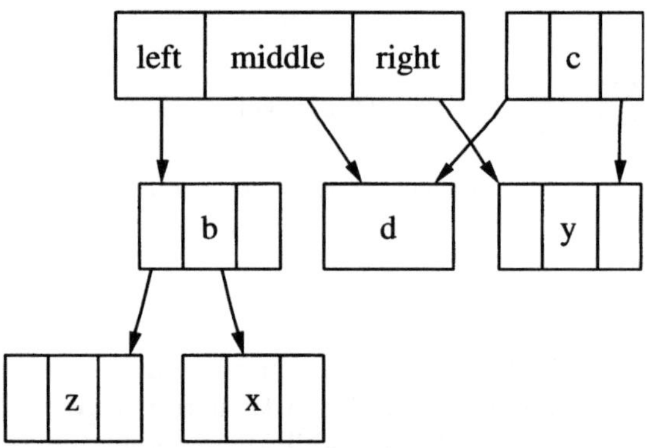

Fig. 3. Records, fields and node ports.

If $e = (u, v)$ is an edge, let Δ_u and Δ_v be the desired horizontal displacements for the edge endpoints from the centers of u and v, respectively. A negative Δ corresponds to the port occurring to the left of the vertex center. We can then modify the optimization problem (3), making the cost of an edge $\Omega(e)\omega(e)|x_u - x_v + d_e|$, where $d_e = |\Delta_v - \Delta_u|$, and with $\delta(e_u) = d_e$ and $\delta(e_u) = 0$, assuming without loss of generality that $\Delta_v \geq \Delta_u$. By applying the construction for G' and using network simplex, we end up with desired horizontal coordinates and port displacements.

Edge Drawing. As a final step, chains of artificial nodes are used to guide the construction of splines, which then replace them. Although we use some special techniques for layered graph, in particular to handle parallel and flat edges, the essence of the approach used in Graphviz will be described below in Section 3.4 concerning the spline path planner.

3.2 Virtual Physical Layouts

For so-called symmetric layouts,[1] Graphviz provides two algorithms using virtual physical models. One is an implementation of the Kamada-Kawai spring layout algorithm [25]. This is a variation on the multidimensional scaling algorithm devised in the statistics community in the 1950's and 1960's [34,35,37], and was first proposed as a graph layout algorithm by Kruskal and Seery [27] in 1978. In addition to the standard model using path lengths in the graph for the difference matrix, our implementation also provides a circuit model based on Kirchoff's laws suggested by Cohen [8]. This encodes the number of paths between two nodes in the distance calculation, and has the effect of making clusters tighter.

A second symmetric layout is provided which implements several of the spring-based force models described in Section 4.5 of the Technical Foundations. For large graphs, it relies on dynamic bins, an extension of the technique proposed by Fruchterman and Reingold [14] and recently adopted by Walshaw [40], to approximate long distance repulsive forces, thereby reducing the running time to roughly linear. In addition, it supports hierarchical clustered graphs using recursion.

Removing Node Overlaps. Virtual physical layout solvers usually assume that nodes are drawn as points and edges as straight lines[2] Problems arise if nodes are drawn as shapes having area, because they often overlap other nodes and edges. If the graph is large or the intention is to just see the "shape" of the graph, such node overlaps are unimportant. For small to medium graphs, however, the user typically does not want nodes occluding each other.

Graphviz has three optional strategies for removing node overlaps. One eliminates them by uniformly scaling up distances between node centers while retaining node sizes [30]. This preserves overall relationships between nodes, but can waste considerable area. A second approach is the force scan method [31] of Misue *et al.* Here, the layout is searched using horizontal and vertical scan passes, and rigid translations of subsets of nodes are performed

[1] In the vernacular, not mathematical, sense.

[2] Incorporating node size into the model without introducing new problems such as overconstraining the layout is a subtle problem (cf. [19]). We have implemented some of the algorithms in the literature which include node sizes as part of the model, and have found that there are situations where overlaps can still occur.

in the scan direction to remove overlaps. This preserves orthogonal ordering while usually, but not always, requiring less space than scaling.

The third technique (Algorithm 2) is a more sophisticated iterative heuristic using Voronoi diagrams, based on work by Lyons *et al.* [29]. The rationale

Algorithm 2: Voronoi adjustment

Input : Layout of vertex set V
Output: New layout of V such that $v \cap u = \emptyset\ \forall v, u \in V$
Construct bounding rectangle containing all nodes
Let C be the number of intersecting pairs of vertices
while $C > 0$ **do**
  Construct Voronoi diagram using vertex centers as sites
  Clip unbounded cells to bounding rectangle
  Move each vertex to the centroid of its cell
  Let C' be the new number of intersections
  if $C' \geq C$ **then**
    Expand bounding rectangle
  end
  Let $C = C'$
end

behind this technique is that if a node is moved in its Voronoi cell, it is still closer to its previous position than any other node, helping to roughly maintain the layout's shape. This method requires the least amount of extra space, but is much more destructive of the shape of the graph and the relative positions of the nodes.

In the implementation, node overlap is computed at the polygon level using a simplified version of the linear algorithm described in O'Rourke [33], preceded by a quick bounding box check. Non-polygonal nodes are approximated by polygons, typically using around 20 sides. In addition, the polygons are scaled up slightly to guarantee that on termination, there will be a clear positive distance between nodes. We use Fortune's $O(n \log n)$ sweepline algorithm [12] to compute Voronoi diagrams on n sites.

Several characteristics of this heuristic deserve further investigation.

- Counterintuitively, it runs faster while producing comparable layouts when all the nodes are moved on every iteration, instead of only moving overlapping nodes.
- It ignores edges. Better layouts could probably be made by incorporating edge information, for example, as part of the original layout.
- Unnecessary distortion of the graph's original shape occurs because the procedure expands the graph to fill the bounding rectangle. It would be interesting to try different bounding polygons, such as convex hulls or star-shaped outlines.

Once node overlaps are removed, the user has the option of avoiding node-edge overlaps by invoking a spline path planner module, as described in Section 3.4; edge-edge intersections are not considered.

3.3 Radial Layout

Graphviz also provides an implementation (Algorithm 3) of a radial layout based on an algorithm of Eades [11] previously adapted by Wills [41]. Given a

---

Algorithm 3: Radial layout

Input : Graph G, vertex $c \in V$, $S > 0$
Output: Radial layout of G with c in the center
Construct rooted spanning tree T with c as root
foreach $v \in V$ **do**
  Let $size_v$ be the number of leaves in subtree of T rooted at v
  Let $parent_v$ be the parent of v in T
  Let $dist_v$ be the path distance of v from c
end
$angle_c = 2\pi$
foreach $v \in V$ **do**
  $p = parent_v$
  $angle_v = (angle_p \cdot size_v)/size_p$
end
$\theta_c = 0$
foreach $v \in V$ **do**
  if $v == c$ **then**
    $\Theta = 0$
  else
    $\Theta = \theta_v - angle_v/2$
  end
  foreach *child* w *of* $v \in T$ **do**
    $\theta_w = \Theta + angle_w/2$
    $\Theta = \Theta + angle_w$
  end
end
foreach $v \in V$ **do**
  $H = S \cdot dist_v$
  $x_v = H\cos(\theta_v)$
  $y_v = H\sin(\theta_v)$
end

---

center node c, the spanning tree is constructed such that, for each node v, the path from v to c in the tree is a shortest path in G. This algorithm is extremely fast, and works well with large graphs, typically representing nodes as points and encoding additional attributes by color. A drawback of this layout is that the effectiveness of the diagram is very dependent on the choice of the center node. If the user does not supply a center, the implementation picks a "most central" node, i.e., one whose shortest distance to a leaf node is maximal. If there are no leaf nodes, a node is picked at random. This procedure is not unreasonable, since these types of radial layouts, especially if the graph is large, are only effective if the input graph is tree-like with low edge density.

3.4 Utility Algorithms

Graphviz implements several general-purpose geometric algorithms to handle tasks which arise in almost all layouts. We discuss two of these here.

Spline Path Planner. Both for reasons of æsthetics and clarity, Graphviz gives the user the ability to draw edges as smooth curves. To accomplish this, we have implemented a general-purpose spline path planner, which will construct a spline curve between two points while avoiding nodes.

The spline path planner is a two-phase heuristic, as given in Algorithm 4. The procedure starts with the desired endpoints of the edge, typically clipped to the boundary of the node shapes, and a polygonal region to which the spline is constrained. The polygon need not be simply connected. The polygon will usually contain at least the nodes of the graph, but may be modified further to additionally constrain the path. The first phase determines a shortest path connecting the two endpoints in the visibility graph of the vertices of the polygon. With a running time of $O(n^3)$ for the visibility graph computation, where n is the number of polygon vertices, this is only practical on modest-sized graphs.

Algorithm 4: Path planning heuristic

Input : Polygonal region P, points s and t in P
Output: B-spline C connecting s and t with C inside P
Construct visibility graph VG induced by s, t and the vertices in P
Find a shortest path L connecting s and t in VG
Construct Bézier curve C connecting s and t and fitting L
if $C \cap ext(P) \neq \emptyset$ **then**
  Adjust initial and terminal tangents
  if $C \cap ext(P) \neq \emptyset$ **then**
    Pick v on L furthest from C
    Replace L by the two paths $[s, v]$ and $[v, t]$ and recurse
  end
end

The second phase takes this piecewise-linear shortest path L connecting the two given endpoints and fits a candidate curve C to the path using the algorithm of Schneider [18]. If the resulting curve remains on or within P, we are done. If not, we perform small adjustments to the tangents at the endpoints, bowing or flattening the curve, and stop if any of these variants work. If none do, we continue by recursion. This is done by picking a point v on L furthest from C, dividing the path at this point into two paths L_1 and L_2, and solving the each path separately. We maintain tangent information at v in order to combine the two solutions into a single B-spline that is C^1-continuous.

Note this technique offers no guarantee that the resulting spline topologically matches the original path, or that any of the path points except the endpoints are included. Our rationale is that the topological equivalence condition is difficult to check and is not usually a problem in practice, and forcing intersection with the path points often causes unwanted inflections in the curve.

In certain situations, the time for the first phase can be significantly improved. If we can guarantee that the polygon is simply connected, we can construct a shortest path using the "funnel" algorithm of Hershberger and Snoeyink [20] in time $O(n \log n)$. This is usually the case in hierarchical layouts, where it is easy to specify the polygonal region as the union of a set of contiguous, isotropic rectangles.

The spline router fits only one edge at a time; unwanted edge-edge intersections or tangencies can arise in routing multiple edges serially, whether between the same or different endpoints. To obtain effective global routing, the calling code needs to tailor the set of obstacles for each edge. Even when this is done, the splines created will typically be affected by the order in which they are created. One reasonable convention is to construct the shorter edges first.

Packing Disconnected Graphs. Most graph layout algorithms assume that the graph is connected. Given a disconnected graph, one can either apply the basic algorithm to each connected component and then arrange the components, or make the graph connected. The first approach is used by the Graphviz hierarchical layout. It aligns the highest rank of each component on a single line, as long as no additional rank constraints have been specified. By default, our implementation of Kamada-Kawai takes the second approach, setting the desired distance between every pair of nodes in separate components to $L/(|E| + \sqrt{|V|} + 1)$, where L is the sum of the lengths of all edges. This is large enough to guarantee that disjoint components do not overlap. Neither of these particular solutions is ideal, the former producing poor aspect ratios when there are many components, while the latter, though producing an attractive layout of central large galaxies surrounded by a ring of smaller systems, wastes a great deal of space.

To avoid these situations as well as to provide a general-purpose technique for combining disconnected graphs, Graphviz has a graph packing library based on the polyomino packing algorithm [13] of Freivalds *et al.* There is an additional benefit of using this approach with Kamada-Kawai, as its basic algorithm has $O(|V|^2)$ complexity. If the graph is of medium size, say around 1000 vertices, but with many small components, applying it to each component and then packing the layouts together can improve the layout time by several orders of magnitude.

3.5 Dynamic *k*-Layered Drawing

While batch layout suffices in many applications, there are others when graphs are intrinsically dynamic and layouts need to be changed incrementally. For example, in an interactive graph editor, users edit graphs with an expectation of layout stability, or perhaps manually adjust the placement of some graph objects while others are being managed automatically. This becomes critical in the context of browsing huge graphs, where the user will need to view adjustable subgraphs or abstractions of a graph through a series of incrementally generated views.

It is possible that, when a small change is made to a graph, a static layout could be replaced, perhaps with the aid of some animation, by a new layout, provided the algorithm is stable under small changes. Typically, though, static algorithms are designed to perform global optimizations, and small changes in the graph can produce dramatic changes in the layout. The central problem, then, is how to make dynamic graph layouts which present readable, æsthetically-pleasing layouts, at each stage close to what one would obtain from a static algorithm, while highlighting changes and preserving a human's sense of context.

Dynagraph serves as the incremental version of Graphviz. The algorithms maintain a model graph with layout information, and accept a sequence of insert, modify or delete subgraph requests, with the subgraphs specifying the nodes and edges involved. The algorithms then adjust the model graph to reflect the layout changes, and generate a sequence of corresponding change messages by which the application can alter its version of the graph.

To give a flavor of the algorithms in Dynagraph, we focus on its incremental version [32] of a Sugiyama-type layout. This is a good example, since the standard static layout consists of 3 phases, with each phase performing a global optimization and with the output of one phase highly dependent on its input from the previous phase. After preprocessing the change sequence, handling requests which can be folded or canceled, the incremental layout still relies on the 3 standard passes.

It first handles ranks, reassigning levels to the nodes to maintain the hierarchy, preserve stability, and minimize total edge length, prioritized in that order. It employs the same network simplex algorithm used in the static case (Section 3.1), but with additional constraints to enforce stability. The added variables and constraints penalize level assignments by their variance from some given assignment, usually the previous layout. Adjusting the penalty edge weights changes the tradeoff between minimizing edge length and maintaining geometric stability. Note also that there is no attempt to check for cycles in an earlier pass; when an edge causing a cycle is encountered during ranking, the edge will be reversed.

After all nodes have been assigned a new rank, the algorithm updates the configuration, converting long edges into chains of nodes as usual. It first moves the pre-existing nodes or node chains to match the new ranks just assigned. Then it moves edges by moving the chains to the new ranks, lengthening or clipping them as necessary.

At this point, the model graph has incorporated all of the requested changes. However, as might be expected, the edges in the layout probably have more crossings and bends than necessary. The next step is to reduce edge crossings. To do this, the algorithm identifies the neighborhoods of nodes and edges where insertion or modification have taken place, and applies a variant of the static crossing reduction heuristic to them. Aping the static case, the heuristic relies on multiple passes up and down the neighborhood, applying the median heuristic (Section 4.2 of the Technical Foundations) and local transpositions.

As in the static algorithm, the final pass involves computing the horizontal coordinates of the nodes. It again follows the static algorithm used in Graphviz, encoding the coordinates in an integer program which is solved using network simplex. As with ranking, the static constraints are extended and the objective function is modified to penalize changes from the current configuration.

Once all nodes are repositioned, the algorithm recomputes edge routes as necessary. Of course, new edges must always be routed, and existing edges are rerouted if an endpoint has moved, or the edge passes too near another node or edge. Edges are routed and drawn using the Graphviz path planner (Section 3.4).

4 Implementation

The design and implementation of Graphviz reflect the age of the software, with much of the core written in the early 1990's. Most of Graphviz is written in C, as it predates stable, efficient or portable implementations of C++ and Java[3]. The supporting libraries consist of some 45,000 lines of code, but two-thirds of that comes from our use of the GD graphics library [3]. The hierarchical layout requires about 6,000 lines; Kamada-Kawai, 3700; spring embedder for compound graphs, 2500; and radial layout, 400. The lefty graphical editor [26] is written in about 16,000 lines, with an additional 3000 lines of lefty script to tailor it for displaying and editing graphs.

[3] If the choice had to be made now, the same decision might be made for the same reasons.

The Graphviz design incorporates an interface level amenable to stream-processing filters for use with scripting languages. Though a library API as well as interactive GUI interfaces are necessary and provided, we believe a well-designed scripting interface can greatly magnify the usefulness of software. A consideration of the many applications in which Graphviz tools have been used (cf. Section 2, Section 5 and [17]), and the simplicity of creating them, bear this out. Here, we mention a simple example. The hierarchical layout program draws disconnected graphs by placing the top rank of each component on the same rank. If there are a great many components, this produces a very wide but very shallow drawing. If this is unacceptable, a simple solution is to stream the graph into a tool that decomposes the graph into a stream of connected components, which in turn is fed into the layout program. This will layout each component, generating a stream of positioned graphs. This stream can then be fed into a packing filter, which combines each of the individual layouts into single layout with a much better aspect ratio. Finally, this graph can be piped into a tool which renders the drawing in the desired output format.

Another aspect that distinguishes the Graphviz software is its emphasis on providing the user with a rich collection of graphical primitives and output formats. Implementing various layout styles in order to view a graph's abstract features and topology is not enough. Graphviz was engineered to produce concrete pictures, in which the user has a wide choice in how semantic information and contextual attributes can be encoded. There are 24 basic node shapes, with most shapes having additional attributes for further customization. Nodes can also be drawn as records (see Figure 3), basically rectangular arrays of text useful for representing data structures, or from user-supplied bitmaps or PostScript code. The user can chose from about 20 different arrowhead shapes, a variety of line styles for edges, most standard font formats such a Truetype and PostScript fonts, and the standard RGB and HSV color models. Graphviz also supports about two dozen output formats.

4.1 Architecture

Graphviz has a conventional layered architecture. At the center are a collection of libraries. The *libgraph* library provides the fundamental graph model, implementing graphs, nodes, edges and subgraphs, along with their related attributes and functions for file I/O. In turn, this library is built on Vo's *libcdt* [39] for the underlying set operations implemented as splay trees. Auxiliary libraries include the spline path planning library (Section 3.4); a version *libgd* of the GD library, which allows Graphviz to provide bitmap output in many standard formats as well use of the Freetype font engine; and a library for splitting graphs into connected components, and later combining the drawings of components into a single drawing.

At the next level, we have a core graph drawing library. This encapsulates the common parts of all layout algorithms, reading graph input, setting up the common data structures and attributes and, at the end, providing the drivers for the two dozen or so output formats supported by Graphviz. Parallel with the core drawing library are the libraries coding each of the layout algorithms.

The next layer consists of the stand-alone programs. With the given libraries, these are basically just a main routine, which processes the command line flags and arguments, and then calls the appropriate library routines to read, layout and render a graph.

The top layer of interactive graph viewers and editors are built, in the main, from generic language and graphical interfaces [26,28], using the Graphviz layout programs as co-processes.

Dynagraph forms a parallel collection of layers for iterative graph layout algorithms. Most of Dynagraph is written in C++, and makes extensive use of C++ templates for code reuse. At the lowest level, Dynagraph creates a C++ API for *libgraph.* Higher layers define algorithms which produce standard layouts such as hierarchical and symmetric drawings, but rely on incremental techniques so that small changes to a graph produce small changes to the drawing. For Dynagraph, software to render graphs in a variety of concrete formats is unimportant. Rather, Dynagraph defines a graph editing protocol [32], which can be used by an application to feed incremental graph changes to the Dynagraph layout engines and, in return, receive descriptions of the incremental changes required in the drawing.

5 Examples

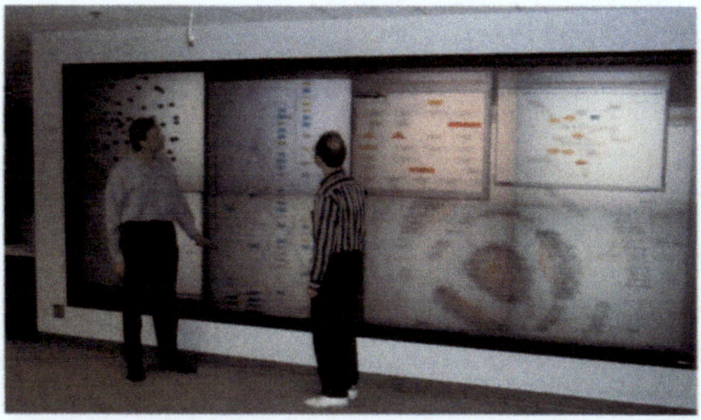

Fig. 4. Information visualization with graph drawings on a 10 megapixel display wall. The displays include maps of virtual private networks, a section of the public Internet, and software engineering diagrams. The visualizations are an important complement to conventional text and statistical displays for exploring large, semistructured information sets.

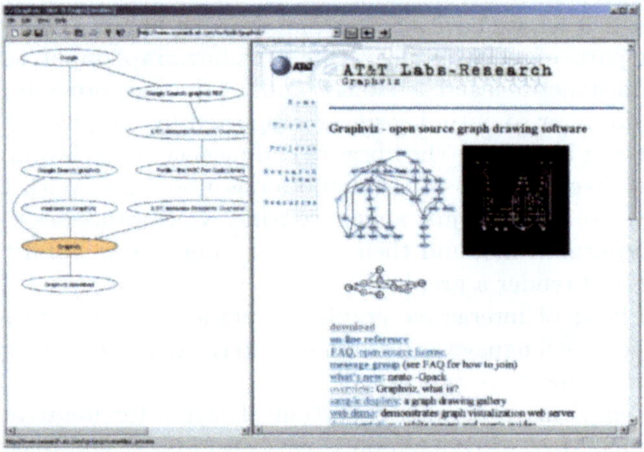

Fig. 5. Sample Histograph session. The right pane is a web browser; the left pane is a clickable history of the pages visited which is extended incrementally. The application illustrates integration of dynamic graph layout with other interactive tools.

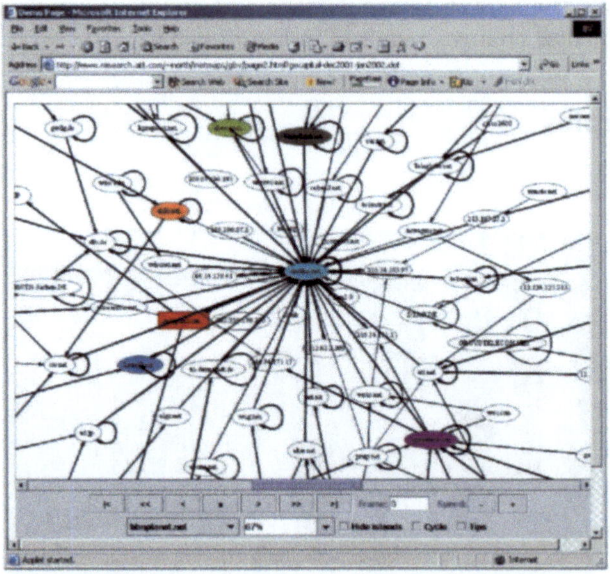

Fig. 6. Internet traceroute map viewer (courtesy of David Dobkin and John Mocenigo). The viewer plays an animation of routes from about 100 traceroute servers worldwide to a predefined list of target hosts. The routes are collected daily. The user interface is based on Grappa, the Java client from Graphviz, with added controls for animation playback and graph search.

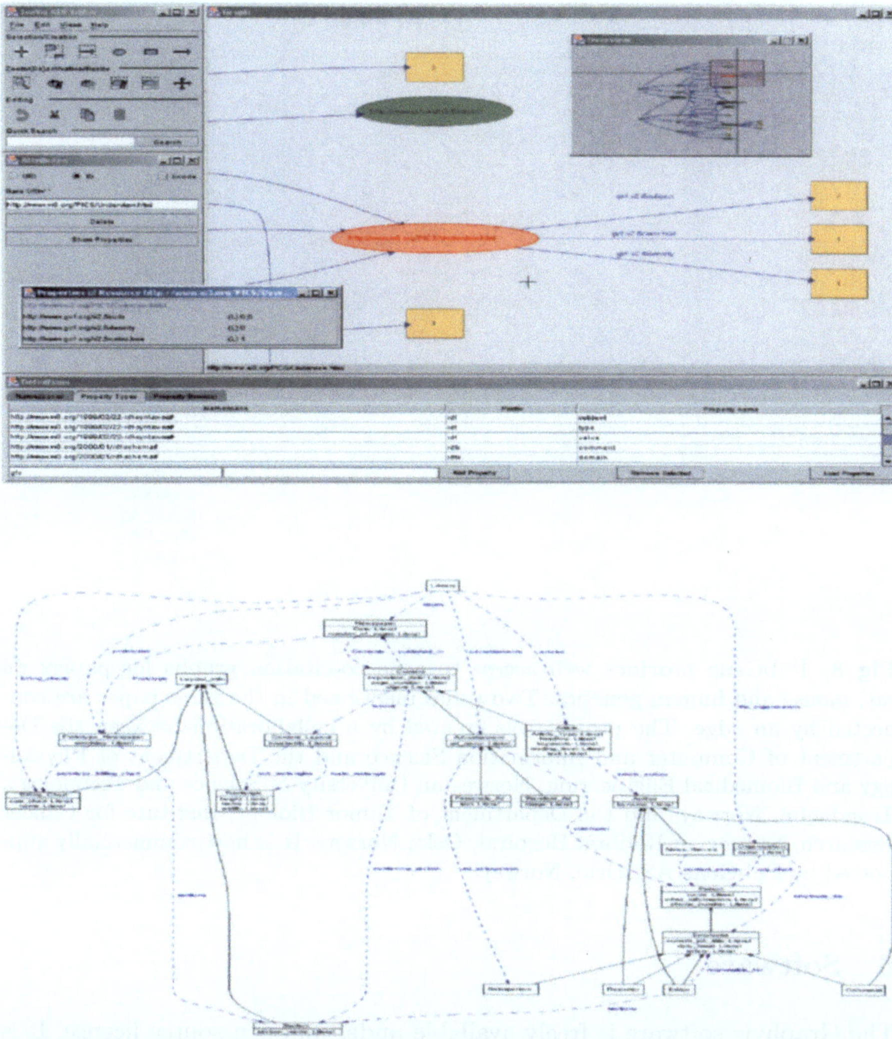

Fig. 7. Views from the IsaViz and RDFSViz RDF visualization tools (courtesy Emmanual Pietriga, W3C, and Michael Sintek, FRODO project at DFKI Kaiserslautern, respectively). IsaViz **(a)** is an RDF browsing and authoring tool which includes a 2.5D viewer based on the Xerox Visual Transformation Machine and is built on the Jena Semantic Web Toolkit from HP Labs and the Xerces XML parser from the Apache XML project. RDFSViz **(b)** is a schema ontology visualization tool built on the Java RDF API from Sergey Melnik at Stanford University and Xerces. It has become part of a related tool, OntoViz, from the Stanford Medical Informatics project Protege 2000, with more than 5000 registered users.

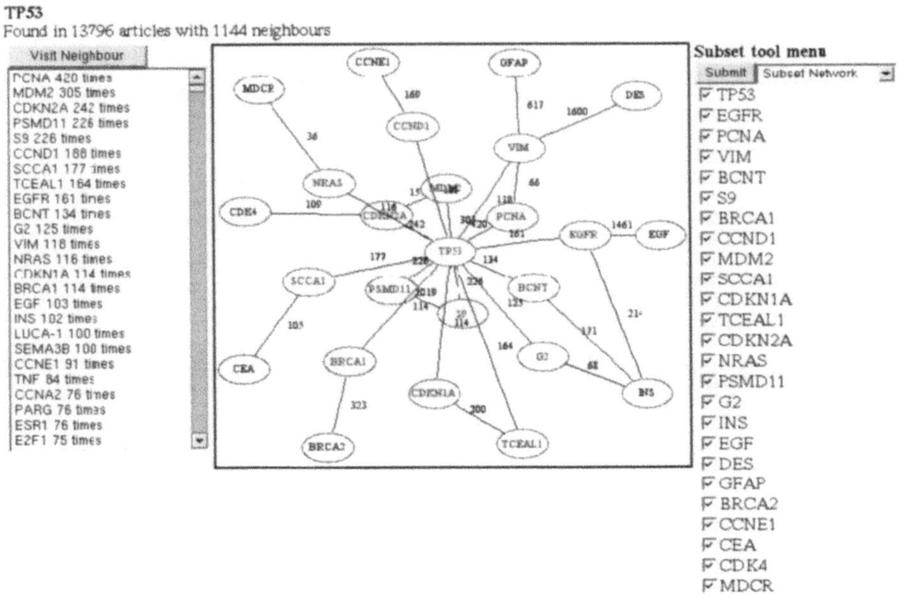

Fig. 8. PubGene provides web access to gene co-citation graphs for papers on rat, mouse and human genetics. Two genes mentioned in the same paper are connected by an edge. The project was created by a collaboration between the Department of Computer and Information Science and the Department of Physiology and Biomedical Engineering, Norwegian University of Science and Technology, Trondheim, Norway, and the Department of Tumor Biology, Institute for Cancer Research/Norwegian Radium Hospital, Oslo, Norway. It is now commercially supported by PubGene AS, Oslo, Norway.

6 Software

The Graphviz software is freely available under an open source license. It is available at `www.graphviz.org` and at `www.research.att.com/sw/tools/graphviz`. In addition to software, the latter site also provides documentation, sample layouts and links to various sites describing libraries or packages incorporating uses of Graphviz.

References

1. Barnson, M. P. (2002) The Bugzilla guide. `www.bugzilla.org/docs/html/`
2. Bond, G. W., Cheung, E., Purdy, K. H., Ramming, J. C., Zave, P. (submitted) An open architecture for next-generation telecommunication service. ACM Transactions on Internet Technology

3. Boutell, T. (2002) GD graphics library. www.boutell.com/gd/
4. Chen, Y. F., Gansner, E. R., Koutsofios, E. (1998) A C++ data model supporting reachability analysis and dead code detection. IEEE Transactions on Software Engineering **24** (9), 682–693
5. Chen, Y. F., Koutsofios, E. (1997) WebCiao: A website visualization and tracking system
6. Chvátal, V. (1983) *Linear Programming.* W. H. Freeman, New York
7. (2002) Gnucleus: An Open Source Gnutella Client. www.gnucleus.net
8. Cohen, J. (1987) Drawing graphs to convey proximity: an incremental arrangement method. ACM Transactions on Computer-Human Interaction **4** (11), 197–229
9. Cook, W. J., Cunningham, W. H., Pulleyblank, W. R., Schrijver, A. (1998) Combinatorial Optimization. John Wiley and Sons
10. de Icaza, M. (2001) The mono project: An overview. developer.ximian.com/articles/whitepapers/mono/
11. Eades, P. (1992) Drawing free trees. Bulletin of the Institute for Combinatorics and its Applications **5**, 10–36
12. Fortune, S. (1987) A sweepline algorithm for Voronoi diagrams. Algorithmica **2**, 153–174
13. Freivalds, K., Dogrusoz, U., Kikusts, P. (2002) Disconnected graph layout and the polyomino packing approach. In: P. Mutzel et al. (eds.) Graph Drawing '01, Lecture Notes in Computer Science 2265, Springer-Verlag, 378–391
14. Fruchterman, T. M. J., Reingold, E. M. (1991) Graph drawing by force-directed placement. Software – Practice and Experience **21** (11), 1129–1164
15. Gansner, E. R. (2002) The DOT language. www.research.att.com/~erg/graphviz/info/lang.html/
16. Gansner, E. R., Koutsofios, E., North, S. C., Vo, K.-P. (1993) A technique for drawing directed graphs. IEEE Transactions on Software Engineering **19** (3), 214–230
17. Gansner, E. R., North, S. C. (2000) An open graph visualization system and its applications to software engineering. Software – Practice and Experience **30**, 1203–1233
18. Glassner, A. S. (ed.) (1990) An algorithm for automatically fitting digitized curves. Graphics Gems, Academic Press, 612–626
19. Harel, D., Koren, Y. (2002) Drawing graphs with non-uniform vertices. In: Proceedings of Advanced Visual Interfaces (AVI'02), ACM Press, 157–166
20. Hershberger, J., Snoeyink, J. (1991) Computing minimum length paths of a given homotopy class. In: Proceedings of the 2nd Workshop Algorithms Data Structure, Lecture Notes in Computer Science 519, Springer-Verlag, 331–342
21. Holzmann, G. J. (1997) The model checker SPIN. IEEE Transactions on Software Engineering **23** (5), 279–295, spinroot.com/spin/whatispin.html/
22. Isaksson, B. (2001) DNS Bajaj. www.zonecut.net/dns/
23. Jenssen, T. K., Laegreid, A., Komorowski, J., Hovig, E. (2001) A literature network of human genes for high-throughput analysis of gene expression. Nature Genetics **28**, 21–28, www.pubgene.com
24. Johnston, P. (2002) Syntacs translation toolkit. inxar.org/syntacs/
25. Kamada, T., Kawai, S. (1989) An algorithm for drawing general undirected graphs. Information Processing Letters **31**, 7–15
26. Koutsofios, E., Dobkin, D. (1991) LEFTY: A two-view editor for technical pictures. In Graphics Interface '91, 68–76

27. Kruskal, J., Seery, J. (1980) Designing network diagrams. In: Proceedings of the First General Conference on Social Graphics, 22–50
28. Lee, W., Barghouti, N., Mocenigo, J. (1997) Grappa: A graph package in Java. In: G. Di Battista (ed.) Graph Drawing '97, Lecture Notes in Computer Science 1353, Springer-Verlag, 336–343
29. Lyons, K., Meijer, H., Rappaport, D. (1998) Algorithms for cluster busting in anchored graph drawing. Journal of Graph Algorithms and Applications **2** (1), 1–24
30. Marriott, K., Stuckey, P. J., Tam, V., He, W. (in press) Removing node overlapping in graph layout using constrained optimization. Constraints, 1–31
31. Misue, K., Eades, P., Lai, W., Sugiyama, K. (1995) Layout adjustment and the mental map. Journal of Visual Languages and Computing **6** (2), 183–210
32. North, S. C., Woodhull, G. (2001) Online hierarchical graph drawing. In: P. Mutzel, M. Jünger, S. Leipert (eds.) Graph Drawing '01, Lecture Notes in Computer Science 2265, Springer Verlag, 232–246
33. O'Rourke, J. (1994) Computational Geometry in C. Cambridge University Press, Cambridge
34. Sammon, Jr., J. W. (1969) A nonlinear mapping for data structure analysis. IEEE Transactions on Computers **18**, 401–409
35. Shepard, R. N. (1962) The analysis of proximities: multidimensional scaling with an unknown distance function. Psychometrika **27**, 125–140; 219–246
36. Thain, D. (2000) netmap. `www.cs.wisc.edu/~thain/projects/netmap`
37. Torgeson, W. S. (1965) Multidimensional scaling of similarity. Psychometrika **30**, 379–393
38. van Heesch, D. (2002) Doxygen. `http://www.stack.nl/~dimitri/doxygen/`
39. Vo, K.-P. (1997) Libcdt: A general and efficient container data type library. In: Proceedings of Summer '97 Usenix Conference
40. Walshaw, C. (2000) A Multilevel Algorithm for Force-Directed Graph Drawing. In: J. Marks (ed.) Graph Drawing '00, Lecture Notes in Computer Science 1984, Springer-Verlag, 171–182
41. Wills, G. (1997) Nicheworks – interactive visualization of very large graphs. In: G. Di Battista (ed.) Graph Drawing '97, Lecture Notes in Computer Science 1353, Springer-Verlag, 403–414
42. Wong, L. (2001) A protein interaction extraction system. In: Pacific Symposium on Biocomputing 6, 520–531

AGD – A Library of Algorithms for Graph Drawing

Michael Jünger[1], Gunnar W. Klau[2], Petra Mutzel[3], and René Weiskircher[3]

[1] University of Cologne, Department of Computer Science, Pohligstraße 1, D-50969 Köln, Germany
[2] Konrad–Zuse–Zentrum für Informationstechnik Berlin, Takustraße 7, D-14195 Berlin, Germany
[3] Vienna University of Technology, Institute of Computer Graphics and Algorithms, Favoritenstraße 9–11, A-1040 Wien, Austria

1 Introduction

The development of the AGD software, an object-oriented C++ class library of **A**lgorithms for **G**raph **D**rawing, has started in 1996. AGD is a general purpose graph drawing tool suited for beginners as well as for advanced users. It contains a variety of layout algorithms leading to different layout styles.

However, the primary goal of development has been to provide users with a toolbox for creating their own implementations of graph drawing algorithms according to their specific needs. Since, in many cases, users want the layouts to satisfy application-specific requirements that are not foreseen in generic graph drawing methods. AGD is designed in such a way that it is easy to add user-specific changes to the layout algorithms.

Another important goal of AGD was to bridge the gap between theory and practice in the area of graph drawing. E.g., for drawing general graphs, Batini *et al.* [3,2] suggested a method based on planarization which often leads to good drawings for many applications. However, until 1996, no publically available software layout tool used the planarization method. The reason for this was twofold: On the one hand, a lot of expertise is necessary concerning planarity testing algorithms, combinatorial embeddings, planar graph drawing algorithms, and (often $\mathcal{NP}$-hard) combinatorial optimization problems. On the other hand, great effort is needed to implement all necessary algorithms and data structures, since the planarization method consists of various phases that require complex algorithms.

Recently, major improvements have been made concerning the use of the planarization method in practice (e.g., [32,19,26–28]). Today, there exist some (publically available) software libraries using the planarization method successfully for practical graph layout [1,22,23]. In AGD, the planarization method is implemented in a modular form, so that it is easy to experiment with different approaches to the various subtasks of the whole approach. This enables experimental comparisons between various algorithms in order to study and understand their impact on the final drawing. Not only in graph drawing, the empirical study of combinatorial algorithms is getting increasing attention.

Also the Sugiyama-style method for drawing graphs with preferred direction is rather a methodological frame than a fixed algorithm. For each phase layer assignment, crossing minimization, and coordinate assignment, a variety of possible implementations exists. AGD allows users to simply switch among a variety of implementations, and gives software programmers the possibility to introduce new algorithms.

Another reason for building AGD was our intention to show how mathematical methods can help to produce good layouts. Many of the optimization problems in graph drawing are $\mathcal{NP}$-hard. However, this does not mean that it is impossible to solve them in practice. AGD shows that problem instances can often be solved to provable optimality within short computation time by using polyhedral combinatorics and branch-and-cut algorithms.

2 Applications

We can distinguish two groups of users of AGD: The first group uses only the algorithms that are already implemented without making any changes or extensions while the second group writes new modules in order to change the behavior of the drawing algorithms already contained in AGD. The first group only needs the executables of the demo programs. The `agd_demo` executable contains only algorithms working without additional software packages while `agd_opt_demo` contains the exact optimization algorithms that only work on systems where ABACUS [35] and CPLEX are installed.

Both demo programs have graphical user interfaces that are based on the class `graph_win` of the LEDA-library [43]. This class already contains methods for loading and storing graphs in different formats and also for creating and manipulating them. The demo programs extend the menus of `graph_win` by the methods implemented in AGD for generating and drawing graphs. Since `graph_win` allows drawings to be exported in PostScript format, drawings generated using AGD algorithms can easily be used as illustrations in documents.

The demos thus constitute a very general graph drawing environment. Data we collected from people who downloaded the demos show a diverse range of applications. In the field of biology, AGD is used to visualize metabolic networks, protein interactions, gene regulatory networks, and plant distributions. In social science, uses include drawing genealogical trees, collective labor agreements and net structures in cognitive models. Other applications include the visualization of neural networks, electrical grids, flowcharts and the dependency graph of university courses.

The disadvantage of the generality of the demos is that they are not suitable for applications where the drawings have to meet a very restrictive set of requirements. Therefore, the second group of users writes new modules or classes that are derived from AGD-classes to modify the behavior of the algorithms that already exist in the library. In this way, users can address their specialized layout needs.

AGD is also used as a platform for research in the area of graph drawing, e.g., [15,38]. Because of its modular construction, researchers can concentrate on the innovative part of their drawing algorithm while leaving standard tasks to the algorithms implemented in AGD. One example is the comparison of different methods for the compaction of orthogonal drawings done by Klau *et al.* [38]. It was only necessary to implement the different compaction methods that should be compared as AGD-modules, while the computation of the orthogonal representation for each graph and the visualization of the computed drawing was left to the corresponding classes already implemented in AGD. This enabled the authors to save more than half of the programming work compared to starting the project from scratch.

3 Algorithms

AGD contains a variety of implementations of methods for drawing graphs with the planarization method (see Section 3.1). A basic ingredient to the planarization method are planar graph drawing methods. AGD includes implementations of many different planar graph drawing algorithms, some of which can be combined with the planarization method (see Section 3.2). Relatively new are orthogonal planar drawing methods for clustered graphs (see Section 3.3). For Sugiyama-style layout, AGD contains many different implementations of the phases layer assignment, crossing minimization, and coordinate assignment (see Section 3.4).

3.1 Algorithms for Planarization

In this section we will mainly focus on the planarization method and its implementation in AGD. General graphs can also be drawn using force-directed methods. Indeed, most available software tools for graph drawing use force-directed methods. These are especially useful for drawing very sparse, tree-like graphs. AGD contains implementations of the spring-embedder algorithm by Fruchterman and Reingold [20], and the algorithm by Tutte [51]. However, for many applications, e.g., data base visualization or software design, the planarization method leads to much nicer layouts. E.g., in general the planarization method leads to grid drawings having a small number of edge crossings.

AGD contains a very flexible implementation of the planarization method (`PlanarizationGridLayout`). So far, all planar layout routines in AGD generate grid drawings, i.e., the computed coordinates are integer. This is supported with the `GridLayoutModule`. The AGD modules involved in the planarization method are shown in Figure 1.

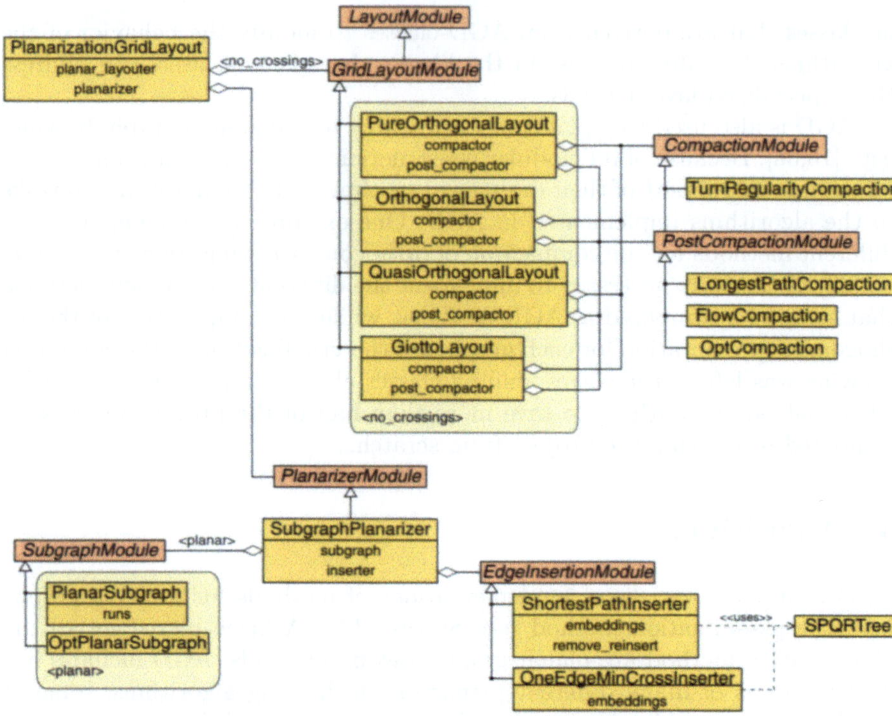

Fig. 1. Modules for the planarization method.

In the planarization phase, any procedure transforming the given graph G into a planar graph G' is allowed. One can imagine that a method generating a random or a force-directed layout and then substituting the crossings by artificial vertices could be a `PlanarizerModule`. AGD offers the possibility of adding and creating any new method for planarizing a graph via substituting edge crossings by artificial vertices.

Our experiments have shown that, in order to keep the number of crossings small, it is advantageous to use planarization via edge removal (`Subgraph Planarizer`). AGD contains a heuristic `PlanarSubgraph` [30] based on PQ-trees that achieves good results in practice, and a branch-and-cut algorithm `OptPlanarSubgraph` to solve this $\mathcal{NP}$-hard problem to optimality [32]. Any other planar subgraph heuristic can easily be added to AGD.

For the edge re-insertion phase, AGD contains the standard procedure `ShortestPathInserter` described in Algorithm 2, Section 4.3 in the Technical Foundations, as well as the optimal embedding re-insertion algorithm `OneEdgeMinCrossInserter` (Algorithm 3, Section 4.3 in the Technical Foundations) [28]. All edge insertion modules provide optional heuristics that can improve the quality of the solution significantly. The two algorithms that fix an embedding allow calling the algorithm for several randomly generated embeddings and select the best solution. The number of embeddings is controlled by the parameter `embeddings`. Generating random combinatorial embeddings requires computing the SPQR-tree for each biconnected component [9]. AGD provides a linear-time implementation of SPQR trees [27] in the class `SPQRTree`. Experiments show that significant improvements are achieved if, in a postprocessing step, a set S of edges is removed from the graph and reinserted [34,53]. In each such step, the number of crossings can only decrease. All three edge insertion algorithms support this heuristic that is controlled by the parameter `remove_reinsert`. Possible settings are `none` (skip postprocessing), `inserted` (apply postprocessing with all reinserted edges), and `all` (apply postprocessing with all edges in the graph).

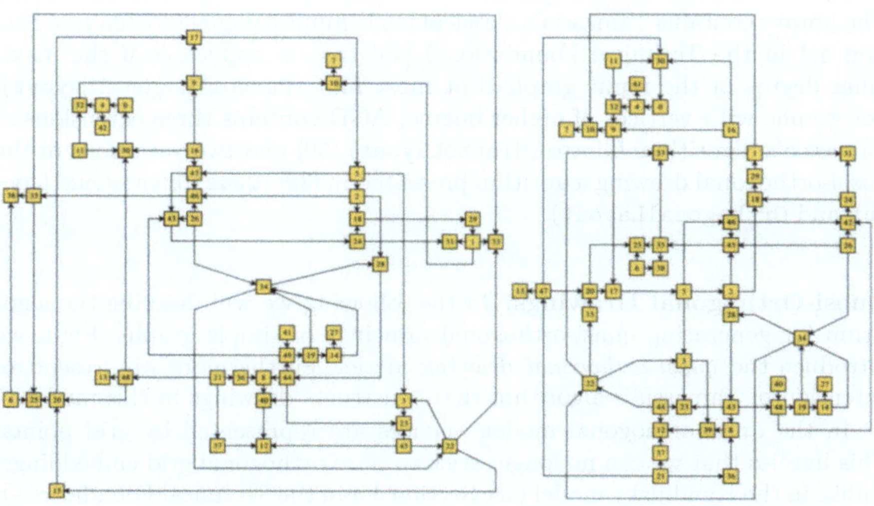

(a) Fixed embedding (b) Optimal embedding

Fig. 2. The influence of the combinatorial embedding.

Figure 2(a) shows a graph for which the standard iterative edge insertion leads to 14 crossings if a random combinatorial embedding is chosen. In this case the drawing has a grid size of 22×22. However, when taking the optimum one edge insertion module and adding the remove and reinsert algorithm for all edges, the resulting drawing has only 11 crossings and has size 16×22 (see Figure 2(b)). This is a good example that shows how the size of the drawing increases with the number of crossings.

3.2 Planar Graph Drawing Algorithms

The planarization phase leads to a planar graph G' that contains artificial vertices. Now, any planar graph drawing algorithm may be used for G'. Replacing all artificial vertices with edge crossings in a drawing of G' results in a drawing of the input graph G. We prefer to use orthogonal or quasi-orthogonal algorithms because, in this case, an edge crossing is drawn as two crossing horizontal and vertical line segments.

In orthogonal graph drawing, an important goal is to keep the number of bends small. Many minimum cost flow-based algorithms are available for this task (see Figure 1). In a first step (bend minimization) a flow in an underlying network determines the shape of the orthogonal drawing. A second step (compaction) deals with assigning the coordinates to the vertices and bends. The library contains Tamassia's classical bend-minimizing algorithm (see Section 4.4 in the Technical Foundations) [49] that is applicable if the maximum degree of the input graph is at most four (`PureOrthogonalLayout`). For graphs with vertices of higher degree, AGD contains three extensions of Tamassia's algorithm: Giotto (`GiottoLayout`) [50] and two variations of the quasi-orthogonal drawing algorithm presented in [39] (`QuasiOrthogonalLayout` and `OrthogonalLayout`).

Quasi-Orthogonal Drawings. In the following we will describe the algorithm for generating quasi-orthogonal drawings of simple graphs. First, we introduce the *quasi-orthogonal* drawing model. Furthermore we present an extension of Tamassia's algorithm that constructs drawings in this model.

In the quasi-orthogonal model, vertices are represented by grid points. This implies that we can no longer stick to pure orthogonal grid embeddings. Unlike in the Kandinsky model (see Section 4.4 in the Technical Foundations), vertices and edges share a common grid in the quasi-orthogonal model. These two requirements enforce some edges to leave the grid lines. We require, however, that 4-planar subgraphs are still drawn according to the pure orthogonal standard. We call vertices with degree greater than four *high-degree vertices*. Our proposal is to allow the first segment of any edge leaving a high-degree vertex to run diagonally through the grid. The following definition provides a formal description of the quasi-orthogonal standard:

A *quasi-orthogonal grid embedding* of a planar graph $G = (V, E)$ is a function Γ that maps V to points in the grid and E to sequences of segments whose endpoints lie on the grid. The following properties hold:

(Q1) $\Gamma(v) \neq \Gamma(w)$ for $v, w \in V, v \neq w$.
(Q2) The endpoints of $\Gamma(e)$ are $\Gamma(v)$ and $\Gamma(w)$ for all $e = (v, w) \in E$.
(Q3) For two different edges e_1 and e_2 the paths $\Gamma(e_1)$ and $\Gamma(e_2)$ do not intersect except possibly at their endpoints.
(Q4) $\Gamma(G \setminus \{v \in V \mid \deg(v) > 4\})$ is an orthogonal grid embedding.

Notice that property (Q4) of this definition ensures pure orthogonal grid embeddings for 4-planar graphs. This implies that every orthogonal grid embedding is also a quasi-orthogonal grid embedding. Figure 3 shows an example for a drawing respecting the properties of the above definition.

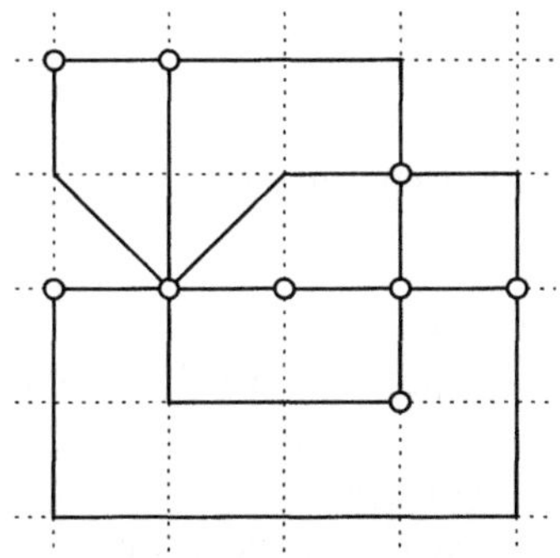

Fig. 3. Quasi-orthogonal grid embedding of a 6-planar graph with 7 bends.

In the following we describe an algorithm that computes quasi-orthogonal grid embeddings for simple planar graphs, see also [39] and [37]. Similar to the related *Giotto* algorithm, high-degree vertices v are replaced by faces f_v with $\deg(f_v) = \deg(v)$. The vertices on the boundary of such a representative face f_v correspond to the adjacencies of the former vertex v, reflecting the order of the neighbors. We call these special faces *cages*, in a later phase of the algorithm every high-degree vertex will be placed in its corresponding cage. Unlike in *Giotto*, we do not prescribe on which side of f_v the edges adjacent to v have to leave. We refer to the transformation as T_1 (see Algorithm 1 and Figure 4).

Algorithm 1: Transformation T_1

Input : Planar graph $G = (V, E)$, vertex $v \in V$
Output: Transformed graph G (v is replaced by a cage)
for *all edges* $e = (v, w) \in E$ *adjacent to* v **do**
  Split edge (v, w)
end
for *all faces* f *adjacent to* v **do**
  Link pair of new vertices in f by an edge
end
Delete v and incident edges

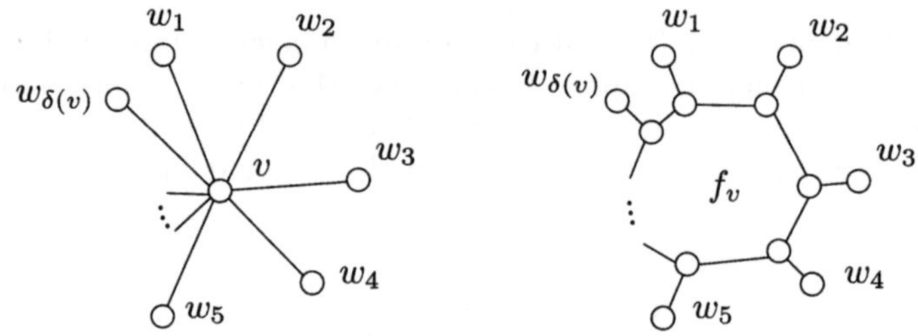

Fig. 4. Transformation T_1: Replacing a high-degree vertex v by a cage f_v.

After applying $T_1(G, v)$, the newly created face f_v represents the former vertex v. Notice that v has been replaced by a structure of $\deg(v)$ vertices, each of which has exactly three neighbours. Let $\widetilde{G}$ be the graph that results from applying T_1 to every high-degree vertex in G. In the following analysis, V_i denotes the set $\{v \in V \mid \deg(v) = i\}$. It is obvious that T_1 does not change the planarity of the graph and that the resulting number of vertices of $\widetilde{G}$ is in $O(|V|)$ since T_1 introduces for each edge in E at most two new vertices. Furthermore one can easily verify that the inverse operation of transformation T_1 results in the original graph.

Now we can apply Tamassia's algorithm for 4-planar graphs to $\widetilde{G}$. Since $|\widetilde{V}| = O(|V|)$, the asymptotical notion of running time does not change.

If we, however, do not distinguish between cages and normal faces, the result is a pure orthogonal grid embedding in which the cages have arbitrary rectilinear shape. Since we want to place the high-degree vertices inside their corresponding cages, it would not be a good idea to let the shapes of the cages get too complicated. Therefore we force cages to be of rectangular shape by modifying the network of Tamassia's original algorithm. We then show that our modifications indeed achieve the desired results and that our formulation always provides a solution meeting our constraints.

A rectilinear polygon Π has rectangular shape if neither of the angles inside Π exceeds 180°. We exploit this fact to formulate a modification of network N as introduced in Section 4.4 of the Technical Foundations. Consider the set of elements $R = \{r \in H(f) \mid f \text{ is a cage}\}$. For every element $r \in R$ we must ensure $a_r \leq 180$ and $s_r = 0^*$. These two constraints guarantee that there will be neither a concave angle nor a concave bend in a cage. In [11] a similar method is proposed resulting in drawings according to the *Giotto* standard. In this approach the angles a_r are forced to be equal to 180°; this leads to an increased total edge length compared to our approach.

Notice that the first requirement ($a_r \leq 180°$) is automatically satisfied. Each vertex v bounding a cage has degree $\deg(v) = 3$ and thus can only form angles of at most 180°. We formulate the second constraint by deleting certain arcs in N. We have to avoid a flow $\chi_{(u_g, u_f)}$ in the case that f represents a cage. Deleting the arc (u_g, u_f) makes such a flow impossible.

We have now modified the network of Tamassia's algorithm for 4-planar graphs so that each legal flow in it corresponds to an orthogonal representation with rectangular cages. The following lemma states that these modifications have no influence on the feasibility of the minimum cost flow problem:

Lemma 1. *The minimum cost flow in the modified network corresponds to an orthogonal representation with the minimum number of bends under the constraint that every cage has a rectangular shape.*

Proof. Let N be the modified network. The modification concerns only the arcs in A_F. To prove the lemma we only have to show that the conservation rule at nodes $u_f \in U_F$ still holds. Therefore we consider three cases:

1. Face f is a cage.
   The incoming flow is $\sum_{u_v} \chi(u_v, u_f)$, the outgoing flow is $\sum_{u_g} \chi(u_f, u_g)$. There are exactly four angles of 90° in the cage occurring either at vertices or at bends. Thus
   $$|\{u_v \mid \chi(u_v, u_f) = 1\}| + \sum_{u_g} \chi(u_f, u_g) = 4 .$$
   We get
   $$\sum_{u_v} \chi(u_v, u_f) - \sum_{u_g} \chi(u_f, u_g) = 2\deg(f) - |\{u_v \mid \chi(u_v, u_f) = 1\}| - \sum_{u_g} \chi(u_f, u_g)$$
   $$= 2\deg(f) - 4 = b_{u_f} .$$
2. Face f is the neighbor of a cage.
   According to their construction, cages can never be neighbors to other cages, neither can they enclose other faces. For this reason the demand of u_f can be satisfied by adjacent normal faces.
3. Face f is neither a cage nor a neighbor of a cage.
   In this case there is no difference from the unmodified network. Conservation is guaranteed. □

We now construct an initial orthogonal embedding Γ for the auxiliary graph $\widetilde{G}$ with one of the methods for the compaction phase of the topology-shape-metrics method (see Section 4.4 in the Technical Foundations). During this step we ensure that both the height and the width of a cage measure at least two grid units which can easily be incorporated in any of the compaction methods. At this point, we want to reverse the changes of transformation T_1. Therefore, we define a second transformation T_2 (see Algorithm 2) that operates on grid embeddings and places the high-degree vertices in their cages. The aim is to minimize the number of bends arising at the boundary of a cage during the process of connecting a high-degree vertex v with its adjacent edges. Let $w_1, \ldots, w_{\deg(v)}$ be the vertices on the boundary of the corresponding cage f_v and let $\Gamma(f_v)$ characterize the set of grid points covered by f_v. Using straight line edges for the connection of v with its neighbors, we can save at most four bends. For the detailed and somewhat tedious description of finding the best grid point for v, see [37]. A final compaction step might help to further reduce the area of the drawing.

Algorithm 2: Transformation T_2.

Input : Orthogonal drawing Γ, cage f_v with boundary $w_1, \ldots, w_{\deg(v)}$
Output: Γ in which f_v is replaced by the appropriate vertex v

```
Place v in Γ(f_v) // creating a minimum number of bends in Γ(f_v)
for i = 1 to deg(v) do
 |  Connect v with w_i
end
```

The method is summarized in Algorithm 3. Procedure `tamassia_mod` refers to the modified bend minimizing algorithm of Tamassia (see Section 4.4 in the Technical Foundations for a description of the original algorithm) where each cage is forced to be of rectangular shape.

Algorithm 3: Quasi-orthogonal drawing algorithm.

Input : Planar graph $G = (V, E)$ with planar embedding P
Output: Quasi-orthogonal grid embedding Γ of G

$\widetilde{G} = G$
while $\exists$ *vertex* $v \in \widetilde{V}$ *with* $\deg(v) > 4$ **do**
  | $\widetilde{G} = T_1(\widetilde{G}, v)$
end
$\widetilde{\Gamma} = \text{tamassia\_mod}(\widetilde{G}, \widetilde{P})$
$\Gamma = \widetilde{\Gamma}$ **for** *all faces* $f \in \widetilde{F}$ *if* f *is a cage* **do**
  | $\Gamma = T_2(\Gamma, f)$
end
Return Γ

Compaction Algorithms. The AGD library contains several algorithms for the compaction phase within the topology-shape-metrics approach. Construction heuristics assign coordinates to vertices and bends of a given orthogonal representation that encodes the shape of a planar orthogonal drawing. Improvement heuristics operate directly on a layout and try to decrease its total edge length and area. This division is reflected in the library: The user chooses a construction method (from `CompactionModule` or `PostCompactionModule`) and optional improvement heuristics (from PostCompactionModule). The former transforms the orthogonal representation by introducing artificial edges and vertices. By changing the options of the compaction algorithms, there are different techniques available for this transformation. AGD's constructive heuristics include longest path-based or flow-based compaction with rectangular dissection (LongestPathCompaction and FlowCompaction) [49] and two variants of a flow-based compaction technique based on the property of turn-regularity (TurnRegularityCompaction) [4]. For the improvement phase, AGD offers iterative application of compaction with longest path or flow computations (LongestPathCompaction and FlowCompaction) as used in the area of VLSI-design, see, e.g., [41]. In addition, AGD provides an implementation of the integer linear programming-based approach by Klau and Mutzel (OptCompaction) [40] that produces an optimum drawing in terms of minimum total length or maximum edge length.

The modular design of the compaction phase proved very useful in a recent experimental study [38]. All combinations of constructive and improvement heuristics could easily be compared against each other and against the optimum values provided by the integer linear programming-based algorithm. One of the main insights of this study has been that flow-based compaction should always be used as an improvement method. Figure 5 shows the output of two different compaction strategies and a corresponding optimum solution.

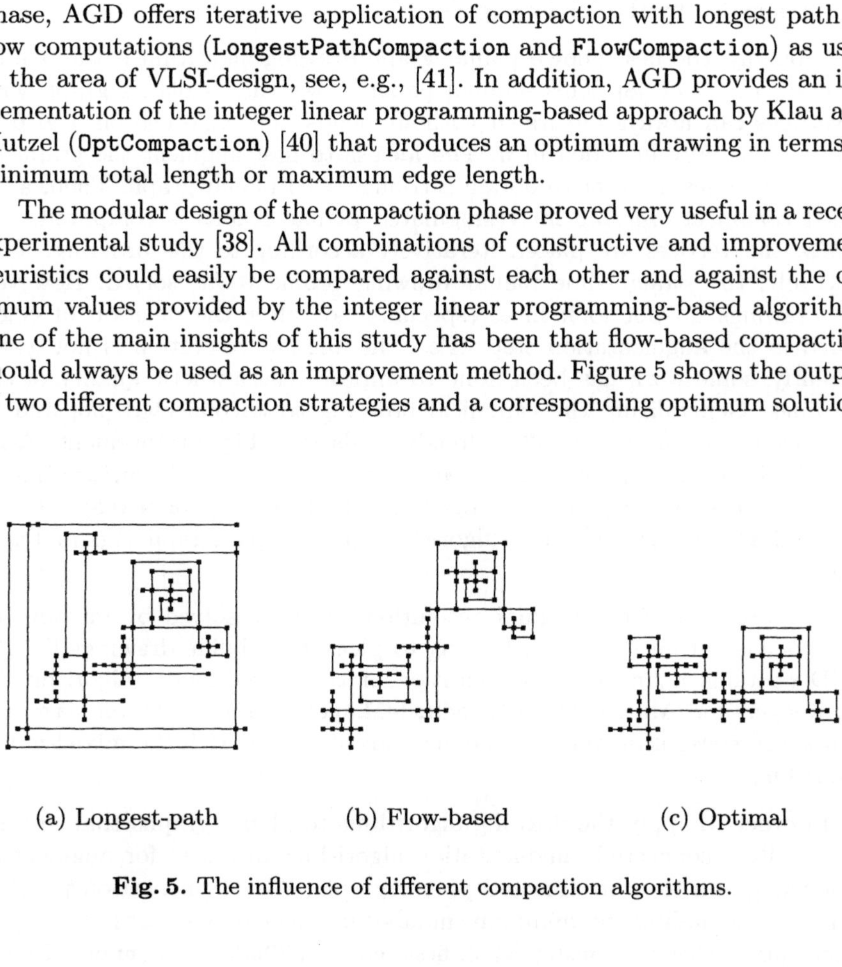

(a) Longest-path (b) Flow-based (c) Optimal

Fig. 5. The influence of different compaction algorithms.

Alternative Planar Drawing Algorithms. In addition to the orthogonal and quasi-orthogonal planar drawing algorithms described above, the following planar drawing algorithms are contained in AGD (the corresponding AGD modules are shown in Figure 6).

AGD contains an implementation of the Kandinsky algorithm `Kandinsky Layout` described in Section 4.4 of the Technical Foundations [19] that is not yet available as a module in the planarization method, but can be used for planar graphs with arbitrary vertex degrees. Unlike other flow-based orthogonal drawing methods, the Kandinsky algorithm places vertices and bends as points on a coarse grid and routes the edges in a finer grid as sequences of horizontal and vertical line segments. A variant of the algorithm uses a common grid for vertices and edges. Vertices are represented as boxes whose size is bounded by the vertex degree.

Probably, the best known planar graph drawing algorithm is the one by de Fraysseix *et al.* [8]. This seminal paper shows that a planar graph with n vertices can always be drawn without bends and crossings on a grid of size polynomially bounded in n. The idea is to first augment the graph by additional edges in order to obtain a triangulated planar graph. Then, a so-called *canonical ordering* for triangulated planar graphs is computed, and finally, the vertices are placed iteratively according to this ordering. Theoretically, the straight-line planar drawing problem was solved. However, the drawings do not look nice, especially not after the deletion of edges added in the augmentation step. Also, the angular resolution is not good. Recently, some work has been done to improve the æsthetic quality of the drawings. Generalizing the canonical ordering to triconnected [36] and to biconnected planar graphs [25] already leads to a big improvement. AGD provides implementations of all three canonical orderings (`CanonicalOrder`) and the corresponding placement algorithms (`FPPLayout`, `ConvexLayout`, and `PlanarStraightLayout`). The algorithms of this paragraph run in linear time.

The problem of the angular resolution has been solved by introducing some bends within the edges, leading to pleasant polyline drawings [36,26]. AGD contains a linear implementation of the mixed-model algorithm by Gutwenger and Mutzel [26] (`MixedModelLayout`). Figure 11 on page 168 shows a screenshot of AGD displaying a graph drawn with the mixed-model algorithm.

In order to apply the drawing algorithms to planar graphs that are not necessarily biconnected, augmentation algorithms are used for augmenting a planar graph to a biconnected planar graph. The augmentation problem consisting of adding the minimum number of edges is $\mathcal{NP}$-hard. AGD provides a simple heuristic using depth-first-search (`LEDAMakeBiconnected`), the 5/3-approximation algorithm by Fialko and Mutzel [18] (`PlanAug`) that in most cases yields a solution that is very close to an optimum solution, and a branch-and-cut algorithm for exact optimization (`OptPlanAug`) [44,31,17].

In addition, AGD contains linear implementations of two algorithms for producing convex drawings of triconnected planar graphs (`ConvexLayout` [36] and `ConvexDrawLayout` [6]), generalizations of these algorithms to general

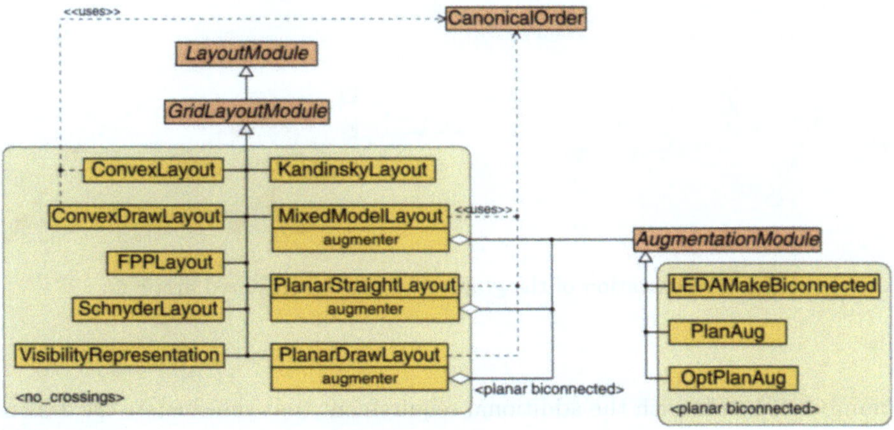

Fig. 6. Modules for drawing planar graphs.

planar graphs [25] (`PlanarDraw Layout`), and an algorithm for producing weak visibility representations [47] (`VisibilityRepresentation`).

3.3 Algorithms for Planar Cluster Drawings

Recently, we integrated planar cluster drawing algorithms into the library. In the following we describe our approach in more detail. We use the notation of Sections 2.5 and 3.3 in the Technical Foundations. A grid drawing of a clustered graph is called *orthogonal* if the underlying graph is drawn orthogonal and the cluster regions are drawn as rectangles where the corners lie on integer grid points.

Given a *c*-planar embedding of $C = (G, T)$ (e.g., obtained via the cluster planarity algorithm described in [16]), we apply a modified version of Tamassia's algorithm to obtain an orthogonal grid drawing of C.

To make use of Tamassia's algorithm, we generate the graph G' from C as follows: We start with a *c*-planar embedding of C. Beginning with the leaves of T, we traverse the cluster tree from bottom to top (level order traversal). For a non-trivial cluster $\nu \in T$ we insert an artificial vertex on every incident edge of ν and afterwards connect the artificial vertices by virtual edges along the cluster boundary (see Figure 7). This information is given by the c-planar embedding. It is obvious that this operation preserves the given *c*-planar embedding.

Then we apply the modified algorithm of Tamassia to G'. In order to achieve rectangular regions in the final drawing, we need to modify the flow network. Notice that the representation of the regions of the cluster in G' are very similar to the *cages* that have been introduced in the description of the quasi-orthogonal drawing algorithm (see Section 3.2). We can use almost the same modification of Tamassia's network in order to guarantee the minimum

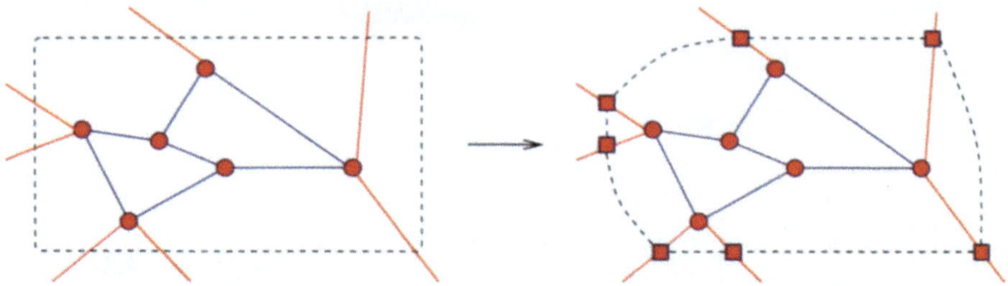

Fig. 7. Generation of the graph G' from the clustered graph C.

number of bends with the additional requirement that the clusters are drawn as rectangular regions.

Finally, we construct an orthogonal grid drawing of C from the orthogonal grid drawing of G'. It is obvious that we can use the positions of the original vertices and edges of C that are not incident to clusters of C. In the drawing, we replace each path containing artificial vertices and representing an original edge of G incident to a cluster with the drawing of a single edge. We also replace the virtual edges representing the cluster boundaries by rectangles. Since the corners of these rectangles correspond to bends in the virtual edges, they are positioned on integer grid points. The result is an orthogonal grid drawing of C. An example is shown in Figure 8.

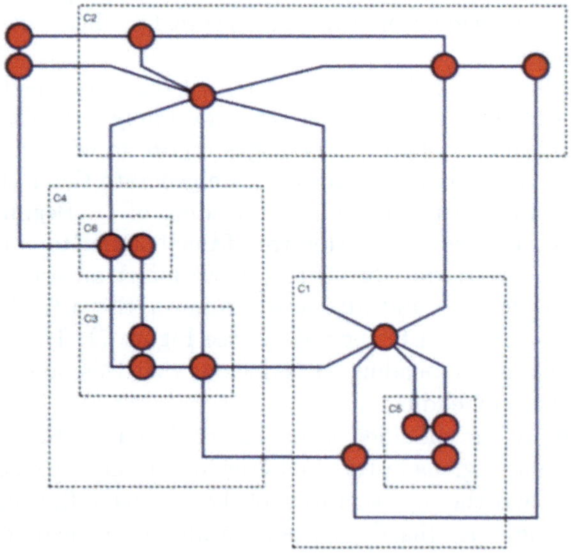

Fig. 8. Example for a drawing of a clustered graph produced by the algorithm.

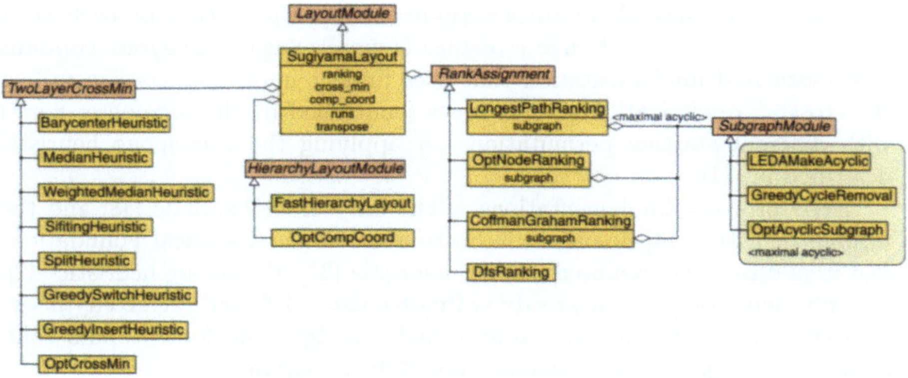

Fig. 9. Modules for Sugiyama-style layout.

Let $h(T)$ be the height of the cluster hierarchy T. Then the running time of the drawing algorithm is $O(\tilde{n}^{\frac{7}{4}}\sqrt{\log \tilde{n}})$ where $\tilde{n} = O(|V|h(T))$.

3.4 Algorithms for Sugiyama-Style Layout

AGD provides a flexible implementation of the *Sugiyama algorithm* [48] represented by the module `SugiyamaLayout` that consists of three phases. For each phase, various methods have been proposed in the literature. The available AGD modules and their dependencies are shown in Figure 9.

In the first phase, handled by modules of type `RankAssignment`, the vertices of the input graph G are assigned to layers. If G is not acyclic, then we compute a maximal acyclic subgraph and reverse the edges not contained in the subgraph. AGD contains two linear-time heuristics for solving the $\mathcal{NP}$-hard maximal acyclic subgraph problem (`LEDAMakeAcyclic` based on depth-first-search and a greedy algorithm (`GreedyCycleRemoval`) [13]), as well as a branch-and-cut algorithm (`OptAcyclicSubgraph`) [24] that is able to solve the problem to provable optimality within short computation time.

Currently, AGD contains the following algorithms for computing a layer assignment for an acyclic graph in which the edges are directed from vertices on a lower level to vertices on a higher level. `LongestPathRanking` is based on the computation of longest paths and minimizes the number of layers (height of the drawing), `OptNodeRanking` minimizes the total edge length [21] (here the length of an edge is the number of layers it traverses plus 1), `CoffmanGrahamRanking` computes a layer assignment with a predefined maximum number of vertices on a layer (width of the drawing) [7], and `DfsRanking` simply uses depth-first-search and handles general graphs (see Section 4.2 in the Technical Foundations). If edges traverse at least one layer, they are split by inserting additional artificial vertices such that edges connect only vertices on neighboring layers.

The second phase determines permutations of the vertices on each layer such that the number of edge crossings is small. `SugiyamaLayout` contains a sophisticated implementation that uses further improvements like calling the crossing minimization several times (controlled by the parameter `runs`) with different starting permutations, or applying the `transpose` heuristic described in [21].

AGD provides implementations of the barycenter heuristic [48] and the median heuristic [14] described in Section 4.2 of the Technical Foundations and in addition the weighted median heuristic [21], the sifting heuristic [42], the split heuristic [12], the greedy switch heuristic [12], and the greedy insert heuristic [12]. Furthermore, a branch-and-cut algorithm for optimum solutions based on [33] is implemented (texttttOptCrossMin).

AGD contains two implementations for the final coordinate assignment phase. The first (`OptCompCoord`) tries to let edges run as vertical as possible by solving a linear program presented in Section 4.2 of the Technical Foundations, the second (`FastHierarchyLayout`) proposed by Buchheim *et al.* [5] guarantees at most two bends per edge and draws the whole part between these bends vertically. Figure 10 shows two Sugiyama-style layouts of the same graph for which different algorithms for the coordinate assignment phase have been used: the method proposed in [5] (top), and the LP-based approach (bottom).

Some more specific classes of graphs require algorithms that exploit their special structure. E.g., trees can be drawn nicely in AGD using the algorithm by Reingold and Tilford [46] and Walker [52] (see Section 4.1 in the Technical Foundations). Moreover, upward planar *st*-digraphs can be drawn by the algorithm suggested in [10].

4 Implementation

AGD [1] is an object-oriented C++ class library, which is based on the two libraries LEDA [43] and ABACUS [35]. LEDA provides basic data types and algorithms, e.g., the data type for the representation of graphs. ABACUS is a framework for the implementation of branch-and-cut algorithms. The ABACUS library is only used by branch-and-cut algorithms, whereas the whole basic functionality of AGD is independent of ABACUS. Therefore, we split the library into two parts, the basic part **AGD** and the part **AGDopt** that contains all ABACUS dependent classes. This makes it possible to use a subset of the algorithms in AGD without having an ABACUS installation – a LEDA installation is sufficient in this case.

The most important design feature in AGD for algorithm engineering is the representation of algorithms as classes that provide one or more methods for calling the algorithm. Thus, a particular instance of an algorithm is an object of that class, which can also maintain optional parameters of the algorithm as member variables. Algorithms providing basically the same

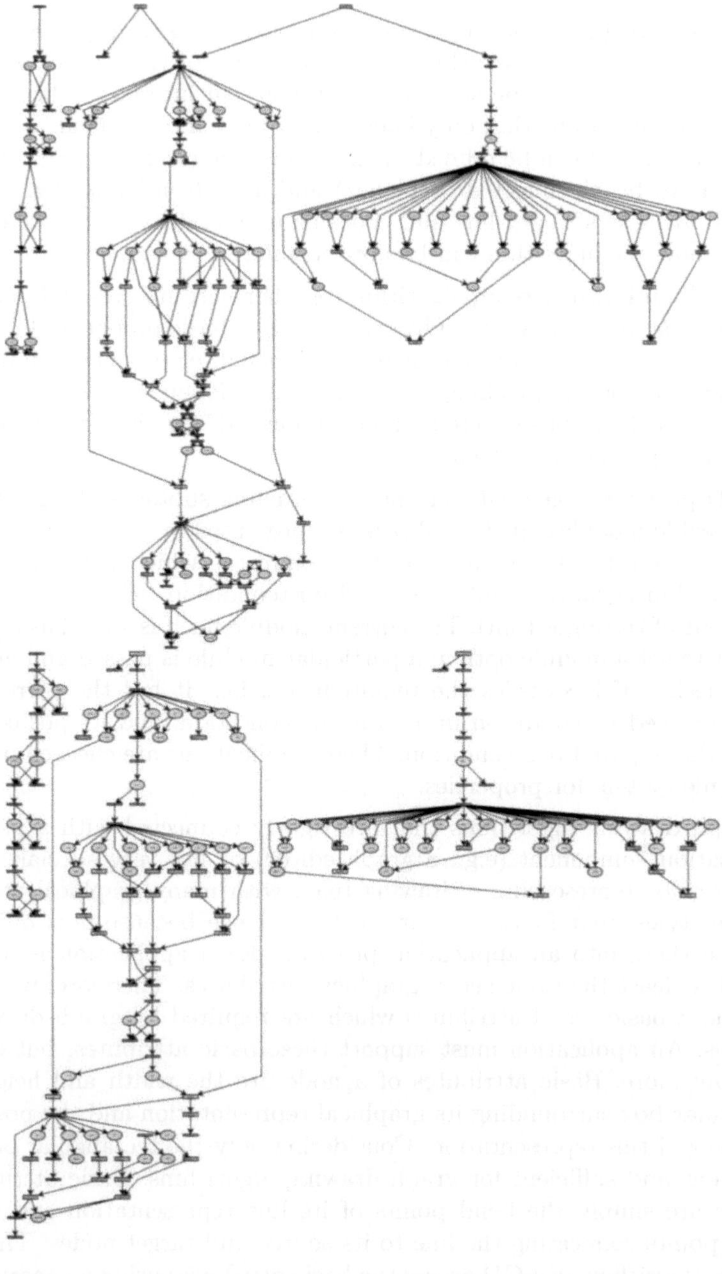

Fig. 10. Two Sugiyama-style layouts of the same graph drawn with different modules for the coordinate assignment phase.

functionality (e.g., computing a subgraph or drawing a graph) are derived from a common base class, which we call the *type* of the algorithm, i.e., algorithms of the same type support a common call interface. This allows to write generic functions that only know the type of an algorithm. The type is rather general, but can be refined by declaring a *precondition* (e.g., the input graph has to be biconnected or planar) and a *postcondition* (e.g., the produced drawing is straight-line and contains no crossings). The precondition specifies how the algorithm can be applied safely.

We call an instance of an algorithm together with its pre- and postcondition a *module*. Pre- and postconditions are sets of basic properties (e.g., properties of graphs like planar, acyclic or biconnected, or properties of drawings like orthogonal or straight-line). AGD maintains dependencies between these properties, such as "biconnected implies connected", or "a tree is a connected forest", in a global rule system.

AGD provides a general concept for modeling subtasks of algorithms as exchangeable modules. Such a subtask is represented by a *module option* that knows the module type, a guaranteed precondition (which always holds when the algorithm is called), and a required postcondition (which must hold for the output of the algorithm). The current module itself is stored as a pointer. In order to set a module option, a particular module is passed and automatically checked if it satisfies the requirements, i.e., it has the correct type, the guaranteed precondition implies its precondition, and its postcondition implies the required postcondition. These implications are checked using the global rule system for properties.

Graph drawing algorithms that are tightly connected with a particular visualization component (e.g., a graph editor) or use very specialized data structures for representing a drawing (e.g., with many graphical attributes like line styles, text fonts, ...) are of limited use because it is difficult to integrate them into an application program. Each application is forced to support at least the same set of graphical attributes. Therefore, we decided to define a basic set of attributes which are required by graph drawing algorithms. An application must support these basic attributes, but can also use many more. Basic attributes of a node are the width and height of a rectangular box surrounding its graphical representation and the position of the center of this representation. Considering only the rectangular outline is convenient and sufficient for graph drawing algorithms. Basic attributes of an edge are simply the bend points of its line representation and the two anchor points connecting the line to its source and target nodes. The graph drawing algorithms in AGD access the basic attributes using a generic layout interface class. For a particular visualization component, an implementation is derived from the generic class and some virtual functions are overridden. The implementation class is responsible for storing the attributes. When a graph drawing algorithm is called, an object of this implementation class is passed and used by the algorithm to produce the layout.

An implementation of the generic layout interface for LEDA's graph editor GraphWin is already part of AGD, as well as a simple data structure for storing a layout. The latter is particularly useful for testing algorithms when it is not necessary to display the computed layout. AGD comes with the demo programs agd_demo, agd_opt_demo, cluster_demo, and spqr_viewer based on GraphWin, that realize a graph editor with sophisticated layout facilities. The programs allow to experiment with the various algorithms of AGD, i.e., changing options and using different algorithms for subproblems. They can also be extended and adapted by developers, since their source code is part of AGD. The program agd_server, written by Stefan Näher, is also part of the AGD package. The server allows to use AGD algorithms via a file or socket interface. The program reads the graph in GML format [29] from a given input file and loads the AGD options that specify the layout algorithm from a second file. Then, the selected algorithm is applied and the result is written back to the input file, again in GML format.

The following code fragment gives a programming example with AGD. It shows how to set the planarizer option for the planarization layout.

```
OptPlanarSubgraph optSub;
OneEdgeMinCrossInserter optInsert;
optInsert.removeReinsert(EdgeInsertionModule::all);

SubgraphPlanarizer planarizer;
planarizer.set_subgraph(optSub);
planarizer.set_inserter(optInsert);

PlanarizationLayout plan;
plan.set_planarizer(planarizer);
```

We use a subgraph planarizer called planarizer and set its subgraph option to a module for computing an optimal planar subgraph and its edge insertion option to the OneEdgeMinCrossInserter with the removeReinsert option set to all. Finally, we call the planarization layout algorithm plan for a graph myGraph with the layout information myLayout (containing information on the size of the vertices, the position of the vertices, and the position of the bend points):

```
plan.call(myGraph,myLayout);
```

5 Examples

Figure 11 shows a screenshot of AGD displaying a graph with 62 vertices and 89 edges drawn with the planar mixed model drawing algorithm (see Section 3.2).

Figure 12 shows a quasi-orthogonal drawing (see Section 3.2) of a data base graph from the literature [45] generated by AGD.

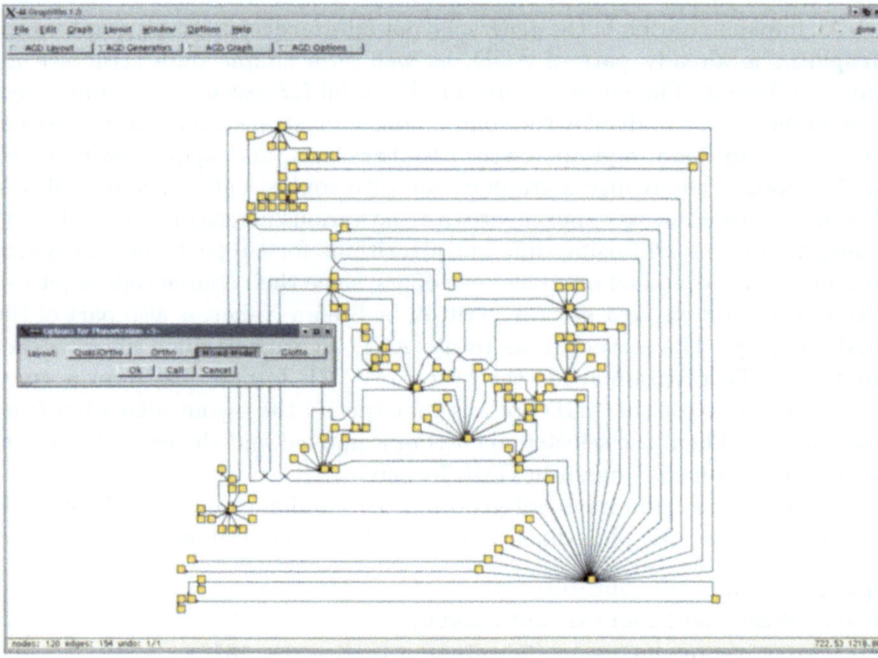

Fig. 11. A screenshot of AGD showing a mixed-model drawing and its options.

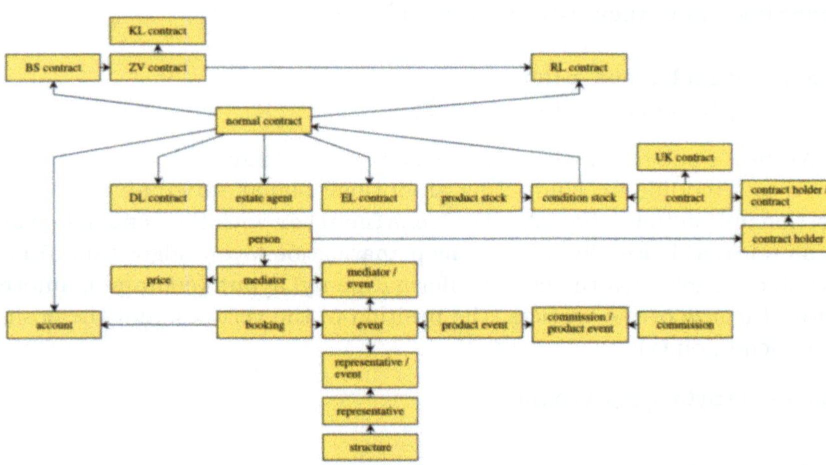

Fig. 12. A quasi-orthogonal drawing of a data base graph.

6 Software

AGD is freely distributed for non-commercial use to universities and academic institutions from the AGD home page (`http://www.ads.tuwien.ac.`

at/AGD/) as platform-dependent binary packages containing precompiled libraries and executable demos. The demos can be used without any additional software or tools. The same holds for the AGD server. This program is command line based and reads a graph from a file. Depending on the parameters given in the command line, a new layout is computed and written into an output file. The library is based on LEDA (currently versions 4.1 and 4.3) [43].

The AGD library comes in two versions, a standard version that fits the need of most users, and the version **agd_opt** with additional layout and optimization algorithms that need special purpose optimization software, namely ABACUS (version 2.3) and the LP-solver CPLEX (**http://www.ilog.com**). ABACUS is currently distributed via OREAS (**http://www.oreas.com**) and will soon become open source. The following list shows the currently available distributions.

Linux

- Standard AGD-R: g++ 3.2, LEDA 4.4
- Standard AGD-R: g++ 2.95.3, LEDA 4.1
- AGD-R OPT: g++ 2.95.3, LEDA 4.1, ABACUS 2.3, CPLEX 6.5+
- The AGD server program
- Demo programs

Windows 95/98/NT

- Standard AGD-R: MS Visual C++ 6.0 (multi-threaded), LEDA 4.1
- The AGD server program
- Demo programs

Acknowledgments

The AGD system, as it is today, is by far not the product of the authors of this paper. It benefits from software contributions and advice of many additional supporters, in alphabetical order: David Alberts, Dirk Ambras, Philipp Blauensteiner, Ralf Brockenauer, Christoph Buchheim, Markus Chimani, Matthias Elf, Sergej Fialko, Carsten Gutwenger, Stefan Hachul, Karsten Klein, Gunter Koch, Michael Krüger, Thomas Lange, Sebastian Leipert, Dirk Lütke-Hüttmann, Stefan Näher, Merijam Percan, Christof Spanring, and Thomas Ziegler. We gratefully acknowledge the fruitful cooperation.

References

1. AGD User Manual (Version 1.2) (2000) Max-Planck-Institut Saarbrücken, Technische Universität Wien, Universität zu Köln, Universität Trier. See also **http://www.ads.tuwien.ac.at/AGD/**

2. Batini, C., Nardelli, E., Tamassia, R. (1986) A layout algorithm for data flow diagrams. IEEE Transactions on Software Engineering **SE-12** (4), 538–546
3. Batini, C., Talamo, M., Tamassia, R. (1984) Computer aided layout of entity relationship diagrams. Journal of System and Software **4**, 163–173
4. Bridgeman, S., Di Battista, G., Didimo, W., Liotta, G., Tamassia, R., Vismara, L. (2000) Turn-regularity and optimal area drawings of orthogonal representations. Computational Geometry: Theory and Application **16** (1), 53–93
5. Buchheim, C., Jünger, M., Leipert, S. (2000) A fast layout algorithm for k-level graphs. In: J. Marks (ed.) Graph Drawing '00, Lecture Notes in Computer Science 1984, Springer-Verlag, 229–240
6. Chrobak, M., Kant, G. (1997) Convex grid drawings of 3-connected planar graphs. International Journal of Computational Geometry and Applications **7** (3), 211–224
7. Coffman, E. G., Graham, R. L. (1972) Optimal scheduling for two processor systems. Acta Informatica **1**, 200–213
8. De Fraysseix, H., Pach, J., Pollack, R. (1990) How to draw a planar graph on a grid. Combinatorica **10** (1), 41–51
9. Di Battista, G., Tamassia, R. (1996) On-line planarity testing. SIAM Journal on Computing **25** (5), 956–997
10. Di Battista, G., Tamassia, R., Tollis, I. G. (1992) Area requirement and symmetry display of planar upward drawings. Discrete and Computational Geometry **7**, 381–401
11. Doorley, M. (1995) Automatic Levelling and Layout of Data Flow Diagrams. PhD thesis, University of Limerick, Ireland
12. Eades P., Kelly, D. (1986) Heuristics for reducing crossings in 2-layered networks. Ars Combinatoria **21** (A), 89–98
13. Eades, P., Lin, X. (1995) A new heuristic for the feedback arc set problem. Australian Journal of Combinatorics **12**, 15–26
14. Eades, P., Wormald, N. (1986) The median heuristic for drawing 2-layers networks. Technical Report 69, Department of Computer Science, University of Queensland
15. Eschbach, T., Günther, W., Drechsler, R., Becker, B. (2002) Crossing reduction by windows optimization. In: M. T. Goodrich and S. G. Kobourov (eds.) Graph Drawing '02, Lecture Notes in Computer Science 2528, Springer-Verlag, 285–294
16. Feng, Q. W., Cohen, R. F., Eades, P. (1995) Planarity for clustered graphs. In: P. Spirakis (ed.) Algorithms – ESA '95, Third Annual European Symposium, Lecture Notes in Computer Science 979, Springer-Verlag, 213–226
17. Fialko, S. (1997) Das planare Augmentierungsproblem. Master's thesis, Universität des Saarlandes, Saarbrücken
18. Fialko, S., Mutzel, P. (1998) A new approximation algorithm for the planar augmentation problem. In: Proc. Ninth Annual ACM-SIAM Symp. Discrete Algorithms (SODA '98), San Francisco, California, ACM Press, 260–269
19. Fößmeier, U., Kaufmann, M. (1996) Drawing high degree graphs with low bend numbers. In: F. J. Brandenburg (ed.) Graph Drawing '95, Lecture Notes in Computer Science 1027, Springer-Verlag, 254–266
20. Fruchtermann, T. M. J., Reingold, E. M. (1991) Graph drawing by force-directed placement. Software – Practice and Experience **21**, 1129–1164

21. Gansner, E. R., Koutsofios, E., North, S. C., Vo, K. P. (1993) A technique for drawing directed graphs. IEEE Transactions on Software Engineering **19**, 214–230
22. Graph Drawing Toolkit: An object-oriented library for handling and drawing graphs. `http://www.dia.uniroma3.it/~gdt`
23. Gelfand, N., Tamassia, R. (1998) Algorithmic patterns for orthogonal graph drawing. In: S. Whitesides (ed.) Graph Drawing '98, Lecture Notes in Computer Science 1547, Springer-Verlag, 138–152
24. Grötschel, M., Jünger, M., Reinelt, G. (1985) On the acyclic subgraph polytope. Mathematical Programming **33**, 28–42
25. Gutwenger, C., Mutzel, P. (1997) Grid embedding of biconnected planar graphs. Max-Planck-Institut für Informatik, Saarbrücken, Germany
26. Gutwenger, C., Mutzel, P. (1998) Planar polyline drawings with good angular resolution. In: S. Whitesides (ed.) Graph Drawing '98, Lecture Notes in Computer Science 1547, Springer-Verlag, 167–182
27. Gutwenger, C., Mutzel, P. (2000) C. Gutwenger and P. Mutzel. A linear-time implementation of SPQR-trees. In: J. Marks (ed.) Graph Drawing '00, Lecture Notes in Computer Science 1984, Springer-Verlag, 77–90
28. Gutwenger, C., Mutzel, P., Weiskircher, R. (2001) Inserting an edge into a planar graph. In: Proceedings of the Ninth Annual ACM-SIAM Symposium on Discrete Algorithms (SODA '2001), Washington, DC, ACM Press, 246–255
29. Himsolt, M. (1997) GML: A portable graph file format. Technical report, Universität Passau, see also `http://www.uni-passau.de/Graphlet/GML`
30. Jünger, M., Leipert, S., Mutzel, P. (1998) A note on computing a maximal planar subgraph using PQ-trees. IEEE Transactions of Computer-Aided Design and Integrated Circuits and Systems **17**, 609–612
31. Jünger, M., Mutzel, P. (1994) The polyhedral approach to the maximum planar subgraph problem: New chances for related problems. In: R. Tamassia and I. G. Tollis (eds.) Graph Drawing '94, Lecture Notes in Computer Science 894, Springer-Verlag, 119–130
32. Jünger, M., Mutzel, P. (1996) Maximum planar subgraphs and nice embeddings: practical layout tools. Algorithmica **16**, 33–59
33. Jünger, M., Mutzel, P. (1997) 2-layer straight line crossing minimization: performance of exact and heuristic algorithms. Journal of Graph Algorithms and Applications **1**, 1–25
34. Jünger, M., Mutzel, P. (2003) Automatic graph drawing: Exact optimization helps! To appear in: M. Grötschel (ed.) The Sharpest Cut – Festschrift zum 60. Geburtstag von Manfred Padberg, MPS-SIAM Series on Optimization
35. Jünger, M., Thienel, S. (2000) The ABACUS system for branch-and-cut and price algorithms in integer programming and combinatorial optimization. Software – Practice and Experience **30**, 1325–1352
36. Kant, G. (1996) Drawing planar graphs using the canonical ordering. Algorithmica, Special Issue on Graph Drawing **16** (1), 4–32
37. Klau, G. W. (1997) Quasi–orthogonales Zeichnen planarer Graphen mit wenigen Knicken. Master's thesis, Universität des Saarlandes, Saarbrücken
38. Klau, G. W., Klein, K., Mutzel P. (2001) An Experimental Comparison of Orthogonal Compaction Algorithms. In: J. Marks (ed.) Graph Drawing '00, Lecture Notes in Computer Science 1984, Springer-Verlag, 37–51

39. Klau, G. W., Mutzel, P. (1998) Quasi–orthogonal drawing of planar graphs. Technical Report MPI-I-98-1-013, Max–Planck–Institut für Informatik, Saarbrücken
40. Klau, G. W., Mutzel P. (1999) Optimal compaction of orthogonal grid drawings. In: G. Cornuejols, R. E. Burkard, and G. J. Woeginger (eds.) Integer Programming and Combinatorial Optimization (IPCO '99), Lecture Notes in Computer Science 1610, Springer-Verlag, 304–319
41. Lengauer, T. (1990) Combinatorial Algorithms for Integrated Circuit Layout. John Wiley & Sons, New York
42. Matuszewski, C., Schönfeld, R., Molitor, P. (1999) Using sifting for k-layer crossing minimization. In J. Kratochvil (ed.) Graph Drawing '99, Lecture Notes in Computer Science 1731, Springer-Verlag, 217–224
43. Mehlhorn, K., Näher, S. (1999) The LEDA Platform of Combinatorial and Geometric Computing. Cambridge University Press
44. Mutzel, P. (1995) A polyhedral approach to planar augmentation and related problems. In P. Spirakis (ed.) Algorithms – ESA '95, Third Annual European Symposium, Lecture Notes in Computer Science 979, Springer-Verlag, 494–507
45. Rauh, O., Stickel, E. (1997) Fallstudien zum Datenbankentwurf. Th. Gabler, Wiesbaden
46. Reingold, E., Tilford, J. (1981) Tidier drawing of trees. IEEE Transactions on Software Engineering **7**, 223–228
47. Rosenstiehl, P., Tarjan, R. E. (1986) Rectilinear planar layouts and bipolar orientations of planar graphs. Discrete and Computational Geometry **1** (4), 343–353
48. Sugiyama, K., Tagawa, S.,Toda, M. (1981) Methods for visual understanding of hierarchical system structures. IEEE Transactions on Systems, Man, and Cybernetics **11**, 109–125
49. Tamassia, R. (1987) On embedding a graph in the grid with the minimum number of bends. SIAM Journal on Computing **16** (3), 421–444
50. Tamassia, R., Di Battista, G., Batini, C. (1988) Automatic graph drawing and readability of diagrams. IEEE Transactions on Systems, Man, and Cybernetics **18**, 61–79
51. Tutte, W. T. (1963) How to draw a graph. In: Proceedings of the London Mathematical Society, Third Series **13**, 743–768
52. Walker II, J. Q. (1990) A node-positioning algorithm for general trees. Software – Practice and Experience **20**, 685–705
53. Ziegler, T. (2001) Crossing minimization in automatic graph drawing. Doctoral Thesis, Technische Fakultät der Universität des Saarlandes

yFiles – Visualization and Automatic Layout of Graphs

Roland Wiese[1], Markus Eiglsperger[2], Michael Kaufmann[2]

[1] yWorks GmbH, Sand 13, 72076 Tübingen, Germany
[2] Wilhelm-Schickard-Institut für Informatik, Universität Tübingen, 72026 Tübingen, Germany

1 Introduction

Viewing, editing, optimizing, layouting and animating – these are the general tasks for a software packet for the visualization of graph-like structures.

An extensive and reliable visualization system is crucial in application areas such as software engineering, database management and database modeling, WWW visualization, bio-informatics, business process engineering and networking. From the aspect of rapidly increasing amount of data and information, it becomes even more important.

Numerous tools have been developed for special purpose applications. These tools often lack extensibility and are hard to maintain. A major goal for us has been to keep the architecture flexible and extensible, so that additional features can be easily added and tools from diverse application areas can be realized.

Although most relational data can be modeled perfectly as graphs, in general however, this modeling step does not imply a useful view for these data. An automatic edit and layout facility which is user-friendly, customizable and is designed to be reusable and extensible provides the necessary basis to build applications that handle complex data and dependencies. This was the main challenge when we started the *yFiles* project.

yFiles has been designed and realized as a Java® -based library for the visualization and automatic layout of graph structures. Figure 1 shows the structure of the library and the main components.

Conceptually, the *yFiles* library consists of three cooperating components:

The *yFiles Basic component* contains essential classes and data structures. It provides very efficient implementations of advanced data structures like graph, trees and priority queues. It furthermore makes available a wide variety of graph and network algorithms.

The *Viewer/Editor component* is built upon the Basic component. It provides a powerful graph viewer component and other Java-Swing based graphical user interface (GUI) elements. Although it provides a wide range of functionality, the user interface has been kept intuitive and easy-to-use. The component is showcased in the yEd [27] graph editor demo application.

The *yFiles Layout component* is also build upon the Basic component. It provides a large suite of graph layout algorithms. Some of them are described in the Section on layout algorithm. Diverse layout styles like hierarchical, orthogonal or specified aspect ratio, circular are supported by easy to integrate components that can be configured by an application programmers interface (API) to suit most layout demands.

The Layout as well as the Viewer/Editor component can be used as independent building blocks. The components have been designed to integrate easily into any Java-based application that either needs a viewer component or layout algorithms for graph structures or both.

Based on the single components, extension packages in different directions are available and can be added, like support for different data formats or special applications like biochemical networks.

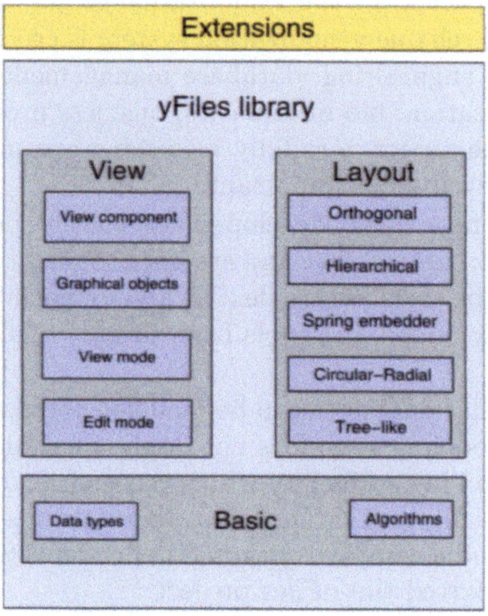

Fig. 1. The main components of the *yFiles* library.

In the following, we give an overview on areas of possible and realized applications and the main layout algorithms as well, we provide a closer look to the main components of the *yFiles* library and describe some prototypical applications.

2 Applications

Meanwhile, *yFiles* has been successfully employed to numerous application domains and, thus, has already proved the high achievements of flexibility and usefulness.

The applications domains of the users include

- Bio-informatics
  - Metabolic and regulatory pathways
  - Protein interaction networks
  - Phylogenetic trees
- Data bases
  - Schema and meta-data visualization
  - Data mining
- Computer and telecommunication networks
  - Systems management
  - Network topology
- Software engineering
  - UML class diagrams
  - parallel execution graphs
- Business applications
  - Business process modeling
  - Work-flow management
  - Customer relationship management
- Knowledge representation
- Analysis of link structures of the WWW
- Social networks
- Animation of algorithms

In the section on Examples, we will describe some of the applications in more detail. A list of reference users can be found at `http://www.yworks.com/en/company_references.htm`.

3 Algorithms

In this section we give an overview of the layout algorithms contained in *yFiles*. We will describe our algorithm that supports the circular-radial layout style and the concept for orthogonal layout in more detail while we review the remaining algorithms and the special features only shortly.

3.1 Circular-Radial Layout

The original circular layout style assumes that the graph is partitioned into clusters, the nodes of each cluster are placed on the circumference of an embedding circle, and each edge is drawn with a straight line [24].

It has found more and more applications in network design and development, especially in the area of computer and telecommunication networks, but also in social networking [18].

The layout style has been introduced by Madden *et al.* [6,15] to the graph drawing community. The method used is a comparably simple heuristic. Six and Tollis [23,24] adapted the style but developed a scientific framework for the approach. Their main idea is to display each biconnected component in a circular way, and the block-tree, i.e., the tree of biconnected components, of the graph as a radial tree of such circles.

The framework of Six and Tollis can be summarized as follows: The graph $G = (V, E)$ is decomposed into the biconnected components which form the resulting block tree. For the articulation nodes v which are not adjacent to a bridge between two components, v is assigned to one of the components. The nodes of each single component are placed on a circle such that the distance between neighboring nodes is fixed. This determines the circumference of each component, which is represented as a single super-node of large size in the following. Next an adoption of the algorithm for radial tree layout (Section 4.1 in the Technical Foundations) [4] taking into account the super-nodes, which usually have different sizes, gives the final layout of the whole structure. In radial tree layouts, the non-root nodes are placed in concentric cycles around the root.

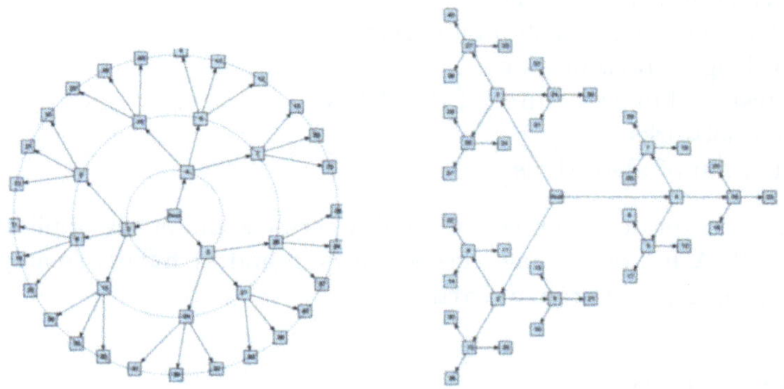

Fig. 2. Comparing the traditional way and the new recursive way for circular-radial layout.

Note that some rotations are also necessary in order to obtain a nice final drawing. Further note that the circular drawing of each component can be enhanced by various techniques for crossing reduction [22,23]. We extended the framework in the following way:

As before, the idea is to take the block tree of biconnected components and layout the root component R in a circular way. Then *recursively* layout the subtrees T adjacent to the root R. The layouts of the subtrees are approximately represented by round super-nodes of a size according of the size of the layout. To find appropriate positions for these super-nodes, the available space around the layout of R is partitioned by straight lines starting from the center of the layout of R. These lines define certain sectors, the so-called wedges [24]. The size of the wedges is chosen appropriate to the size of the super-nodes, while the position of the wedge relative to the layout of R is chosen such that afterward the layout of T, here represented by a super-node, can be attached directly to its articulation point in R.

This recursive concept is very flexible and often provides a much better use of the area as shown in Figure 2 where the two layouts for the same ternary tree are displayed for comparison. Note that for the recursive layout style the used area is linear in the size of the tree while for the traditional radial layout the area is quadratic. In Figure 3, a more complex example shows the organizational group structure of the PCs and workstations within our institute. The recursive nature of the sub-layouts is clearly visible.

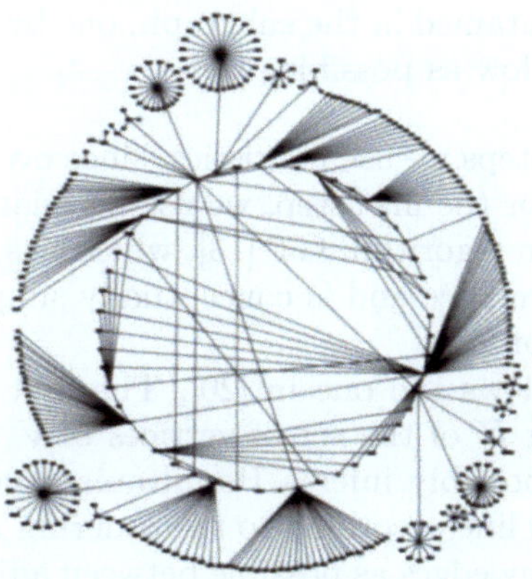

Fig. 3. A more complex example for our circular layouter.

3.2 Orthogonal Layout

For our orthogonal layout, we follow the topology-shape-metrics approach which has been developed by Tamassia. Our algorithm is based on the `Kandinsky` framework. The basics of this approach have been described in Section 4.4 of the Technical Foundations, we shortly review the necessary concepts. Then we show how we extended the paradigm in all three phases: planarization, orthogonalization and compaction.

Planarization. The planarization serves as the first phase in the topological-shape-metrics approach, and it computes a planarized topological representation of the input graph. In a planarized representation, all edge crossings have been replaced by dummy nodes such that a planar graph embedded in the plane appears which then can be used as input for the second phase. Since we want to include more flexibility in our approach, we might require that some of the edges are drawn upward. In contrast to the setting in Section 4.3

of the Technical Foundations, we consider mixed upward planar graphs (see Section 3.2 in the Technical Foundations), where some of the edges are required to have the upward property. We first handle the directed edges, and afterwards the undirected ones.

The basic strategy is derived from techniques for the planarization of undirected graphs: A detailed description together with experimental results can be found in our contribution for the special issue on WADS'01, to appear in the Journal of Graph Algorithms and Applications [8].

- Construct a mixed upward planar subgraph
- Determine a mixed upward embedding of this subgraph
- Insert edges not contained in the subgraph, one by one, keeping the number of crossings as low as possible.

For all these three steps we use heuristics, since even the subproblems are $\mathcal{NP}$-hard in general. For the first step, we use a variant of the Goldschmidt-Takvorian planarization algorithm GT [13], which has been demonstrated to have a very nice performance and is conceptually simple. We shortly review the main components of GT.

Our description follows the one in [20]. The first phase of GT consists of devising an ordering Π of the set of vertices of V of the input graph G. This ordering should possibly infer a Hamiltonian path. The vertices of G are placed on a vertical line according to the ordering Π obtained in the first phase, such that as many edges as possible between adjacent vertices can also be placed on the line. All other edges are drawn as arcs either right or left of the line. In the second phase we determine for each side of the line a set of non-intersecting arcs. If two edges cross when they are drawn on the same side of the line depends exclusively on the node order calculated in the first phase.

The *conflict graph* has a vertex for every edge in G and two vertices are adjacent if the corresponding edges cross with respect to Π. It follows directly from its definition that the conflict graph is an *overlap graph*, i.e., a graph whose vertices can be represented a intervals, and two vertices are adjacent if and only if the corresponding intervals intersect but none of the two is contained by the other. A induced bipartite subgraph of the conflict graph represents a valid planar subgraph. Since finding a maximal induced bipartite subgraph is $\mathcal{NP}$-complete even for overlap graphs GT uses a heuristic. This heuristic calculates two disjoint independent sets of the conflict graph, which together are a bipartite subgraph of the conflict. A maximum independent set of an overlap graph can be calculated efficiently with the algorithm of Asano, Imai and Mukaiyama [1].

The variant including upwardness observes the direction of the edges. The vertex order must ensure that no directed edge has a target vertex which is in the order before the source vertex. Our algorithm is a variation of a topological sorting algorithm and constructs such an ordering incrementally [8].

After having computed a planar subgraph, we insert the remaining edges respecting their directions. The insertion algorithm tries to minimize the number of additional crossings. We first insert the directed edges, then the undirected edges. Here an interesting effect occurs during the insertion of directed edges. While in the undirected case the edges which are not part of the planar subgraph in the first step can be inserted independently of each other, this is different in the directed case. Here we cannot insert an edge into the drawing without looking at the remaining edges which have to be inserted later. The reason for this is that introducing dummy nodes in the graph introduces changes the ordering of the vertices of the graph. This may introduce directed cycles if an edge is added later. We therefore construct a special routing graph which uses layering to ensure that no cycles are created. In Figure 4, we indicate a critical configuration creating new cycles and the solution by the corresponding routing graph.

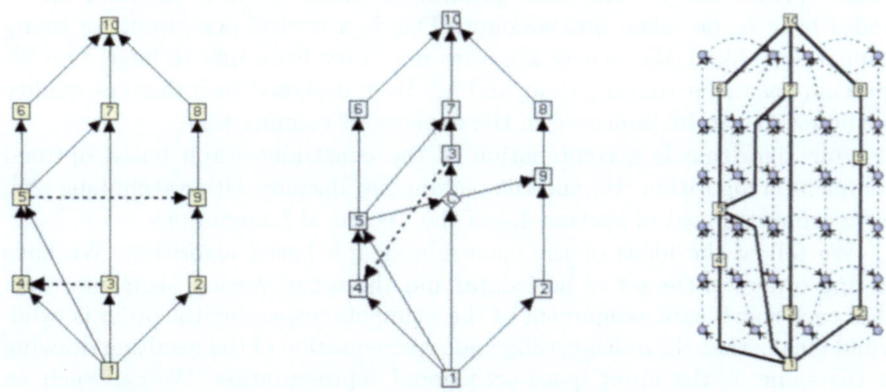

(a) (b) (c)

Fig. 4. Edge insertion: Critical configuration and the routing graph.

Next we apply a local optimization method for an upward planarization to improve the routing of the edges. This method removes a path representing an edge from the planarization. For the removed edge we try to find a better routing. If we succeed, we change the planarization according to the new routing, otherwise we do not change the planarization. We iterate this local optimization until we either do not make any further improvements or a maximal number of iterations has been performed. In a final step the undirected edges are inserted by an algorithm similar to Algorithm 2 in Section 4.3 of the Technical Foundations, which calculates the shortest path in the dual graph of the subgraph.

Orthogonalization and Bend Minimization. In the orthogonalization phase, we use the Kandinsky model with vertices of specified size. Fößmeier

[11] has given a full description of the algorithm for bend-minimization in the Kandinsky model. Since the extension of the min-cost flow algorithm as described in Section 4.4 of the Technical Foundations to the new model is highly complicated, non-trivial and partially not practicable, we apply a flow heuristics to keep our approach simple and robust. Robustness is necessary since very often additional constraints like upwardness, relative positioning etc. are required. Our heuristic essentially consists of a greedy path search for the flows keeping the costs as low as possible. The results of this approach are very satisfactory.

We described a lot of the ideas how to enhance the basic scheme by various constraints in [7] but since this approach is based on linear programming, we decided not to include the concept in *yFiles* by now.

Compaction. Here, we shortly review our compaction algorithm. For a detailed version see [8]. The most prominent feature is that the sizes of the nodes have to be taken into account. This is a critical constraint for many applications like UML, where the sizes may vary from tiny to huge. Our algorithm has linear running time, and has been designed such that the quality of the result can be improved in the expense of running time.

Our algorithm is a combination of the constraint-graph based optimal compaction algorithm [16] and the rectangular decomposition technique [26], both are mentioned in Section 4.4 of the Technical Foundations.

We follow the ideas of the constraint-graph based algorithm: We have to find orders of the set of horizontal and the set of vertical segments, such that each coordinate assignment of the segments respecting the order is valid. Valid means that the quasi-orthogonal representation of the resulting drawing is the same as the input quasi-orthogonal representation. We call such an order *complete.*

A quasi-orthogonal representation defines implicitly a partial order for the horizontal and the vertical segments, which all complete orders must contain. Unfortunately these orders are not necessarily complete. We denote these orders in *constraint graphs*: the vertical constraint graph and the horizontal constraint graph. Klau and Mutzel proposed a branch-and-cut algorithm which extends the constraint graphs such that the resulting complete ordering implies a drawing which has minimal total edge length. Unfortunately, this approach has exponential worst-case running time, since the problem is $\mathcal{NP}$-hard (see Section 4.4 in the Technical Foundations).

We use an alternative approach which simulates the well-known rectangular decomposition technique, but not by subdividing more complicated faces into rectangles by additional edges but by adding corresponding edges to the constraint graph. The resulting algorithm has linear running time, but produces no longer drawings with minimal edge length.

To guarantee the prescribed side lengths of each vertex, we replace each non-dummy vertex by a rectangular face. Each edge adjacent to the node has a node on the border of this face. Also four corner nodes replacing the four corner bends are created. The result is a 4-graph with a simple orthogonal representation. Then the total order in the constraint graph has to be determined obeying the length constraints on the new faces that replace original vertices. This is particularly difficult, since by those length constraints, there might be negative cycles in the constraint graph, such that a completion of the constraint graph might still imply a non-feasible solution, see part *c* of Figure 5. In [8], we describe how we technically get around this problem and report on experiments of running times.

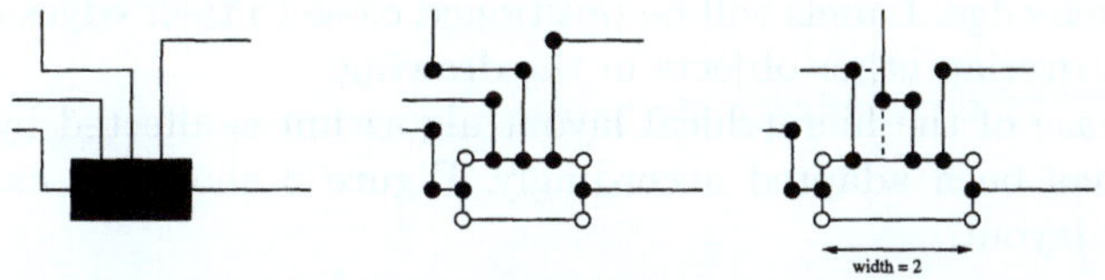

(a) (b) (c)

Fig. 5. Transformation of a node into a face and an invalid compaction.

We found it very pleasant to place the edges near the center of the node. Especially, placing the sole non-bending edge on a vertex side in the center of the node yields nice drawings. This port assignment can be easily achieved by adding edges into the constraint graphs which point from the bottom, resp. left, segment of the vertex to the according segment of the edge.

To improve an existing drawing, we can apply one-dimensional compaction, known from VLSI-design (see, e.g., [19]), as post-processing. We can reuse for this case the compaction algorithm; we only have to replace the rectangle decomposition step by a separation function based on the visibility of segments in the input drawing.

3.3 Layered Layout

Here we follow the traditional Sugiyama-approach (see Section 4.2 in the Technical Foundations). For each phase of the algorithm we provide multiple alternatives:

Layer assignment: longest path layering, network flow (simplex), fixed
Crossing minimization: barycenter and median heuristics
Coordinate assignment: linear segments (at most 2 bends), pendulum [21], network flow (simplex)

Optionally edges can be routed orthogonally.

Unique extensions are support for port constraints, arbitrary layer assignments, node grouping and integrated edge labeling.

Port constraints allow to specify for each edge the side of the node to which it connects. Additionally the port coordinates for the final drawing can be specified. For example port constraints can be used to force each edge to leave its source node at the bottom side and enter its target node at the top side, regardless of the relative position of the nodes. Arbitrary layer assignments also include non-hierarchical cases where nodes connected with each other reside on the same layer. Applications for this feature are commonly found in interactive settings. Grouping allows to partition the nodes within each layer into several groups. Nodes within the same group will be placed in a block within each layer. The layout algorithm can position an arbitrary number of labels for each edge. Labels will be positioned close to their edges and so that they do not overlap other objects in the drawing.

Each phase of the hierarchical layout algorithm is affected by these features and has been adapted accordingly. Figure 6 shows an example of a hierarchical layout.

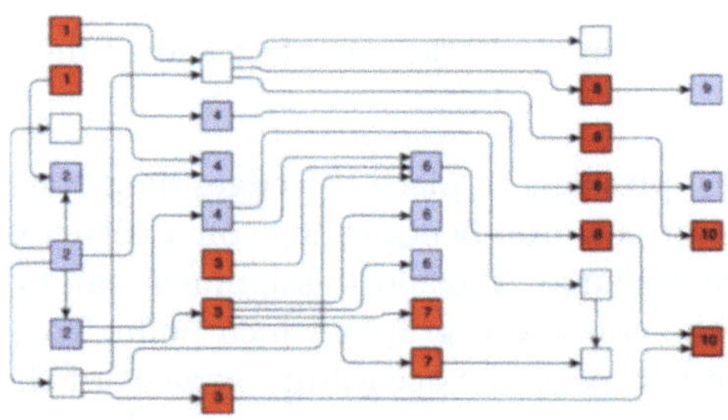

Fig. 6. An example for the hierarchical layout, enriched by a fixed layer assignment and grouping of nodes. The red and bluish nodes form a group, white nodes do not belong to any group. Note that because of the fixed layer assignment, the diagram contains edges with endpoints in the same layer.

3.4 Force-Directed Approach

The algorithm based on the force-directed paradigm follows the ideas described in Section 4.5 of the Technical Foundations. It supports individual edge lengths and layout of subgraphs. Furthermore the running time of the algorithm can be limited by a time bound. An interesting and very fast alternative by [17] which follows the idea to start with a coarse representation of the input graph and use iterative refinement, has recently been included in the collection of layout algorithms.

3.5 Tree Layout

For trees, we have realized the Reingold-Tilford approach (Section 4.1 of the Technical Foundations), and some more advanced algorithms that should demonstrate the ability and flexibility of the system. Here, a hv-like drawing style [3] where the child nodes are placed to the right as well as below the corresponding parent node should be mentioned. This variant allows to specify the aspect ratio of the layout area and in that sense, it provides an essential improvement of the use of the area and aspect ratio compared to the conventional tree drawing approaches. In Figure 7, we give an example comparing a traditional 'Reingold-Tilford tree' layout with the new hv-like layout.

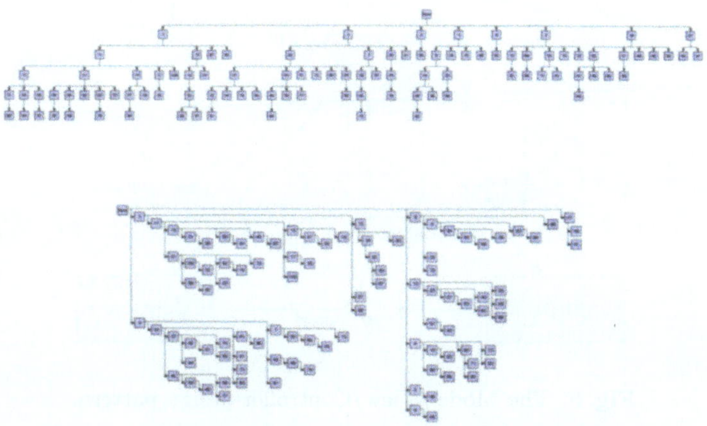

Fig. 7. A traditional Reingold-Tilford tree layout in orthogonal style, and a more advanced hv-like version realized within our library.

4 Implementation

In this section, we take a closer look to the three cooperating components of the library:

4.1 Basic Component

The Basic component contains the following algorithms and data structures:

- Data structures: graph, linked list, stack, queue, priority queue
- Graph traversal: Dfs, Bfs
- Graph connectivity: connected, biconnected
- Node orderings: st-ordering, topological sorting
- Shortest Paths: Dijkstra, Bellman-Ford
- Minimum Spanning Tree: Prim, Kruskal
- Network flow: Max flow, Min-cost flow
- Rank Assignment: Simplex method

The most important data structure is the graph data structure. Essentially all algorithms act on this data structure. The Viewer/Editor component and the Layout component use extended versions of it.

4.2 Viewer/Editor Component

The editor/viewer fully supports the complete set of graphical attributes necessary for effective graph visualization. The viewer architecture adheres to the model-view-control design pattern, cf. Figure 8.

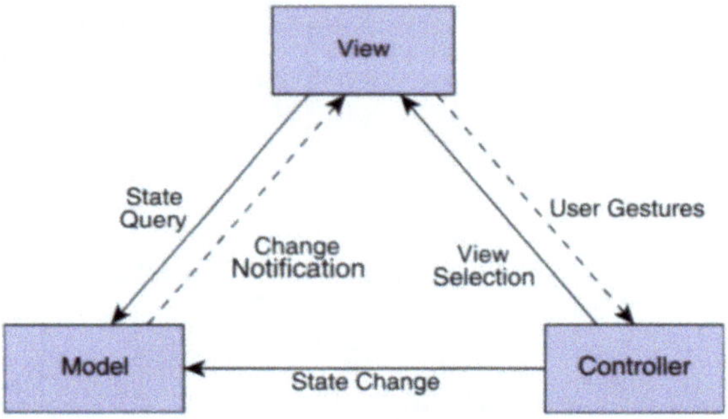

Fig. 8. The Model/View/Controller design pattern.

Decoupling the *model* (i.e., the graph) from the *view* allows to represent a single graph in multiple views at the same time, e.g., in a detailed view and an overview that allows panning the view-port of the main view.

The *view* component itself is a Java-Swing based component that can easily be added to any application GUI. It supports features like zooming, scrolling, layout morphing and rendering at different levels of detail.

The appearance of nodes and edges is defined by so called realizer classes. Default node realizers can represent nodes as colored shapes or images. Default edge realizers can represent edge paths as polylined, splined or arcs with graphical arrow and port augments if desired. All realizers can manage one or more multi-line labels.

Since certain application types like UML tools require a special graphical representation of nodes and edges, it is possible to define customized graphical representations of all graph features.

All graph features can be equipped with one or more labels. For each label there is an associated label model and label position. Each label model defines a set of symbolic label positions which are available within that model. Label models are an elegant way to constrain the set of available label positions for graph features that an automatic labeling algorithm can choose from. The labeling algorithms are adapted versions of the well-known labeling algorithm by Christensen, Marks and Shieber [2].

The *control* defines the way in which a user can interact with the view and the underlying model. The graph viewer can be extended to a graph editor by connecting specialized controls to the view.

We call these controls *view modes*. A view mode defines the way a user can interact with the viewer. Each view mode itself can temporarily activate minor view modes which are responsible for specialized interaction scenarios like creating an edge, opening a pop-up menu or drawing a rubber-band box for object selection. This way, it is quite easy to define a customized view mode by plugging together a set of available minor view modes.

4.3 Layout Component

Currently *yFiles* includes graph layout algorithms for the following styles: Hierarchical, tree, force-directed, circular-radial and orthogonal. These algorithms are mostly tuned variants of published algorithms [21], [10], [12], [24], the basic variants have been reviewed in Section 4 of the Technical Foundations. The implementation of the algorithms is guided by the principles of *robustness* and *efficiency*. All algorithms (except the tree layouter) make no assumptions about the input graph. The algorithms can handle graphs which contain an arbitrary number of self-loops, multiple edges, connected components, etc.

Besides layout algorithms which assign coordinates to edge paths and nodes, *yFiles* also supports the automatic assignment of edge and node label coordinates [2].

Both layout and labeling algorithms can be customized to a high degree. Customization can be done by either setting layout parameters or by exchanging certain stages of an algorithm by customized code.

The ability to customize and combine the different layout algorithms and styles has proved to provide a high flexibility and user-friendliness.

4.4 File Formats

The following file formats for graphs are supported by *yFiles*:

- The ygf file format is the native format of *yFiles*. It is extensible and stores all graphical features supported by *yFiles*.
- The GML file format, which is a text based format widely used in the graph drawing community [14].
- The GraphML file format, a non-proprietary XML-based format which has currently been developed and introduced (`www.graphdrawing.org`), and which is gaining increasing popularity from the community.

Furthermore, images of graphs can be exported in the following formats:

- The SVG format is a popular XML-based scalable vector graphics format.
- jpg and gif are standard image based export-only formats.

5 Examples

In this section, we demonstrate the large diversity of possible applications of our library by giving some examples that have been developed using *yFiles*.

5.1 yEd - Graph Editor

yEd [27] is a powerful graph editor that is written entirely in the Java programming language. It can be used to quickly generate drawings and apply automatic layouts to all kinds of diagrams and networks. It is built using Swing components, i.e., it will run on any platform for which there is a suitable Java Runtime Environment available. yEd has an intuitive user interface, that complies with the Design Guidelines for Java Applications. Among its various features are:

- Undo-ability support
- Clipboard facility
- Keyboard shortcuts for most of the functions.
- A help system

Figure 9 gives an impression of the user interface of yEd.

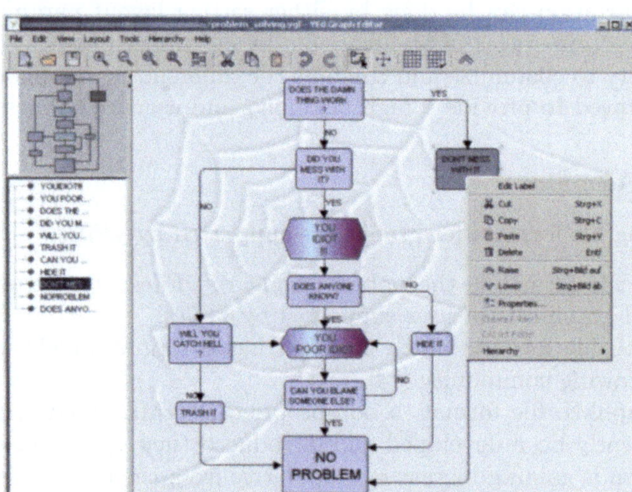

Fig. 9. Screen-shot of the yEd graph editor.

5.2 JarInspector - UML Class Diagrams

JarInspector [9] is an application that displays automatically generated UML class diagrams, mainly using a combination of techniques we discussed in the section on orthogonal layout algorithms. It can be downloaded at [28].

The program should not be considered as a full-featured reverse engineering tool. Its main aim is to show how automatic layout can be used in the scenario of software engineering,

The program takes Java byte-code as input, either from a Java archive (jar) or from class files stored in a directory hierarchy, and generates an UML model from it, which contains the following information:

- Each class or interface defined in the byte-code,
- all generalization relationship between classes/interfaces,
- all package dependencies, and
- associations which are defined by a field of a class.

The content of the generated UML model can be browsed interactively by the user. For each selected view of the model, a diagram is generated and layouted automatically. The layout of the diagram obeys standard æsthetic criteria for class diagrams. The inheritance relation between classes is drawn upward, in a tree-like fashion, while non-inheritance edges are drawn to minimize crossings and bends. In Figure 10, a screen-shot of the JarInspector application shows the layout of a UML class diagram.

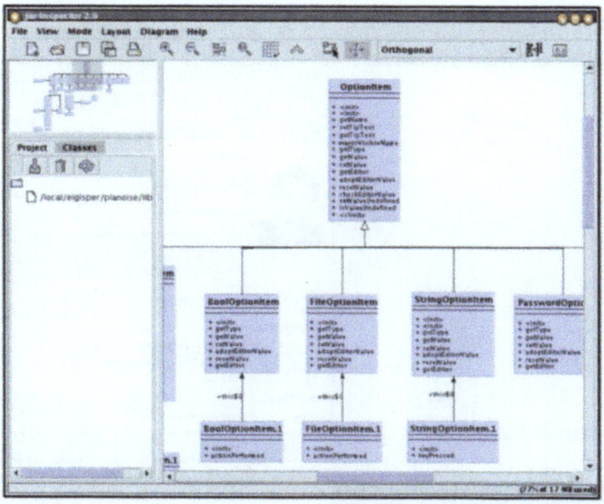

Fig. 10. Screen-shot of the `JarInspector` application.

5.3 yWeb - User-Driven Interactive Site-maps

In this project, we developed an application for the automatic generation of interactive navigational site-maps. As the basis for visualization and interaction we analyze usage data to find popular paths traveled by users through a web-site.

The technique is part of our site-map system called *yWeb* [5,29]. Usage-based site-maps provide an alternative view of a web locality by enhancing frequently used paths between web pages. The popular path map can therefore be seen as a result of collaborative filtering action that distinguishes possibly interesting content from the huge number of nodes available in a web locality.

Our popular path layout was our first excursion into the realm of usage-based layouts. It proved to be of special interest by providing information about the close external neighborhood of a web locality by visualizing the external referers which provide a rich contextual cue for the respective site nodes. Another distinguished feature was the dynamic filtering technique that allows the user to select the map's level of granularity by modifying the number of visible paths while preserving the mental map. Figure 11 shows a layout of the site-map of our university group, with emphasis on the home-page of Markus Eiglsperger.

We have performed tests on a variety of very different data sets which showed the robustness of our approach [5]. The examined localities include university departments, commercial sites, online magazines, download sites and private home-pages.

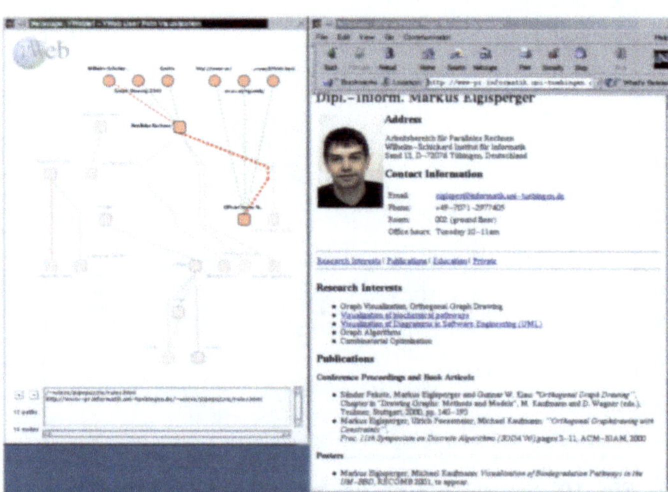

Fig. 11. A display of the site-map of the web site of our working group, highlighted are the most popular user paths to the home-page of Markus Eiglsperger.

5.4 yWays - Interactive Visualization of Metabolic Pathways

yWays is a library for the visualization of metabolic networks. It is built upon *yFiles* and provides, like *yFiles*, a view and a layout component.

The usage of yWays as a visualization component is demonstrated in the software BioMiner. BioMiner is a new software system for analyzing and visualizing complex biochemical networks and processes. BioMiner was designed to simplify the implementation of tools for answering a broad range of interesting biochemical questions. At the moment the main feature of BioMiner is finding new metabolic pathways. BioMiner has mainly been developed at the Center of Bio-informatics in Saarbrücken and in our group [25].

The system is designed as a three-tier application. The first tier provides interfaces to existing database. The second tier is responsible for the analysis of biochemical data. The result of the analysis is visualized in the third tier. On the basis of the yWays library, we were able to provide a visualization component for the third tier which nicely meets the requirements of the users.

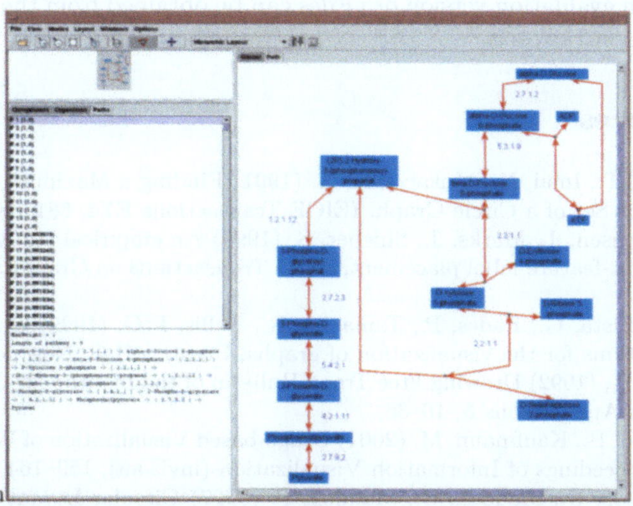

Fig. 12. A screen-shot of the user interface of yWays.

In Figure 12, we give a glimpse of the user interface. The component offers a number of options, among them *reaction clustering* and *show EC numbers/co-compounds on/off*. In the above case, the reactions are clustered and displayed in red. EC numbers are shown next to the respective reaction edge. Co-compounds are hidden. If clustering is disabled, each organism is coded with a certain color used for each reaction that belongs to this organism. Furthermore, different *views* are possible. In the global view, the whole metabolic network (*MG*) is displayed. When the user chooses a pathway from the list of detected pathways, all according reactions are highlighted in the graph. The user can browse through the list to see the differences between the pathways. In the path view, only those reactions and substrates are shown that actually belong to the chosen pathway. Further sub-windows show, among other things, the pathway as a list in the form substrate – EC number – substrate, the list of organisms, the list of all compounds with s and t being marked, an overview window, a reaction window where a selected reaction is shown in detail, and a compound window with detailed informations for a chosen compound. The user can select from different layout algorithms and a number of different parameters. Also the graph can interactively be rearranged.

6 Software

The library runs on all Java2 platforms, currently including Linux, Solaris, HPUX, MacOS X, and Microsoft Windows (95/98/2000/NT/XP).

By now, the *yFiles* library is a commercial product distributed by yWorks GmbH. An evaluation version of *yFiles* can be obtained from the yWorks web page `www.yworks.com`.

References

1. Asano, T., Imai, H., Mukaiyama, A. (1991) Finding a Maximum Weight Independent Set of a Circle Graph. IEICE Transactions **E74**, 681–683.
2. Christensen, J., Marks, J., Shieber, S. (1995) An empirical study of algorithm for point-feature label placement, ACM Transactions on Graphics **14** (3), 203–232
3. Di Battista, G., Eades, P., Tamassia, R., Tollis, I. G. (1999) Graph Drawing: Algorithms for the visualization of graphs. Prentice Hall, New Jersey
4. Eades P., (1992) Drawing Free Trees, Bulletin of the Institue for Combinatorics and its Applications **5**, 10–36
5. Diebold, B., Kaufmann, M. (2001) Usage-based Visualization of Web Localities. In: Proceedings of Information Visualization (invis.au), 159–164
6. Dogrusöz, U., Madden, B., Madden, P. (1997) Circular Layout in the Graph Layout Toolkit. In: S. North (ed.) Graph Drawing '96, Lecture Notes in Computer Science 1190, Springer-Verlag, 92–100
7. Eiglsperger, M., Fößmeier, U., Kaufmann, M. (2000) Orthogonal graph drawing with constraints. In: Proceedings of the 11th ACM-SIAM Symposium on Discrete Algorithms, 3–11
8. Eiglsperger, M., Kaufmann, M. (2001) Fast Compaction for Orthogonal Drawing with Vertices of prescribed Size. In: P. Mutzel, M. Jünger, S. Leipert (eds.) Graph Drawing '01, Lecture Notes in Computer Science 2265, 124-138
9. Eiglsperger, M., Kaufmann, M., Siebenhaller, M. (to appear) Automatic layout for UML class diagrams. SOFTVIS'03.
10. Fößmeier, U., Kaufmann, M. (1995) Drawing high degree graphs with low bend numbers, In: F.-J. Brandenburg (ed.) Graph Drawing '95, Lecture Notes in Computer Science 1027, Springer-Verlag, 254–266

11. Fößmeier, U. (1997) Orthogonale Visualisierungstechniken für Graphen, Dissertation, University of Tübingen
12. Frick, A., Ludwig, A., Mehldau, H. (1995) A fast adaptive layout algorithm for undirected graphs. In: R. Tamassia, I. G. Tollis (eds.) Graph Drawing '94, Lecture Notes in Computer Science 894, Springer-Verlag, 388–403
13. Goldschmidt, O., Takvorian, A. (1994) An efficient graph planarization two-phase heuristic. Networks **24**, 69–73
14. Himsolt, M. (1997) GML: A portable Graph File Format. Technical Report, University of Passau
15. Kar, G., Madden, B., Gilbert, R. (1988) Heuristic Layout Algorithms for Network Presentation Services, IEEE Network **11**, 29–36
16. Klau, G. W., Mutzel, P. (1999) Optimal compaction of orthogonal grid drawings. In: Integer Programming and Combinatorial Optimization (IPCO'99), Lecture Notes in Computer Science 1610, 304–319
17. Gajer, P., Kobourov, S. (2002) GRIP: Graph Drawing with Intelligent Placement. Journal of Graph Algorithms and Applications **6** (3), Special Issue on GD '00, 203–224
18. Krebs, V. (1996) Visualizing Human Networks. Release 1.0: Esther Dyson's Monthly Report, 1–25
19. Lengauer, T. (1990) Combinatorial Algorithms for Integrated Circuit Layout. Wiley-Teubner
20. Resende, M., Ribeiro, C. (1997) A GRASP for graph planarization, Networks **29**, 173–189
21. Sander, G. (1994) Graph layout through the VCG tool. Technical Report A03/94, Universität des Saarlandes
22. Six, J. M., Tollis, I. G. (1999) Circular Drawings of Biconnected Graphs. Proc. Alenex '99, Lecture Notes in Computer Science 1619, Springer-Verlag, 57–73
23. Six, J. M., Tollis, I. G. (2000) A Framework for Circular Drawings of Networks. In: J. Kratochvil (ed.) Graph Drawing '99, Lecture Notes in Computer Science 1731, Springer-Verlag, 107–116
24. Six, J.M. (2000) VisTool: A Tool for Visualizating Graphs. Ph.D. Thesis, University of Texas at Dallas
25. Širava, M., et al. (2002) BioMiner – Modeling, Analyzing, and Visualizing Biochemical Pathways and Networks. In: Proceedings of ECCB, Bioinformatics **19** (10)
26. Tamassia, R. (1987) On Embedding a Graph in the Grid with the Minimum Number of Bends. SIAM Jounal on Computing **16** (3), 421–444
27. `http://www.yworks.com/products/yed`
28. `http://www-pr.informatik.uni-tuebingen.de/research/uml/jarinspector.xml`
29. `http://www-pr.informatik.uni-tuebingen.de/research/yweb`

GDS – A Graph Drawing Server on the Internet*

Stina Bridgeman[1] and Roberto Tamassia[2]

[1] Department of Computer Science, Colgate University, Hamilton, NY 13346, USA
[2] Center for Geometric Computing, Brown University, Providence, RI 02912, USA

1 Introduction

Motivated by the wide variety of applications in many different fields, new graph drawing algorithms are continually being developed and implemented. However, there are many barriers in the way of someone wishing to make use of this technology. First, a potential user must know that the technology exists, which often means she must be well-versed in the terminology and literature of the graph drawing community. Then she must locate and install an implementation, which requires that the software creators provided the correct executable for her environment, or that she has the knowledge and tools to build the application from source code. Running the newly-installed program requires sufficient computational resources (CPU power, memory, disk space). Finally, due to the wealth of different graph description formats, it is likely that she must convert her data to the format used by the program. Another translation step may be required at the end, if the program does not output the data in a format she can use. Overall, this process is time-consuming for even an expert user, and may be prohibitively difficult for the casual or novice user.

Furthermore, it can be difficult to reuse graph algorithms and graph drawing algorithms in other contexts — libraries and packages such as LEDA [17], AGD [1] (see the chapter on AGD in this book), and GDToolkit [14] provide collections of graph algorithms, but only programs developed in C++ (or capable of calling a separate executable) can make use of these implementations. Using a particular algorithm in an applet, for example, requires that it be recoded in Java — a potentially non-trivial task, and wasteful since it has already been implemented and thoroughly tested in another package.

A service which aims to remove these obstacles has several requirements:

Ease-of-use: The user interface should be simple and intuitive, and the user should not need to be aware of algorithm details like file formats and command lines.

* The authors would like to thank Gill Barequet, Christian Duncan, Ashim Garg, and Michael Goodrich for their contributions to the Graph Drawing Server and GeomNet, and Rob Mason for the creation of the graph editor applet.

Platform Independence: The service should be available to as many machine architectures as possible, and clients should be able to obtain reasonable performance even with limited resources.

Flexibility: The service should not be limited to only certain types of algorithms, or only certain types of clients.

Authoring: It should be possible to easily integrate existing implementations into the system.

Data Protection: Proprietary client data should be protected from unauthorized access.

Code Protection: Algorithm code should be protected from software piracy.

Security: The service infrastructure should be safe from intruder attacks and unauthorized users.

The Graph Drawing Server (GDS) [8] is a web-based graph drawing and translation service which aims to satisfy these requirements. It uses the ASP model, where application service providers host applications on behalf of remote users. A user needs only a commonly-available web browser to access a variety of algorithms, without having to install any additional software. (Advanced or frequent users can opt to install a client module on their own computers to obtain access to more advanced features.) Few restrictions are placed on the types of software that can be integrated into the service, so that algorithms from many sources can be easily incorporated. Furthermore, the Graph Drawing Server supports a number of different graph description formats and will automatically convert between any of those formats and the format(s) required by requested tools. As a result, once the user's graph data is in a format supported by the service, any of GDS' algorithms can be used without requiring the user to perform further format conversions.

Users interact with the service by sending a request consisting of the graph to be drawn, the algorithm to be run and values for its parameters, the format of the input, and the desired format for the output. Output formats include GIF and Postscript, so that drawings can easily be included in papers and presentations. Requests can be sent using a graph editor applet or a set of forms-based web pages, allowing casual or novice users to make use of the service immediately. For more advanced applications, user programs can make socket or HTTP connections directly to the service. The educational software tool PILOT [9] uses a socket connection to GDS to produce a layout for graph-based problems.

GDS has received over 65,000 requests from 70 countries in six years of operation.

2 Applications

The Graph Drawing Server was designed to be flexible in both the algorithms and interfaces it can support. Potential uses of the Graph Drawing Server include:

Graph Drawing: The service can be used to draw user-supplied graphs with a variety of drawing algorithms.

Translation: The service can be used in a "translation-only" mode to convert between graph descriptions in different formats.

Graph Exploration: Different drawing algorithms can highlight different aspects of a graph's structure, and the Graph Drawing Server makes it easy to try out a variety of algorithms on the same graph.

Demonstration: The service can be used to demonstrate graph drawing algorithms in an educational setting, without requiring setup overhead.

Experimentation: By collecting many algorithms in one place and removing the need to convert graphs into many different formats, the Graph Drawing Server provides an ideal test bed for experimental comparisons of graph drawing algorithms.

Testing and Development: New algorithms can be easily added to the Graph Drawing Server, and once incorporated into the service, they can be used with any of the existing GDS interfaces. This is especially useful for testing algorithms, as GDS' graph editor can then be used to construct test cases and view the results. This can be more convenient than working directly with text-based graph descriptions.

Evaluation: Graph drawing algorithms can be made available to customers on a "try before you buy" basis, without releasing code to customers.

Web Services: Graph drawing algorithms can also be made available to customers on a fee-per-use basis.

Prototyping: User programs can connect to GDS through a socket connection, allowing the service's graph drawing algorithms to be used as subroutines. This allows rapid prototyping of systems requiring a graph drawing component.

The graph drawing algorithms supported by the service are suitable for a variety of applications.

3 Algorithms

The algorithms available through the Graph Drawing Server come from a variety of sources — GDS does not replace existing graph drawing packages, but rather brings them to a wider audience.

GDS currently supports several general-purpose algorithms for orthogonal, hierarchical, and force-directed drawings, plus specialized algorithms for trees and series-parallel digraphs. New algorithms can be easily incorporated into the service.

3.1 Graph Drawing Algorithms

In the following, n is the number of vertices in the graph, e is the number of edges, and c is the number of crossings in the resulting drawing. Figures 4 and 5 show drawings produced by each of the drawing algorithms.

GIOTTO utilizes the topology-shape-metrics approach for constructing an orthogonal drawing. The planarization phase is based on the algorithm of Batini *et al.* described in Section 4.3 of the Technical Foundations. The orthogonalization and compaction phases use the flow-network-based techniques of Tamassia, see Section 4.4 in the Technical Foundations.

Since GIOTTO accepts a general multigraph as input, two pre-processing steps are needed: first, the input graph is augmented as necessary to create a connected graph, and second, vertices with degree higher than four are replaced by a cycle of degree three vertices (see Figure 1(b)). The cycle vertices are allowed to overlap during compaction, and in the final drawing, a single expanded vertex will replace the cycle (Figure 1(c)).

GIOTTO typically produces high-quality drawings with a small area, though the minimum area is not guaranteed. The time complexity is $O((n+c)^2 \log(n+c))$.

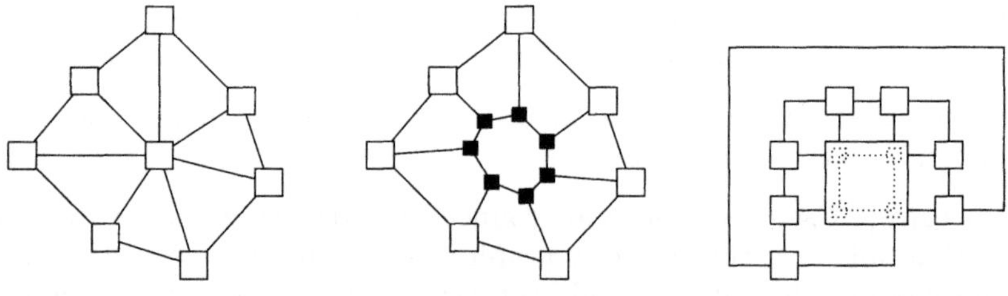

(a) The starting graph.

(b) The high-degree vertex is replaced with a cycle of degree-three vertices.

(c) The final drawing, with an expanded vertex.

Fig. 1. GIOTTO's handling of high-degree vertices. In the final drawing, dotted boxes and lines show the position of the cycle vertices.

BEND-STRETCH differs from GIOTTO only in the orthogonalization step, where it uses the "bend-stretching" heuristic of Tamassia and Tollis [20] to reduce the number of bends. This heuristic makes use of three transformations:

(T1) Two consecutive bends in opposite directions on the same edge can be eliminated. (Figure 2(a))
(T2) If all of the edges incident on a vertex have bends in the same direction, the vertex can be rotated to remove those bends. (Figure 2(b))
(T3) A vertex with a free port on the correct side can be shifted along one of its incident edges to absorb a bend on that edge. (Figure 2(c))

The transformations are applied in order, with each used as often as applicable before the next is tried. While this heuristic does not guarantee a bend-minimal drawing, it does guarantee a (small) constant number of bends per edge. BEND-STRETCH runs in $O(n + c)$ time.

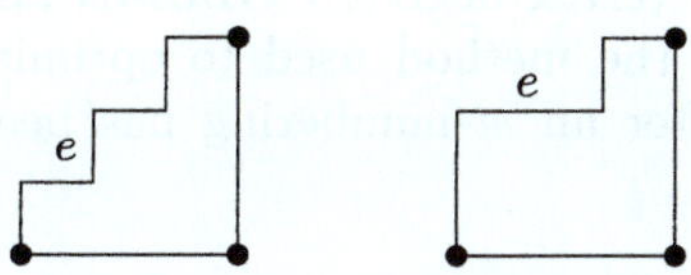

(a) T1. One application removes two bends from edge e; another would remove two more bends.

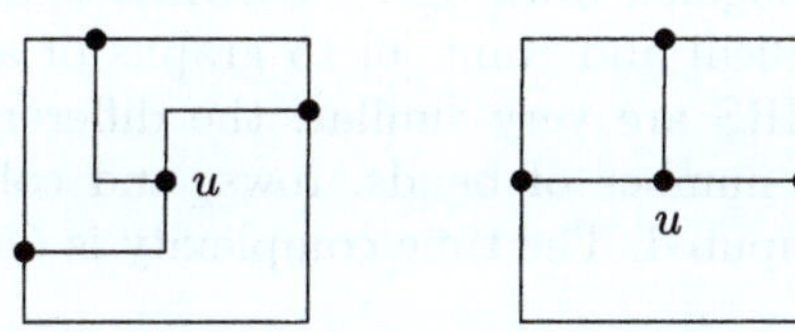

(b) T2. "Rotating" vertex u eliminates one bend from edge adjacent edge.

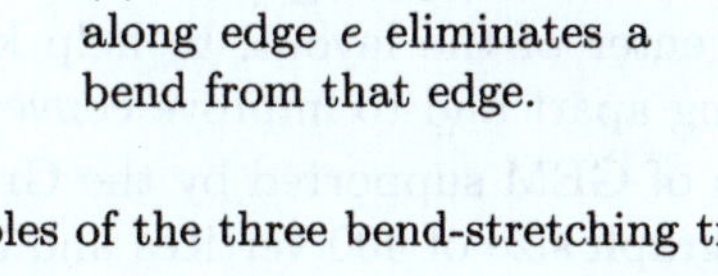

(c) T3. Shifting vertex u along edge e eliminates a bend from that edge.

Fig. 2. Examples of the three bend-stretching transformations.

PAIRS utilizes the incremental construction approach of Papakostas and Tollis [18] for producing orthogonal drawings. PAIRS is limited to graphs of maximum degree four. An *st*-numbering of the graph guides the algorithm.

Graph edges are directed from lower-numbered vertices to higher-numbered vertices. The numbering is first used to identify pairs of vertices so that every degree 3 or degree 4 vertex (other than the source) with at least two outgoing edges belongs to exactly one pair. Each pair results in a "saved" row or column in the final drawing: with a row pair, both vertices are drawn on the same row, or one vertex is drawn on the same row as some other vertex; for a column pair, the vertices are drawn so that at least two different edges can share a column. Once the pairs have been identified, the drawing is constructed by processing vertices in order of the *st*-numbering and placing them according to specific drawing rules. Vertices which are not part of pairs are placed on new rows; vertices which belong to pairs are placed along with the other vertex in the pair, according to the rules for that pair. The result is a drawing with less than n^2 area, a linear number of bends, and at most two bends per edge. The time complexity of the algorithm is $O((n+e)\log(n+e))$.

COLUMN also utilizes the incremental construction approach for producing orthogonal drawings. COLUMN extends the orthogonal drawing algorithm of Biedl and Kant [6] to graphs of arbitrary vertex degree. COLUMN and PAIRS are very similar; the difference is in the method used to optimize the number of bends, rows, and columns after an *st*-numbering has been computed. The time complexity is $O(n + e)$.

GEM [13] uses force-directed layout techniques as described in Section 4.5 of the Technical Foundations. It is designed to achieve good layouts of medium-sized graphs at interactive speeds. Traditional simulated annealing approaches use a global temperature to control how far a vertex can move in a given step; the temperature is gradually cooled so that the drawing converges to a stable state. In addition to a global temperature, GEM allows the temperature of each vertex to be controlled separately. Heuristics are included to detect if a vertex is moving towards its proper location, or if the vertex is involved in an oscillation or rotation. In the first case, raising the vertex temperature can help speed it towards its goal. In the latter cases, lowering the vertex temperature can help damp the oscillation/rotation so the layout converges more quickly. Finally, GEM includes a gravitational force which pulls vertices towards the barycenter of the layout, to help keep loosely connected components from drifting apart and to improve convergence speed.

The implementation of GEM supported by the Graph Drawing Server is limited to a maximum graph size of 400 vertices and 3000 edges.

Sugiyama constructs a layered drawing of a directed graph using the original method of Sugiyama *et al.* as described in Section 4.2 of the Technical Foundations. If the input graph is not directed, it is converted to a directed graph before drawing.

REINGOLD-TILFORD is an adaptation of the Reingold-Tilford binary-tree algorithm (described in Section 4.1 of the Technical Foundations) to handle general trees. Each node is centered above the bounding rectangle of its children. The graph must be directed.

ORTHO-UPWARD produces a straight-line orthogonal upward drawing of a binary tree using the "recursive winding" algorithm of Chan *et al.* [10]. This approach is illustrated in Figure 3. Vertices $v_1, \ldots, v_k$ lie on the longest root-to-leaf path (the "spine") of the tree. Small subtrees T_1 through T_{k-1} are drawn using a simple technique for producing hv-drawings. An hv-drawing is a straight-line grid drawing such that child nodes are either horizontally or vertically aligned with their parent nodes, and the bounding rectangles of the subtrees of each node do not overlap. Larger subtrees T' and T'' are drawn recursively. The dotted outline behind T'' illustrates how the recursively-drawn subtree will be arranged. The result in the final drawing is that the spine of the tree is laid out in an extended S-curve shape (hence the "winding" in the name). ORTHO-UPWARD produces drawings with small area and a good aspect ratio.

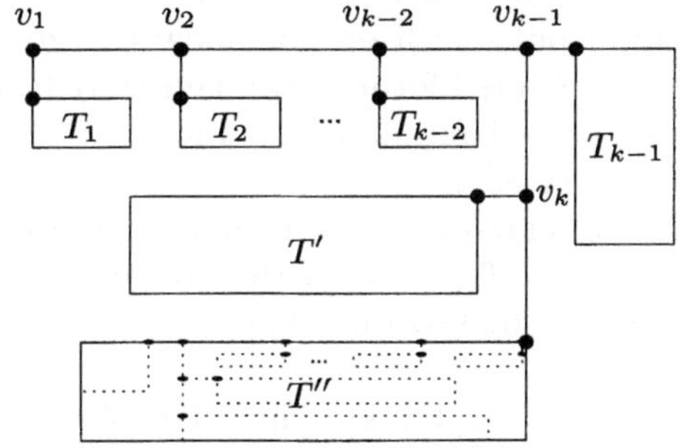

Fig. 3. Recursive winding.

SPD uses the delta-drawing algorithm of Bertolazzi *et al.* [5] to construct an upward drawing of a series-parallel digraph. A series-parallel digraph is a directed graph with the following recursive definition:

- A graph consisting of a source s, and sink t, and a directed edge from s to t is a series-parallel digraph.
- If G' and G'' are series-parallel digraphs, the series composition obtained by identifying the sink of G' with the source of G'' is also a series-parallel digraph.
- If G' and G'' are series-parallel digraphs, the parallel composition obtained by identifying the source of G' with the source of G'' and by identifying the sink of G' with the sink of G'' is also a series-parallel digraph.

The SPD algorithm assumes that the series-parallel digraph does not contain multi-edges. The drawing algorithm is recursive, utilizing the series-parallel decomposition of the digraph. Each subdrawing is placed within a bounding triangle.

3.2 Format Translation

A key component of the Graph Drawing Server is its format translation mechanism. Each graph drawing algorithm supported by the service typically defines its own input/output format, and these formats may be different from the formats requested by the user. The efforts to define a common graph interchange format do not completely solve the problem, since legacy implementations still define their own formats — and the multiple efforts towards standardization are likely to result in multiple "standard" formats. Therefore, there may be a need for translating from one format to another on drawing requests. In addition, the user may explicitly request a translation.

Graph description formats can be grouped into two categories: *graph-oriented* formats, which contain an explicit representation of the graph structure, and *diagram-oriented* formats, which contain a graphical representation of a drawing of a graph but which do not allow the graph structure to be easily extracted. Graph-oriented formats can generally be converted to other graph-oriented formats or to diagram-oriented formats, but diagram-oriented formats can only be converted to other diagram-oriented formats.

Supported diagram-oriented formats include PostScript, GIF, MIF (used by Adobe FrameMaker), and fig (used by the drawing program xfig). Graph-oriented formats supported by GDS include:

GraphML An extensible XML-based format. GraphML [7] consists of a core describing the structural properties of a graph, plus extension packages to add application-specific information such as typed attributes to the graph.

Paren An extensible format consisting of nested lists of keyword-value pairs. The paren format can support arbitrary vertex, edge, and graph-level attributes.

MALF MALF is a modified version of the ALF format supported by the Automatic Layout Facility [4] of Diagram Server [11,12]. The MALF input format supports only the graph structure, with optional vertex names; the MALF output format also includes coordinates of vertices and edge bends.

Edge List (input only) Edge List is currently supported only as an input format. As the format name implies, a graph is specified by listing its edges; vertices are defined implicitly as they are included by an edge. Edge endpoints and the number and coordinates of bends along an edge can be specified. Only vertex names are supported.

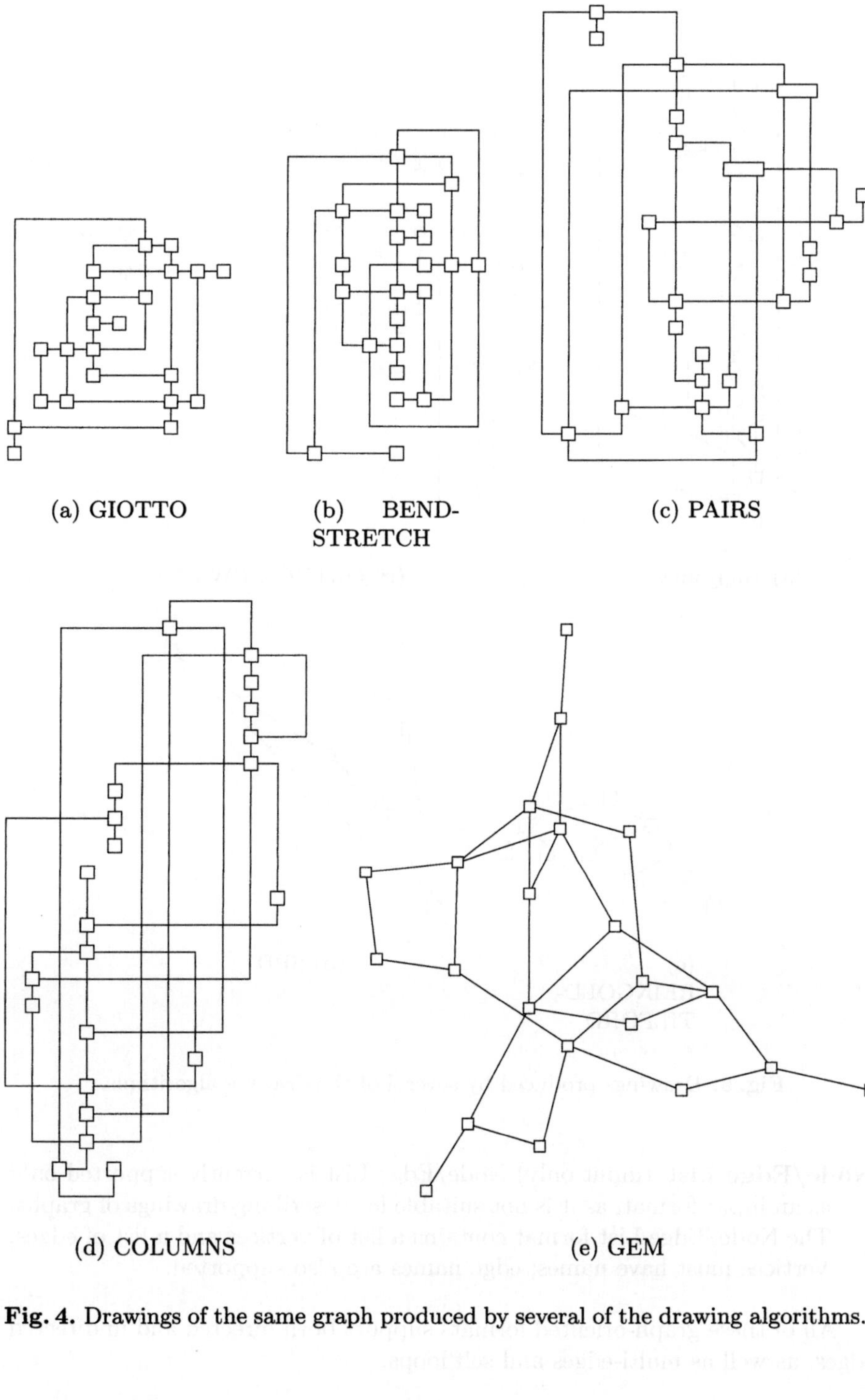

(a) GIOTTO (b) BEND-STRETCH (c) PAIRS

(d) COLUMNS (e) GEM

Fig. 4. Drawings of the same graph produced by several of the drawing algorithms.

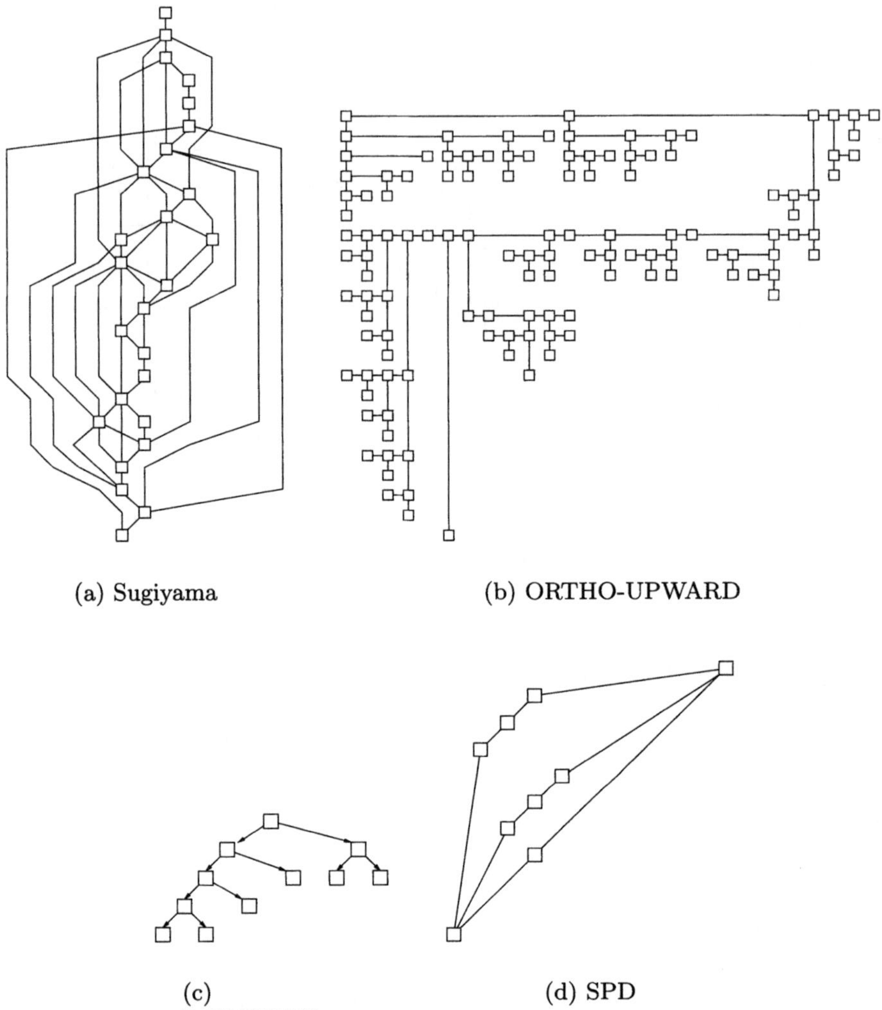

(a) Sugiyama (b) ORTHO-UPWARD

(c) REINGOLD-TILFORD (d) SPD

Fig. 5. Drawings produced by several of the drawing algorithms.

Node/Edge List (input only) Node/Edge List is currently supported only as an input format, as it is not suitable for describing drawings of graphs. The Node/Edge List format contains a list of vertices and a list of edges. Vertices must have names; edge names are also supported.

All of these graph-oriented formats support both directed and undirected edges, as well as multi-edges and self loops.

The request server components of the Graph Drawing Server (Section 4.1) maintain a database of the drawing algorithms and translation functions available through the service. A directed graph, called the translation graph, is used to perform the translation. The vertices and edges of this graph are the formats and translation functions, respectively. To satisfy a translation request, a directed path is found in the graph from the input format to the output format. The translation functions found along the path are called in sequence to perform the translation. A new format can be added to the service by providing translation functions between it and any other already-supported format.

There are several issues which must be addressed by a general-purpose graph format translator.

One is the issue of *structural mismatch.* This occurs when one format supports a graph structure that another does not — for example, one format may support multi-edges while another requires only simple graphs. This type of problem is considered to cause the translation process to fail, and GDS returns a "translation not possible" error message. (We ignore the possibility of encoding the original graph G as some other graph G' which could then be expressed in the desired format, as this encoding is often application-specific. The user can opt to perform the encoding herself, and send the alternate graph to the service for drawing.)

Another issue is *attribute mismatch.* This occurs when the graph structure can be represented by both formats, but one format includes attributes that the other does not. Such attributes commonly include vertex labels, edge labels, colors, and geometric information such as coordinates. The Graph Drawing Server encounters information loss due to attribute mismatch in two ways. First, there are two translation sequences involved in the typical request — one between the user's input format and the algorithm's input format and another between the algorithm's output format and the user's desired output format — and either may consist of more than one step. If any of the intermediate formats is less expressive than the end formats, information is lost. Second, information may be lost if the input and/or output formats used by the algorithm are less expressive than the user's desired formats.

GDS addresses the first problem by carefully choosing the path in the translation graph so as to minimize the information lost. To keep the length of any given path in the translation graph as short as possible and to increase the chances of finding a path in which little or no information is lost, it is envisioned that the translation graph will evolve to contain a tightly-linked core of "powerful" formats, and that application-specific formats would be linked to one of the core formats. Core formats would typically be formats intended as graph interchange formats (e.g., GraphML [7], GXL [21], GraphXML [15], GML [16], or XGMML [19]) because they have been designed to be able to represent a variety of graph structures and attributes. Due to the small number of core formats, it would be feasible to create translation modules for many of the pairwise combinations. As a result, most paths in the translation graph would consist of a single translation into a core format, possibly one core-to-core translation, and finally a translation from a core format to the application's own format. It is expected that the core formats will support most of the attributes present in application-specific formats, so that little information will be lost in this sort of translation sequence.

GDS addresses the problem of information loss due to the algorithm's format being less expressive than the user's format(s) by incorporating a merging step just before the final output is returned to the user. (If the user requests a diagram-oriented format, the merging step is applied to the last graph-oriented format in the translation sequence.) In the merging step, the information from the original input graph description is merged with the current graph description.

It is impractical to create a merging function for every pair of formats. Another solution is to define a "most powerful format" $\mathcal{F}$ which is expressive enough to represent a graph in any other supported format without information loss, and to convert the input graph to this format for merging. Defining such a format is a significant effort, and there is always the possibility that a new format will be added to the service which is not supported by format $\mathcal{F}$. Furthermore, this strategy requires translators to be created to convert any graph format to format $\mathcal{F}$. While these translators can also fulfill one direction of the translation functions required to add a new format to GDS, flexibility is lost by requiring translators between particular formats.

The Graph Drawing Server adopts a middle ground. For the merging step, the user's original input graph is converted to the current format — again using a translation sequence chosen to minimize information loss — and the result merged. This eliminates the need for translators between specific pairs of formats, and requires only one merging function per format. The merging function is also easier to implement, since the graph descriptions being merged are in the same format. The tradeoff is that there is a risk of some information being lost unnecessarily, though if the user requests output in the same format as the original input graph, no information will be lost. Another advantage is that it is still possible to introduce additional translators between specific pairs of formats or to support the "most powerful format" solution, and that such strategies can be applied to every format or just selected ones.

There is an additional complication with merging, because not every attribute from the original input should be preserved. The drawing algorithm may invalidate some of those attributes, either directly or indirectly. In the first case, the algorithm computes new values replacing the old. An example of the latter case is when the user's input contains layout information and an attribute describing the layout as planar, and the requested drawing algorithm produces a new non-planar layout. Since it is not generally possible to determine if a particular drawing algorithm invalidates a particular attribute, GDS allows some of a format's attributes to be designated as "fragile". A fragile attribute is one which may be rendered invalid by a drawing algorithm, such as vertex coordinates or a planar layout. By default, merging functions will not copy fragile attributes from the input graph. Users can override this behavior.

Finally, the merging step assumes that there is some way to identify corresponding vertices and edges. Most formats support some type of vertex name or ID which can be used to identify vertices. Edges can be matched based on the names of their endpoint vertices; for multi-edges, additional techniques may be required if it is necessary to distinguish between them. In the case where there are no vertex names (or the IDs were changed by a drawing algorithm), graph isomorphism routines can be applied to find a correspondence.

4 Implementation

The Graph Drawing Server is a component of GeomNet [2,3], a distributed geometric computing system which provides access to computational geometry and graph drawing algorithms over the Internet. It utilizes the web services framework, where users connect to services running on remote machines rather than installing software packages locally. Clients connect to the Graph Drawing Server via sockets or HTTP, and can include web browsers, custom interfaces designed specifically for providing access to GDS-based algorithms, or application programs which make use of a GDS algorithm as part of their larger working.

The Graph Drawing Server service consists of a network of request servers, code servers, compute servers, and data providers (Figure 6). These components are described in greater detail below.

4.1 Server Components

Request Servers are the only type of GDS server contacted directly by clients. Request servers are responsible for servicing a user's request: they parse the incoming request, determine what translation steps are required, schedule and coordinate the compute servers, code servers, and data servers needed to carry out the task, and finally return the results back to the client. To accomplish this, request servers maintain information about the entire service, including the supported graph description formats, drawing algorithms, and the drawing algorithms' required formats. Request servers also keep track of the available code, compute, and data servers, along with information relevant to scheduling such as the available resources, CPU speed, bandwidth, load, and currently-installed code for each compute server.

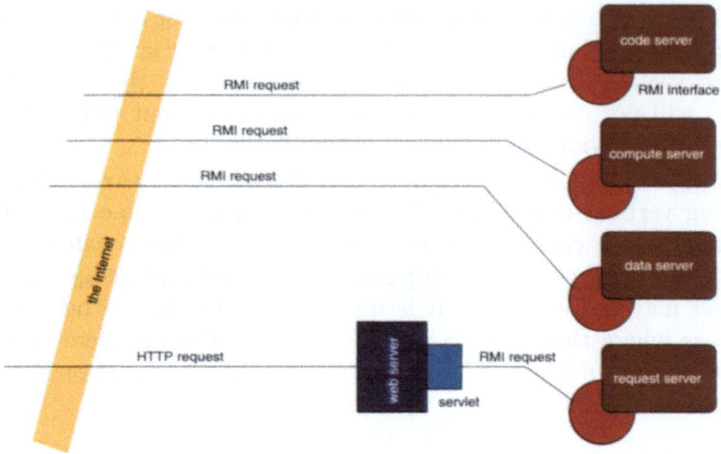

Fig. 6. Architecture of the Graph Drawing Server.

Code Servers are responsible for providing the graph drawing algorithms, translators, and formats supported by the service. The code server stores the source code, Java classes, or executable for each application along with a description file which specifies the application's input and output formats, parameters, and other properties. Different applications may be provided by different code servers.

Compute Servers are responsible for executing code provided to them by code servers. The code server provides a Java "wrapper" which, when executed, results in the necessary files being downloaded from the code server. Compute servers may cache code they are asked to run to avoid having to repeatedly download and install a popular application.

Data Providers provide access to the graph data used and created by drawing algorithms. Data providers provide a standard interface for data access, allowing the system to handle a large variety of different data sources including files, URLs, databases, and Java objects in memory.

Previous versions of the Graph Drawing Server [8] had only a single type of server which performed all of the functions of the request server, code server, and compute server; data was passed as a string or URL. Separating code servers and compute servers allows for greater flexibility. Multiple compute servers can automatically install and run code provided by a single code server, sparing the administrator from having to manually install the application on every compute server which may run it. Clients can also volunteer as compute servers for their own requests, so that a reasonably powerful client with a large amount of data to process can potentially run the computation itself and avoid sending that data over the network.

The GDS server components are implemented in Java, and GDS servers will run on any operating system for which a Java virtual machine exists.[1] Server components interact with each other through Java Remote Method Invocation (RMI). Compatible clients may also use RMI to interact with the service. For clients which cannot or do not wish to use RMI, HTTP-based communication is supported. Java servlets, invoked by the web server, translate the HTTP request into the appropriate RMI call. Secure communications via the Secure Sockets Layer (SSL) is supported to protect proprietary or confidential graph data or algorithm code.

GDS also allows owners of code, computing, and data resources to control access at both the server and individual algorithm levels. Furthermore, since code is allowed to migrate, GDS allows code providers to restrict the compute servers which may run the code to protect against piracy, and allows compute servers to limit what code they run based on its origin to protect the server from unknown code. The Java Authentication and Authorization Service (JAAS) is used, which allows for great flexibility in the selection of particular authentication methods. Individual server administrators can choose the authentication method or methods most appropriate for their systems.

The Java programming language is a natural choice, for several reasons. Because of its portability, a Java-based compute server can be placed on different platforms as needed to support legacy implementations. RMI and object serialization allow mobile code (objects that move from one host to another) and automatically handles loading classes if they are not available on the target host. This facilitates the downloading of code from code server to compute server. The Java language also provides support for safe "sandboxes" in which third-party code can be run — the code can be granted access to system resources such as network connections and the local filesystem based on its origin and/or signer, allowing a code server to execute downloaded code with a maximum of security.

Individual drawing algorithms, translation filters, and client interfaces may be implemented in any language (e.g., C, C++, Java, perl, and, for interfaces, HTML). The only requirements for an application's integration into the Graph Drawing Server are that there is a way to get data into and out of the program in a non-interactive way, and that a GDS server can be run on the platform on which the application runs.

4.2 Clients

Anything with the ability to communicate with a web server can access the basic functionality of the Graph Drawing Server, though Java-based clients can access more advanced features. The Graph Drawing Server currently provides two clients: one based on HTML forms, and a graph editor applet.

[1] Currently Solaris SPARC/x86, Linux x86, Microsoft Windows 95/98/2000/NT 4.0/ME, AIX, HP-UX, IRIX, MacOS, and other platforms.

5 Examples

5.1 Drawing Graphs With the Graph Drawing Server

One advantage of the Graph Drawing Server is that it lets the user easily try a number of different graph drawing algorithms with the same input graph. This is useful in cases where the objective is to obtain a nice drawing of a graph and the most appropriate algorithm is not already known. It can also be useful when exploring an unknown graph, as different algorithms expose different aspect of the graph's structure.

Figure 7(a) shows a graph loaded into the Graph Drawing Server's graph editor applet interface. The graph represents a small hypothetical website belonging to an airline — edges between vertices indicate links between pages. The graph description loaded by the editor contained no layout information, so the editor placed vertices at default (random) locations.

Figures 7(b) and 7(c) show the results of using the GIOTTO and Sugiyama algorithms to draw the graph.

5.2 Translating Graphs With the Forms Interface

Figure 8 shows an example of using the Graph Drawing Server's forms-based interface to convert between different graph description formats. (The forms interface can also be used to execute graph drawing algorithms.) In this case, the graph is being converted from the text-based parenthetic format to the GIF image format.

The original graph description is entered directly into the box provided for that purpose, though it is also possible to specify the input graph via a URL. The desired conversion is specified through a combination of drop-down menus and checkboxes.

The request is then sent to the server, and a results page is returned which displays some processing statistics and provides two alternatives for obtaining the converted file. Both will cause a properly-configured browser to start a helper application as necessary to view the file; the difference is that the first option requires the browser to be configured to recognize a particular filename extension, while the second requires only that the browser be configured to recognize a particular type of file (which may be independent of the file's name).

5.3 Prototyping With the Graph Drawing Server

The Graph Drawing Server can be useful for rapid development of prototypes of systems involving a graph drawing component. Because graph drawing routines can be accessed through GDS, an application developer can easily experiment with a variety of high-quality graph drawing algorithms without a great deal of programming.

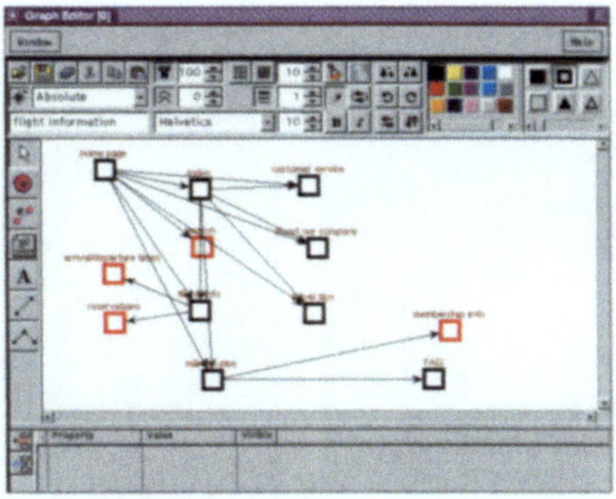

(a) Original graph, with vertices placed randomly.

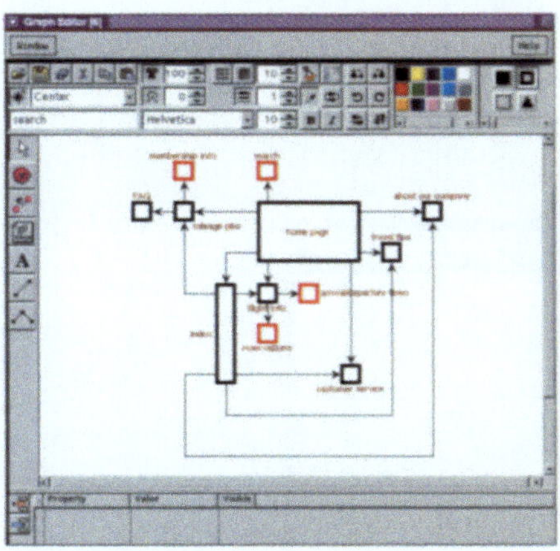

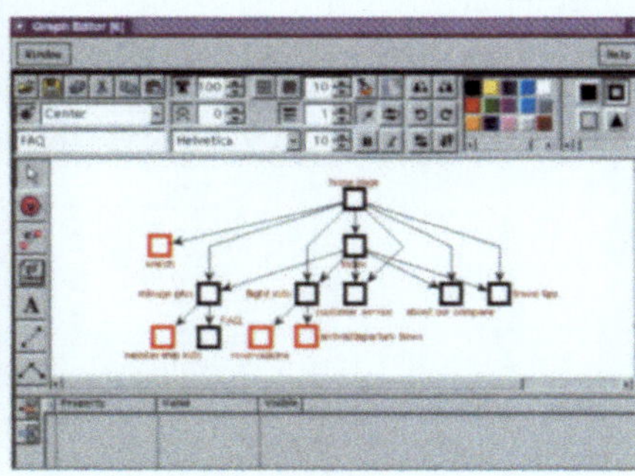

(b) Graph drawn with the GIOTTO orthogonal drawing algorithm.

(c) Graph drawn with the Sugiyama hierarchical drawing algorithm.

Fig. 7. Using the graph editor applet to produce multiple layouts of the same graph.

PILOT [9] is an interactive Web-based educational software tool for testing computer science concepts. It supports automatic generation of random instances of a problem and automatic grading of the student's answer, with useful feedback about where the errors are. For graph-based problems, PILOT's automatic problem generator produces the graph. The Graph Drawing Server is then used to create a layout for the graph so it can be displayed on the screen. Figure 9 shows an example of a problem for Prim's minimum

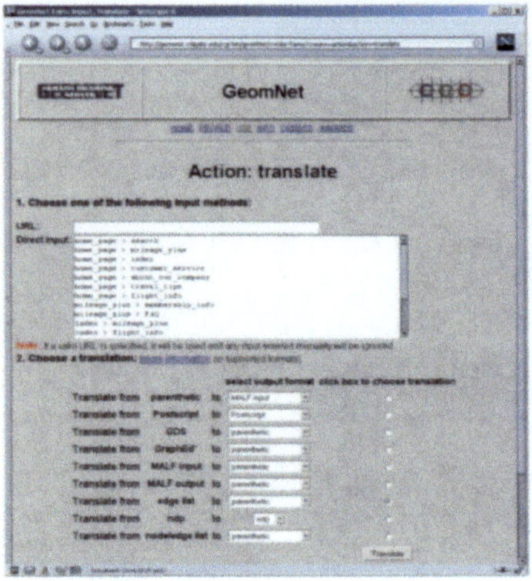

(a) Form for specifying the graph to translate and the formats involved.

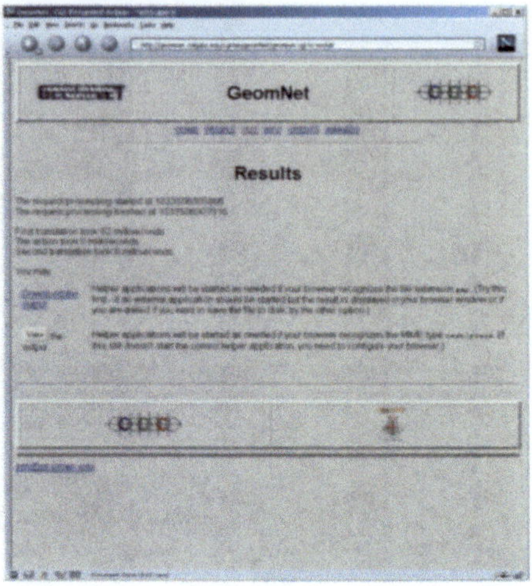

(b) Results page returned by the server.

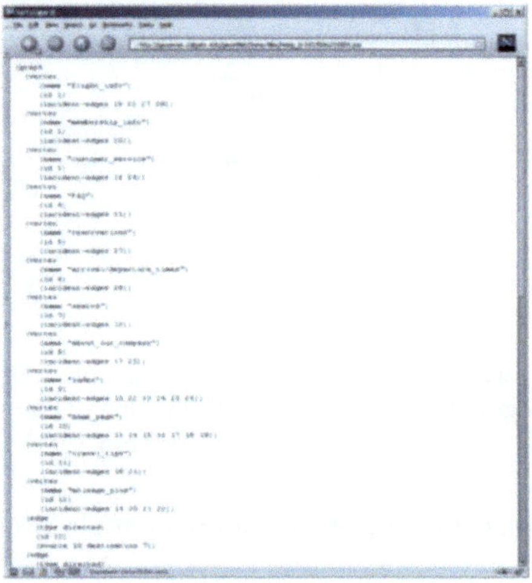

(c) Translated graph description.

Fig. 8. Using the forms interface to convert between graph description formats.

spanning tree algorithm; the highlighted edges and those listed in the "Edge Ordering" box are the student's attempted solution (which consists of the edges in the minimum spanning tree, and the order in which Prim's algorithm added them to the MST). The drawing of the graph was computed by the Graph Drawing Server's Sugiyama algorithm.

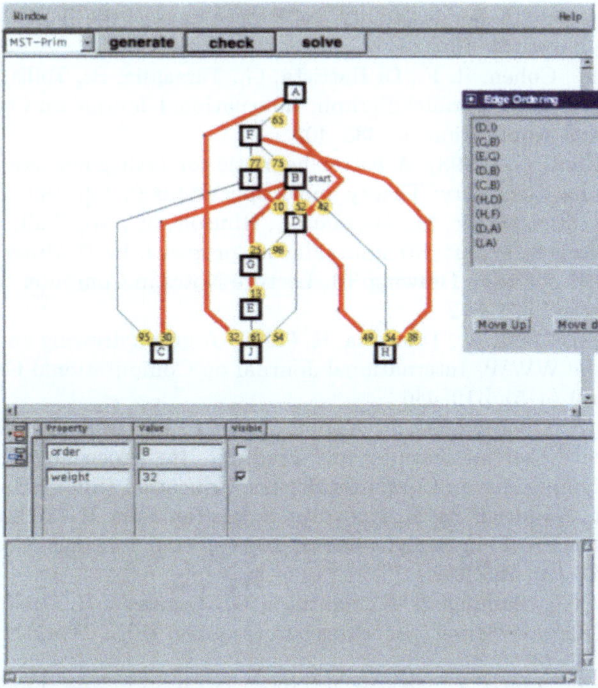

Fig. 9. The educational software tool PILOT, with a graph layout generated by the Graph Drawing Server.

6 Software

The Graph Drawing Server is available on the World Wide Web at `http://geomnet.colgate.edu`.

References

1. Alberts, D., Gutwenger, C., Mutzel, P., Näher, S. (1997) AGD-Library: A library of algorithms for graph drawing. In: Proceedings of the Workshop on Algorithm Engineering, 112–123
`http://www.mpi-sb.mpg.de/AGD/`
2. Barequet, G., Bridgeman, S., Duncan, C., Goodrich, M., Tamassia, R. (1999) GeomNet: Geometric computing over the Internet. IEEE Internet Computing **3** (2), 21–29

3. Barequet, G., Bridgeman, S. S., Duncan, C. A., Goodrich, M. T., Tamassia, R. (1997) Classical computational geometry in GeomNet. In: Proceedings of the 13th Annual ACM Symposium on Computational Geometry, 412–414
4. Beccaria, M., Bertolazzi, P., Di Battista, G., Liotta, G. (1991) A tailorable and extensible automatic layout facility. In: Proceedings of the IEEE Workshop on Visual Languages, 68–73
5. Bertolazzi, P., Cohen, R. F., Di Battista, G., Tamassia, R., Tollis, I. G. (1994) How to draw a series-parallel digraph. International Journal on Computational Geometry and Applications **4**, 385–402
6. Biedl, T., Kant, G. (1998) A better heuristic for orthogonal graph drawings. Computational Geometry: Theory and Applications **9**, 159–180
7. Brandes, U., Eiglsperger, M., Herman, I., Himsolt, M., Marshall, M. S. (2002) GraphML progress report: Structural layout proposal. In: P. Mutzel, M.Jünger, S. Leipert (eds.) Graph Drawing '01, Lecture Notes in Computer Science 2265, Springer-Verlag, 501–512
8. Bridgeman, S., Garg, A., Tamassia, R. (1999) A graph drawing and translation service on the WWW. International Journal on Computational Geometry and Application **9** (4–5), 419–446
9. Bridgeman, S., Goodrich, M. T., Kobourov, S. G., Tamassia, R. (2000) PILOT: An interactive tool for learning and grading. In: Proceedings of the ACM Technical Symposium on Computer Science Education (SIGCSE), 139–143
10. Chan, T. M., Goodrich, M. T., Kosaraju, S. R., Tamassia, R. (2002) Optimizing area and aspect ratio in straight-line orthogonal tree drawings. Computational Geometry **23** (2), 153–162
11. Di Battista, G., Giammarco, A., Santucci, G., Tamassia, R. (1990) The architecture of Diagram Server. In: Proceedings of the IEEE Workshop on Visual Languages, 60–65
12. Di Battista, G., Liotta, G., Vargiu, F. (1995) Diagram Server. Journal of Visual Language Computing **6** (3), 275–298. Special issue on Graph Visualization, I. F. Cruz and P. Eades (eds.)
13. Frick, A., Ludwig, A., Mehldau, H. (1995) A fast adaptive layout algorithm for undirected graphs. In: R. Tamassia, I. G. Tollis (eds.) Graph Drawing '94, Lecture Notes in Computer Science 894, Springer-Verlag, 388–403.
14. GDToolkit. `http://www.dia.uniroma3.it/~gdt/`.
15. Herman, I., Marshall, M. S. (2000) GraphXML — an XML-based graph description format. In: J. Marks (ed.) Graph Drawing '00, Lecture Notes in Computer Science 1984, Springer-Verlag, 52–62.
16. Himsolt, M. (1996) GML: Graph modelling language. Manuscript, Universität Passau, Innstraße 33, 94030 Passau, Germany `http://infosun.fmi.uni-passau.de/Graphlet/GML/`.
17. Mehlhorn, K., Näher, S. (2000) LEDA: A Platform for Combinatorial and Geometric Computing. Cambridge University Press, Cambridge, UK `http://www.mpi-sb.mpg.de/LEDA/leda.html`.
18. Papakostas, A., Tollis, I. G. (1998) Algorithms for area-efficient orthogonal drawings. Computational Geometry: Theory and Applications **9** (1–2), 83–110, special Issue on Geometric Representations of Graphs, G. Di Battista and R. Tamassia (eds.)
19. Punin, J., Wang, Y.-X., Krishnamoorthy, M. XGMML. `http://www.cs.rpi.edu/~puninj/XGMML/`.

20. Tamassia, R., Tollis, I. G. (1989) Planar grid embedding in linear time. IEEE Transactions on Circuits and Systems **CAS-36** (9), 1230–1234
21. Winter, A. (2002) Exchanging graphs with GXL. In: P. Mutzel, M. Jünger, S. Leipert (eds.) Graph Drawing '01, Lecture Notes in Computer Science 2265, Springer-Verlag, 485–500

BioPath – Exploration and Visualization of Biochemical Pathways

Franz J. Brandenburg[1], Michael Forster[1], Andreas Pick[1], Marcus Raitner[1], and Falk Schreiber[2]

[1] Fakultät für Mathematik und Informatik, University of Passau, Innstraße 33, 94032 Passau, Germany
[2] Institute of Plant Genetics and Crop Plant Research (IPK), Corrensstraße 3, 06466 Gatersleben, Germany

1 Introduction

Biochemical reactions in organisms form large and complex networks. Examples are given by the *Biochemical Pathways* atlas [17] and the well known *Boehringer Biochemical Pathways* poster [16], see Figure 1. Biochemists are familiar with visual representations of reactions and reaction networks. Automatic visualizations help in understanding the complex relations between the components of the networks and in extracting information from the data. They are very useful for building sophisticated research tools.

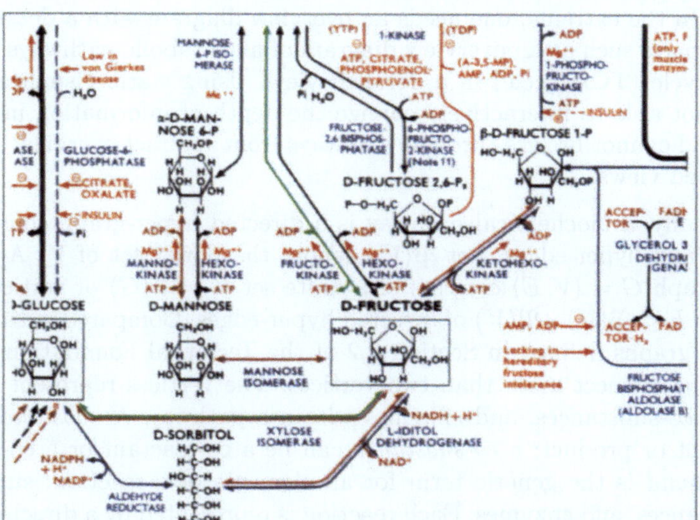

Fig. 1. A cutting of the *Boehringer Biochemical Pathways* poster [16] showing the complexity of the network.

A *pathway diagram* is a visual representation of a reaction network. Pathway diagrams, as in the poster [16], in textbooks on biochemistry, e.g., [22], and in information systems such as *KEGG* [10] are drawn manually. These diagrams represent the knowledge at the time of their generation. Notice that the drawings in textbooks and information systems are created once. They are used very often and they are usually hard-copies. This type of pathway visualization is called *static visualization* [2].

Although static visualization is often used for reaction networks, it has some severe drawbacks. First, static pathway diagrams cannot be updated with a reasonable amount of work. For example, Michal [18] reported that his team spent about one year for the design of the third edition of the *Biochemical Pathways* poster. However, the poster represents only a small fraction of the current knowledge about biochemical reactions and a manual update would be both time consuming and costly. On the other hand, static visualizations are often overloaded with information. A mass of information is given by different text colors and by the style and color of arrows as illustrated in Figure 1. Such visualizations are hard to read, in particular for beginners, and it is difficult to find specific information such as all pathways between two substances. Furthermore, there is no way to specify the amount of detail of each reaction to be displayed. For example, the user cannot choose between the use of enzyme names or enzyme classification numbers [9] in the pathway diagram. Finally, static visualization is restricted to only one level of representation providing either an overview or detailed information. However, there is more knowledge than this aspect and different views are needed. In the extreme, one needs an overview diagram with a detailed view of some parts such as an overview diagram of all catabolic pathways with the citrate cycle (TCA cycle) in a detailed view. Using static visualization the user is not able to interactively change the depth of information in the diagram, and cannot browse through pathways from abstract overview diagrams to detailed views.

Formally, a biochemical pathway is a directed hyper-graph consisting of vertices and hyper-edges. Let $\mathfrak{P}(V)$ denote the power set of V. A directed hyper-graph $G = (V, E)$ consists of a finite set $V = V(G)$ of vertices and a finite set $E \subseteq \mathfrak{P}(V) \times \mathfrak{P}(V)$ of directed hyper-edges. Compared with edges in directed graphs defined in Section 2.2 of the Technical Foundations, hyperedges may connect more than two vertices. The vertices represent the substances, co-substances, and enzymes within a pathway. A *substance* can be a reactant or product; a *co-substance* can be a co-reactant or a co-product. A *compound* is the generic term for all elements of a reaction: substances, co-substances, and enzymes. Each reaction is represented by a directed hyperedge, which connects all compounds of the reaction, see Figure 2(a). More common is the modeling of such relations by directed bipartite graphs, a modeling also used in Petri-net representations of pathways [8,21]. Here the reactions themselves are vertices and edges are binary relations connecting

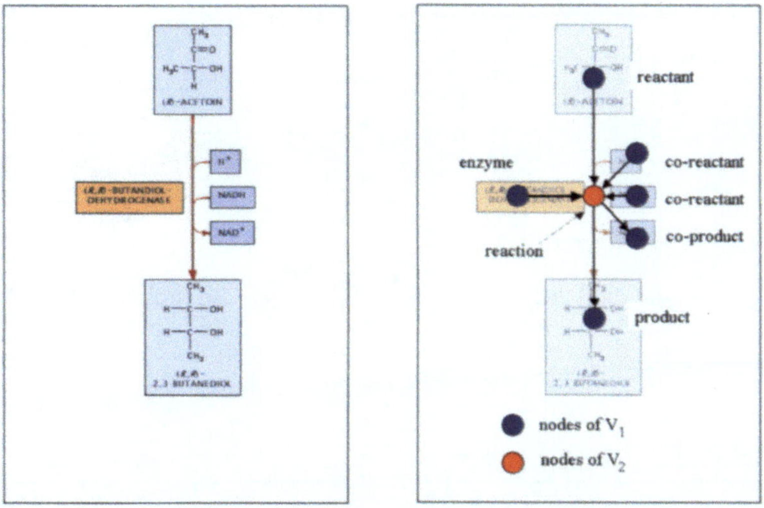

(a) (b)

Fig. 2. The diagram **(a)** shows a biochemical reaction. The connections between enzymes and other compounds are usually displayed by placing an enzyme close to the corresponding hyper-edge. Image **(b)** shows the representation of this reaction as directed bipartite graph.

compounds of reactions with reaction vertices. Without loss of generality, reactions can be represented by directed bipartite graphs, see Figure 2(b). This notation has the advantage that graph algorithms and standard graph drawing techniques can be used.

Our focus is on dynamic visualization in general and on pathway visualization in particular. *Dynamic visualization* is the generation of a diagram on demand at the time the drawing is needed. The placement of objects, e.g., substances or enzymes, and the routing of their connections is a typical graph drawing problem. However, the known graph drawing algorithms are inadequate for visualizing biochemical reaction networks according to the established conventions of biology and chemistry, see Figure 3 for examples. Even combinations of standard graph drawing algorithms [1,13] are insufficient. Some solutions focus only on the placement of the main reactants and products [1], others place co-substances and enzymes in an unusual way like in PFBP [20]. Up to now, the best results have been obtained by using labeling techniques, where the enzymes and co-substances are considered as edge labels and placed separately [13,15]. Nevertheless, these algorithms can produce crossings between co-substances and edges. They also tend to cluster all co-reactants into one vertex and all co-products into another vertex.

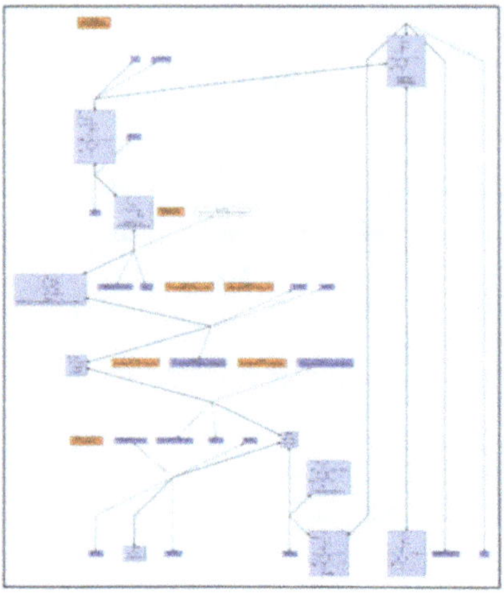

(a)

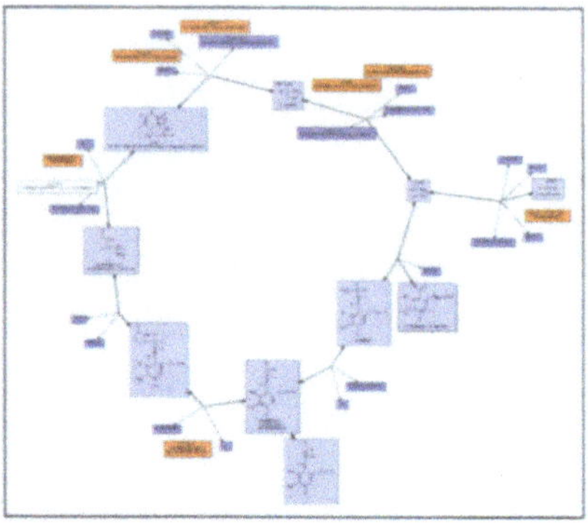

(b)

Fig. 3. Two visualizations of the same biochemical pathway **(a)** using a layered layout technique [23], and **(b)** using a force-directed layout technique [5] (see also Sections 4.2 and 4.5 of the Technical Foundations). These drawings differ very much from typical drawings in biochemical textbooks.

This is unacceptable for some reactions, especially for more complex reaction mechanisms as shown in Figure 4. Furthermore, these drawings of reaction networks often contain many unnecessary edge crossings [13] which reduces their readability.

Interactive navigation through biochemical pathways is a particular advantage of electronic information systems over textbooks and posters. The concept of a hierarchy of reactions is a crucial feature when browsing through reaction networks on different levels of detail. Reactions should be separable into sub-reactions and combinable to pathways. Thus sub-reactions, reactions, and pathways should also be considered as reactions. In some systems this hierarchical organization is realized by linked web pages. The information in *KEGG* [10] is structured by web-links from pathway classes, e.g., carbohydrate metabolism or lipid metabolism, to single pathway diagrams. *UM-BBD* [3] provides a click-able overview picture and a list of pathways organized by functional groups. But it is also necessary to represent this hierarchy in the database. *EcoCyc* and *MetaCyc* [14] represent a hierarchy of reactions by linking pathway objects to objects representing the reactions.

Existing visualization techniques do not meet the conventions of biochemistry; they are far from the typical drawings in textbooks. Moreover, existing databases do not include all relevant information such as the hierarchy of

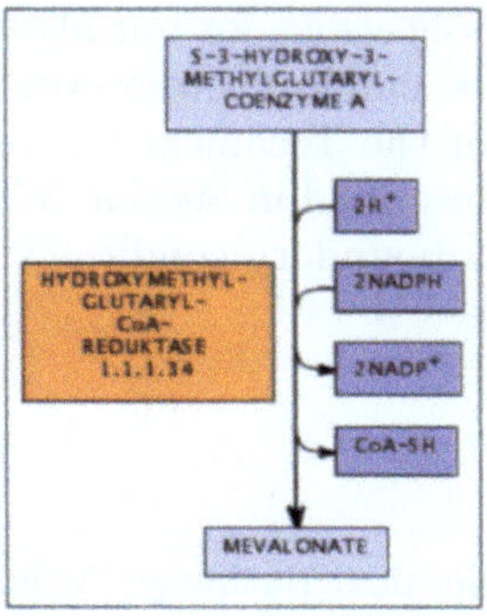

Fig. 4. The order of co-reactants and co-products is crucial for the understanding of the reaction mechanism and should be clearly visualized.

reactions and layout constraints for specific pathways. These constraints are necessary to distinguish pathways like the citrate cycle from arbitrary cycles in the network. Therefore, a new graph drawing algorithm and an adapted database schema are necessary.

The structure of this chapter is as follows. We start with a short overview of the *BioPath* system in Section 2. Section 3 deals with our visualization method. In Section 3.1 we discuss requirements for the visualization of biochemical pathways. We then present a graph drawing algorithm which fulfills these requirements in Section 3.2. Section 4 describes implementation aspects of the *BioPath* system, especially the application server in Section 4.2 and the query engine in Section 4.3. In Section 5 we show examples of the system.

2 Applications

The *Electronic Biochemical Pathways Project* [12] – a joint work of research groups at the universities of Erlangen, Mannheim, Passau and Spektrum Akademischer Verlag – provides convenient electronic access to the growing information of biochemical reactions at a high level of detail. An online exploration tool – *BioPath* [4] – demonstrates the quality of the data, the flexibility of the database schema, and the automatic visualization of pathways. It offers easy access to the information and progressive navigation through pathways. The database contains information about compounds and reactions, especially a hierarchy of reactions. A new graph drawing algorithm for the automatic visualization of pathways visualizes reaction networks according to the conventions of biochemistry. This algorithm and the *BioPath* system can be very useful for the analysis of biochemical pathways. *BioPath* explores all the advantages of an electronic version of the poster [16] over the printed one.

However, the field of applications for our algorithm is not limited to biochemical reactions. It can be employed wherever a Sugiyama style layout as introduced in Section 4.2 of the Technical Foundations is desired. Its comprehensive set of features described in Section 3 is of great value whenever a layout has to meet complex boundary conditions.

3 Algorithms

How shall we draw a biochemical pathway? What are the requirements for a good visualization algorithm? What criteria must be met? These are the crucial questions for the design of a solution that meets the needs of the users. It extends Knuth's question "How shall we draw a tree" to "How shall we draw a biochemical pathway". Knuth proposed to draw trees by layers and top-down, and this has become the common style in Computer Science. Drawing biochemical pathways is much harder, since they are directed hypergraphs. After a thorough analysis and intensive discussions with many experts we propose the following.

3.1 Visualization Requirements

Compounds. The visualization of compounds of a reaction is user-specific. According to existing drawings in the literature, substances should be given by their name or their structural formula or both, co-substances should be displayed using their name or an abbreviation, and enzymes should be represented by their name or their classification number. In *BioPath* the conventions of the poster [16] are used. It displays the names and the structural formulas for substances and the names or abbreviations (e.g., ATP, NADP) for co-substances and enzymes.

The data for the compounds is retrieved from the database. It is transformed into vertices of the graph using varying vertex sizes. The size of the vertex provides the space needed to display the information of the object such as the name or the structural formula. As a consequence, the visualization algorithm must support different vertex sizes.

Reactions. A reaction is visualized by a reaction arrow from the reactants to the products. Enzymes and co-substances are placed on different sides beside this arrow. For co-substances their temporal order, which depends on the reaction mechanism, is important. Therefore they are placed according to this order. Overview diagrams often disregard enzymes and co-substances. Thus the visualization algorithm has to deal with reactions with and without enzymes and co-substances.

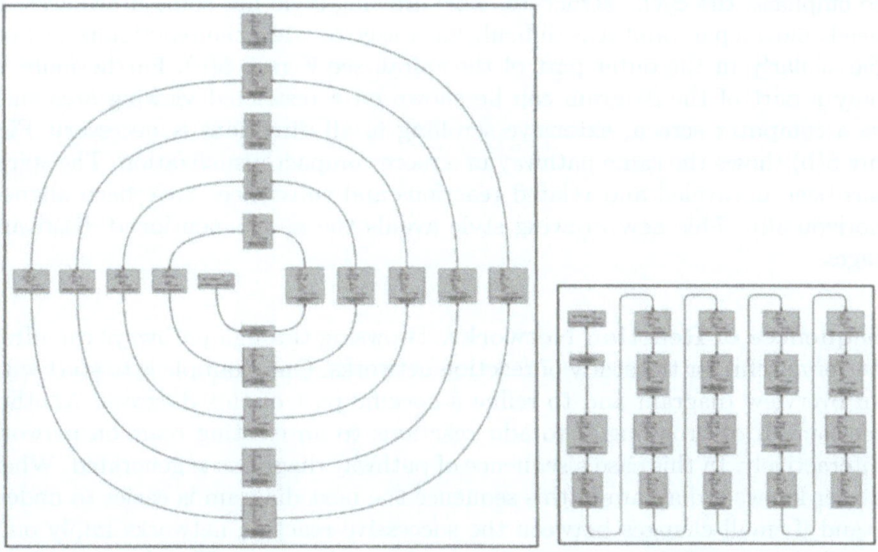

(a) (b)

Fig. 5. Two drawings of an *open cycle* (degradation of fatty acids). For simplicity only the substances are shown. In **(a)** the typical visualization of this pathway as a spiral. In **(b)** the same pathway is shown in a more compact visualization that also emphasizes the corresponding reaction steps and substances.

Reaction Networks. As the temporal order of reactions in the network is crucial, the main direction of reactions should be clearly visible. In *BioPath* the main direction is from top to bottom. This is better than from left to right since it yields more compact representations and a better placement of objects with long textual information.

There is an exception from the top to bottom direction, which is used for the visualization of specific pathways such as the citrate cycle or the fatty acid synthesis. The structure of these cyclic reaction chains should be emphasized. These pathways are characterized by the continuous repetition of a reaction sequence in which the product of the sequence re-enters in the next loop as a reactant. There are two mechanisms. First, the reactant and the product of the reaction sequence are identical from loop to loop (e.g., citrate cycle). This is called a *closed cycle*. Second, the reactant of the reaction sequence varies slightly from the product (e.g., fatty acid cycle). This is called an *open cycle*.

Repetitions in cyclic structures must be clearly visible. In textbooks they are displayed as circles (closed cycles) or as spirals (open cycles). In a spiral equal reaction steps and corresponding substances are placed side by side to emphasis the cyclic structure. This drawing style has some drawbacks. It needs much space and it is difficult for a user to trace the reaction sequence, particularly in the outer part of the spiral; see Figure 5(a). Furthermore, if only a part of the diagram can be shown on a restricted viewing area such as a computer screen, extensive scrolling in all directions is necessary. Figure 5(b) shows the same pathway in a more compact visualization. The spiral has been unraveled and related reactions and substances have been aligned horizontally. This new drawing style avoids the above-mentioned disadvantages.

Sequences of Reaction Networks. Browsing through pathways can often be very useful for the study of reaction networks. One example is to start with an overview diagram and to refine a specific part of this diagram. Another mechanism of browsing is to add reactions to an existing reaction network interactively. In this case a sequence of pathway diagrams is generated. When a user knows a diagram of this sequence the next diagram is easier to understand if small changes between the successive reaction networks imply only small changes of the corresponding pathway diagrams. The drawing of the unchanged part of the network should be preserved, but this is not always possible. For example, there may not be enough space for the insertion of a new reaction. In this case the relative positions of the old objects should be preserved. In graph drawing this technique is called *preserving the mental map* [19].

3.2 The Graph Drawing Algorithm

We model reaction networks as directed bipartite graphs $G = (V_1 \cup V_2, E)$, where substances, co-substances, enzymes, and reactions are represented as vertices $v \in V = V_1 \cup V_2$ and their connections are represented as directed edges $e \in E$; see Figure 2(b). The vertices of this bipartite graph are labeled by the name of the compounds, their role in the reaction (enzyme, substance, or co-substance), their involvement in open or closed cycles, and their rank. The labels are used for the generation of the image of the reaction or reaction network and are translated into associated text, colors, and layout constraints. A layout constraint describes a left-to-right or top-to-bottom relationship and means for example that an enzyme should appear to the left of the reaction arrow.

The visualization algorithm is based on the graph drawing algorithm by Sugiyama *et al.* [23] for the computation of layered layouts of directed acyclic graphs; see Section 4.2 in the Technical Foundations. The main extensions of the algorithm are:

Clustering. *Clustering* means the grouping of disjoint subgraphs into new vertices. Each grouped subgraph can be drawn with its own layout algorithm.

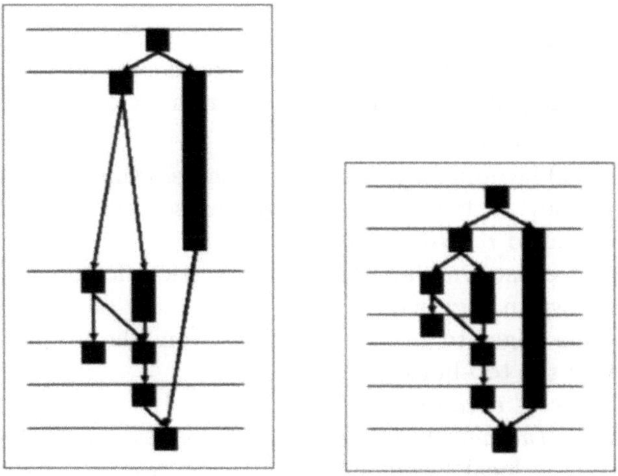

(a) (b)

Fig. 6. Layering mechanisms: **(a)** the typical global layering; **(b)** the local layering. The local layering mechanism considers the vertex sizes correctly and leads to compact placements.

The size of the corresponding new vertex is determined by the space of the drawn subgraph. In this context the routing of edges from vertices of the subgraph to vertices outside the subgraph is a difficult problem.

Vertex Sizes. The Sugiyama algorithm has only a coarse view of the size of vertices. It uses a global layering mechanism by placing all vertices in horizontal layers depending on their topological order. The distance between two layers is defined by the highest vertex of the above layer. Our algorithm is adapted to varying vertex sizes and is extended to a local layering mechanism where all vertices are placed in layers depending only on the placement of all predecessors; see Figure 6.

Layout Constraints. *Layout constraints* are additional application-specific requirements on the placement of objects. The layout algorithm considers the following types of layout constraints: *top-bottom* constraints to place one vertex below another one; *left-right* constraints for the horizontal order of two vertices; *horizontal* constraints to force the same layer for two vertices; and *vertical* constraints to force the same x-coordinate for two vertices. Layout constraints are used to draw open and closed cycles according to the specified requirements, and to preserve the mental map in related drawings. Algorithm 1 shows the main steps of the layout algorithm.

Algorithm 1: Main steps of the layout algorithm.

Input : A directed graph (representing a reaction network) with vertex sizes, vertex types (substance, co-substance, enzyme, reaction) and an indication of open and closed cycles

Output: The drawing of the graph

1 Compute local layouts for co-substances and enzymes of each reaction and cluster these vertices into large vertices, see Figure 7. These large vertices are called *reaction vertices*

2 Insert layout constraints and temporary vertices for open and closed cycles as shown in Figure 8

3 Reverse some edges to remove all cycles from the graph under the restriction of the top-bottom constraints

foreach *reversed edge* **do**

  if *possible (no new cycles occur by the following operations)* **then**

    turn the local layout of the adjacent reaction vertex by 180 degree (this reaction goes now from bottom to top) and change the direction of all edges adjacent to this reaction vertex.

  else

    insert a vertex on each edge adjacent to the corresponding reaction vertex to allow additional bends for these edges.

  end

end

4 Assign vertices to horizontal layers under the restriction of horizontal constraints. All edges should be directed from top to bottom. For each vertex the distance to its predecessors should be minimized. This step computes the y-coordinates of vertices

5 Compute a proper layering by inserting temporary vertices for long spanning edges and long spanning vertices, see Figure 9

6 Permute the order of vertices within each layer to reduce the number of edge crossings in the layered graph such that the left-right and the vertical constraints are fulfilled

7 Compute x-coordinates for the vertices without changing the pre-computed order in the layers and under consideration of the vertical constraints

8 De-cluster reaction vertices, compute an edge routing by using the temporary vertices as additional base points for edges

9 (Additional) Insert constraints for preserving the mental map in the next drawing

It is known that optimization problems connected to some steps are $\mathcal{NP}$-hard [6]; see Section 4.2 in the Technical Foundations. Therefore we use heuristics for these steps. The time critical part of the complete algorithm is step 3 to step 7. Let G be a connected graph, n be the number of vertices and

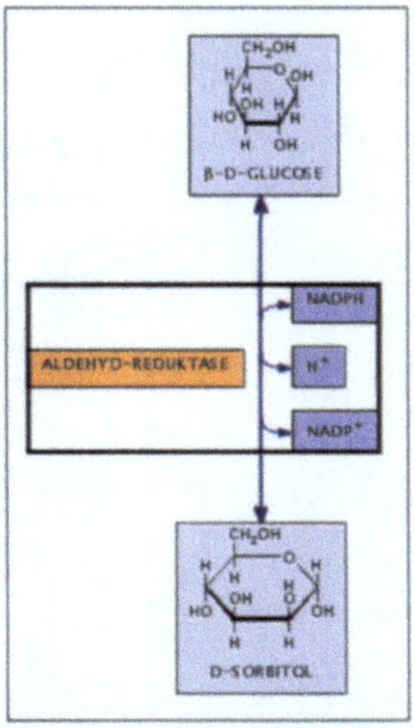

Fig. 7. Clustering of co-substances and enzymes of each reaction into a large vertex (reaction vertex). The positions of the co-substances and enzymes are computed separately. Enzymes are placed to the left of the reaction arrow, co-substances to the right according to their order. This determines the size of the reaction vertex. In the subsequent steps of the layout algorithm the reaction vertex is used instead of the clustered vertices. The order of the co-substances and their current role (co-reactant or co-product) are retrieved from the database.

m be the number of edges of G. For the steps 3, 6 and 7 different heuristics with complexities from linear time to $O(n^4)$ (for step 6) can be chosen, where a higher running time usually gives better results. However, most important are steps 4 and 5, because during these steps up to $n \cdot m$ temporary vertices and edges will be inserted in the graph. This influences the running time of the subsequent steps of the algorithm. The layout algorithm has been tested with more than 200 graphs. These graphs represent reaction networks with up to 50 reactions (or correspondingly up to 300 vertices). Using a standard PC we were able to layout these graphs within a few seconds using the heuristics with the higher complexities.

4 Implementation

4.1 Overview

BioPath is a classical 3-tier web application. See Figure 10 for an architecture overview.

Client Tier. Users access the *BioPath* service using a web browser like Netscape Navigator or Microsoft Internet Explorer. They enter their queries into

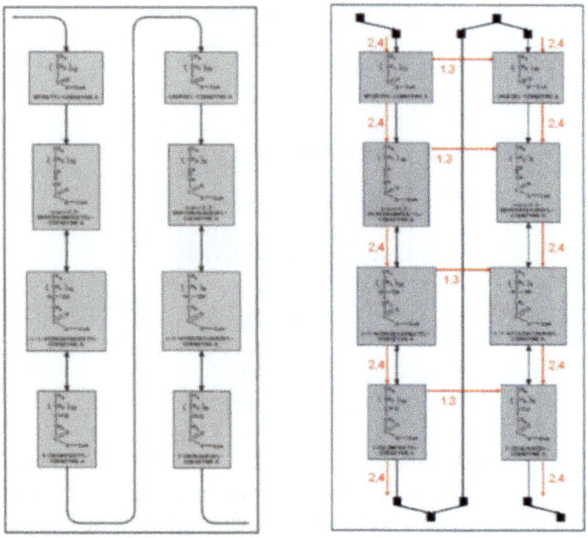

(a) (b)

Fig. 8. Image **(a)** shows the visualization of a part of an open cycle (two loops of the pathway). The diagram **(b)** shows the layout constraints to receive this layout: 1 - Horizontal constraints between corresponding substances in different loops of the pathway. 2 - Top-bottom constraints between consecutive vertices of each loop of the pathway (the vertex at the end of the arrow should be placed below the vertex at the begin of the arrow). 3 - Left-right constraints between vertices in the same layer in neighboring loops. 4 - Vertical constraints between consecutive vertices of each loop to force a vertical placement of vertices. For technical reasons some additional vertices are necessary. For closed cycles similar constraints are used.

HTML forms. The browser passes the query data to the *BioPath* application server by sending a HTTP request. When the application server has finished query processing, the browser displays the returned query results. Clicking on pathway images or on internal links triggers another HTTP request.

Application Tier. The main part of *BioPath* is the application server. It accepts queries, retrieves the corresponding data from the database, computes the result and delivers it to the client tier.

Data Storage Tier. The data of *BioPath* is stored in a relational database management system (currently IBM DB2) using an object oriented schema [11].

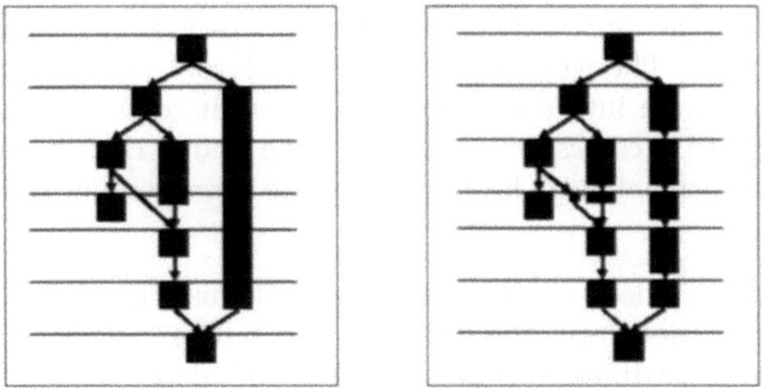

Fig. 9. Image **(a)** shows the assignment of vertices to horizontal layers. Long spanning edges are edges that cross at least one layer, long spanning vertices belong to at least two layers. In image **(b)** these edges and vertices are replaced by chains of temporary vertices.

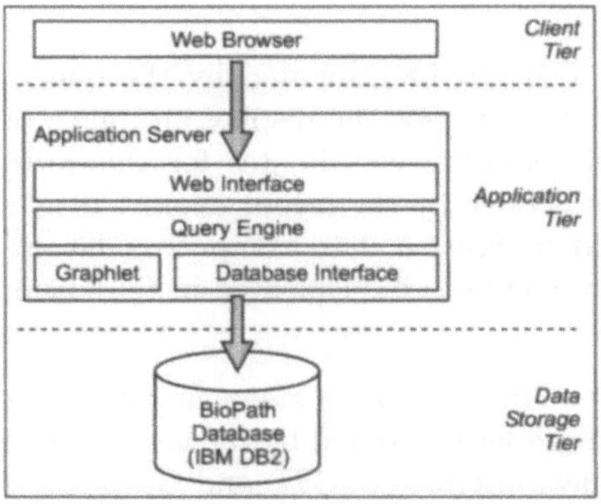

Fig. 10. The *BioPath* system architecture.

4.2 The Application Server

The heart of the *BioPath* system is the application server. It consists of several components, some of which are implemented in Java, some in C++ for execution speed. The communication between the Java and C++ components is done via the Java Native Interface (JNI). The application server has been developed mainly on Linux and Windows in an operating system independent manner, and therefore should be easily portable to any platform for which Java and a recent C++ compiler are available. It contains the following parts.

Web Interface. The web interface is responsible for the communication with the client tier. It receives the query in terms of a HTTP request with associated parameters. It parses the request and triggers the corresponding functionality of the query engine which processes the query and returns the result as a graph. The web interface uses the layout and graphics engine to transform the graph into a picture and delivers it to the client as a GIF or PNG image with a corresponding image map and a HTML page. The web interface is implemented in Java based on the Java Servlet Technology.

Query Engine. The query engine executes the user queries. It extracts the required information from the database and builds a pathway, represented as a graph with attributed vertices and edges. A description is given in Section 4.3. The query engine is implemented in C++ using the "Graph Template Library" (GTL), a C++ library providing a data structure for graphs.

Database Interface. The communication between the query engine and the database is done via the database interface. This encapsulation simplifies adapting *BioPath* to other data sources. The database interface is written in C++.

Layout Engine. The graphs generated by the query engine do not have a geometric representation. For the display an image of the graph must be computed. As a prerequisite, coordinates for the vertices and edges must be calculated. This is done by the layout engine. It uses the graph drawing algorithm described in Section 3 to compute a layout of the biochemical network. The layout engine is implemented in C++ using Graphlet [7].

Graphics Engine. The graphics engine generates images and image maps from the attributed graphs computed by the layout engine. It is implemented in Java using the Java interface of GTL and Graphlet.

4.3 Query Engine

The query engine processes the queries from the web interface, issues database queries, transforms the result and returns the answer to the web interface. The *BioPath* database features an elaborate schema designed by Kanne [11]. It consists of about 115 entities and 70 relations. We concentrate only on the part relevant to the query process.

The biochemical reactions are the main components of the database schema. Each reaction has a set of attributes including the participants, i.e., the substances involved in the reaction. These are classified into enzymes, reactants and products. Reactants and products are further classified into primary and non-primary. Primary reactants and products are used to compose pathways. Non-primary participants have a rank which specifies their relative order in the reaction and is used by the layout engine. The graph representation of the data is described in Section 3.

There are several types of queries. A search query on substances is a standard query for information on a substance, which is passed on directly to the database. The answer is a text or a structural formula as it is stored in the database.

A query on reactions and reaction nets shall return an image. Then the task of the query engine is building a reaction graph. A search-reaction query first collects all participants of the reaction from the database. For each participant the query engine creates a vertex and a vertex for the reaction itself, and labels the vertices with the name of the substance, the role and the rank. Then it adds directed edges between the reaction vertex and the participant vertices. These are directed from the reactant vertices to the reaction vertex and from there to the product vertices. Reactions may be bi-directional, but their internal representation is always one-directional. To show bi-directional edges in the final drawing arrows on both ends of the edge are used.

The search of a reaction net from a source substance to a target substance is finding a sequence of reactions of a predefined maximal length. In *BioPath* two reactions are combined, if a primary product of the first is a primary reactant of the second. This is the common notion of connectivity in such graphs. *BioPath* uses a recursive query to build all sequences starting from the source substance up to a predefined length. It then selects those reaching the target substance. In more detail, this query returns a collection of reactions, which are transformed into labeled graphs as described above. Vertices of primary participants are identified, if they represent the same substance. The so obtained directed graph is returned to the web interface.

5 Examples

BioPath is an online system for the retrieval of information on substances and biochemical pathways. It offers several ways to explore biochemical data and displays the data in the common style as text or graphics.

5.1 Start Page

The start page is shown in Figure 11 and presents general information about the *BioPath* project and the partners, a short introduction, a user guide and a starting point for the exploration of the biochemical data.

The user guide introduces into *BioPath* and explains how to find information about substances, enzymes, pathways, and reactions. It illustrates the visualization of reactions and pathways and displays the main features of *BioPath*.

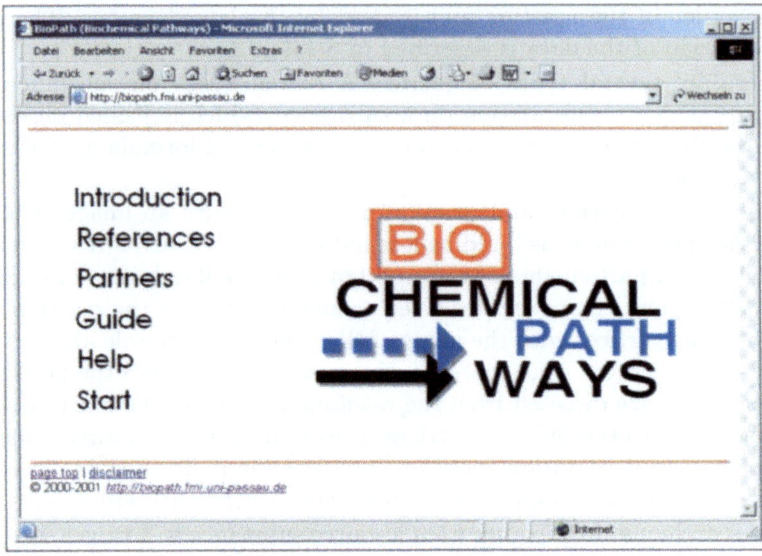

Fig. 11. Start page of *BioPath*.

5.2 Overview Diagram

The overview diagram in Figure 12 has been derived from the overview diagram of the *Biochemical Pathways* atlas [17]. It shows a selection of important biochemical pathways. All colored substances and reactions in the diagram can be clicked to receive more information. This is the only manually made reaction diagram in *BioPath* to ensure similarity to the overview diagram of the atlas.

5.3 Search Substances

Substances can be searched by their name or a part of it, see Figure 13. The result shows biochemical data such as structural and empirical formula, weight, enzyme classification number and charge. Additionally all reactions in which the substance participates as a reactant, a product or an enzyme are listed. Figure 14 is an example for Chlorophyll.

5.4 Search Pathways and Reactions

As shown in Figure 15, pathways can be searched by their name or a part of it. *BioPath* computes a graphical representation containing information like participating enzymes and substances of the reaction or pathway and also shows all pathways the reaction belongs to. As in the overview diagram, displayed substances and reactions can be clicked to receive detailed information.

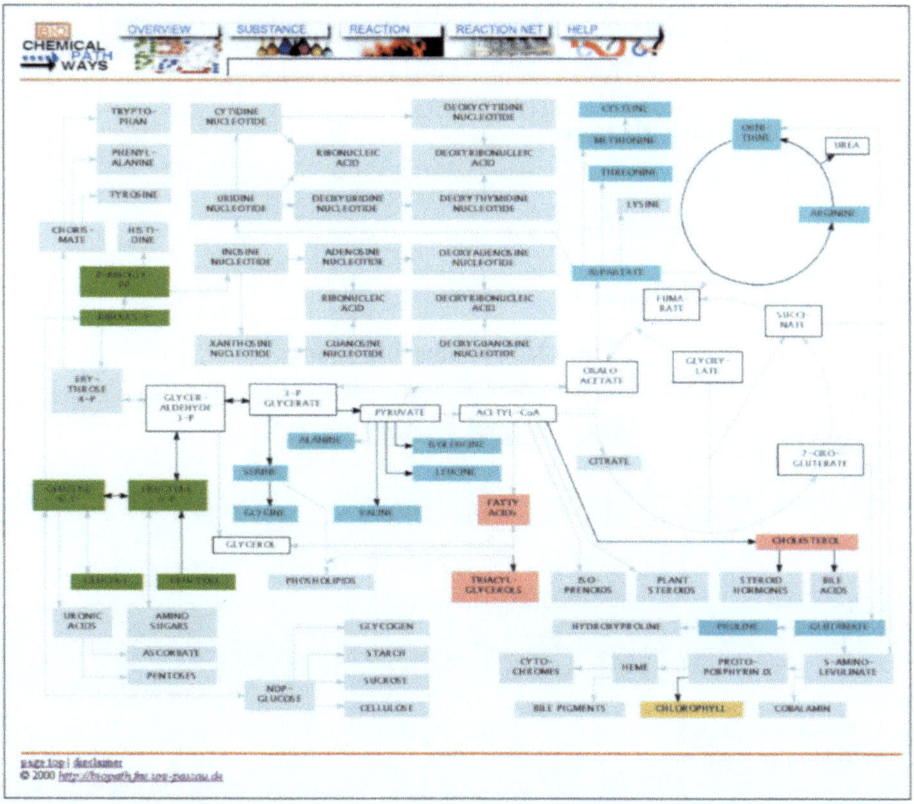

Fig. 12. The overview diagram is a starting point for exploration of the pathways.

5.5 Search Reaction Net

The most advanced feature of *BioPath* is the search for a reaction net between two substances. The query panel is shown in Figure 16. *BioPath* searches all sequences of reactions between two substances up to a given length. Figure 17 shows the result of the query "Search the reaction net between *Maltose* and *D-Gluconate* up to length 10". The search can be restricted to a single pathway and in depth. The later is also used to speed-up the search time and database queries. The depth counts the number of intermediate substances.

The usability of *BioPath* is limited by the given data on substances, reactions, and reaction nets, which is only an excerpt of the information on the poster or in the atlas or in commercial databases. However, this does not restrict our general approach.

6 Software

BioPath is accessible via `http://biopath.fmi.uni-passau.de`.

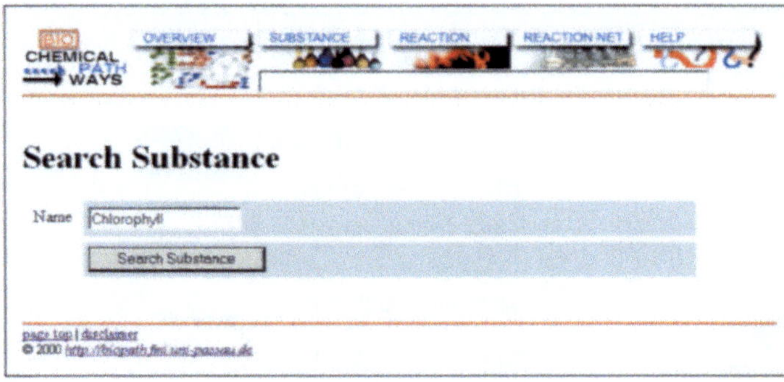

Fig. 13. Searching a substance.

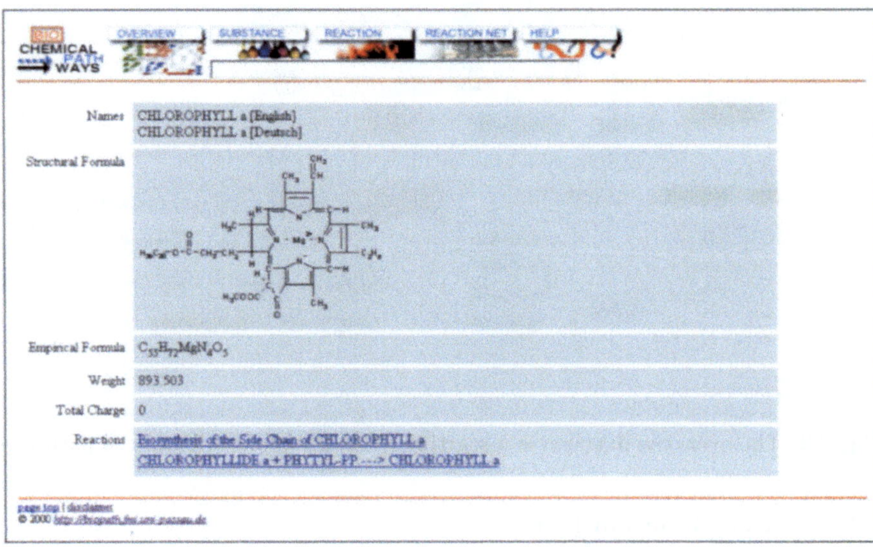

Fig. 14. Information about Chlorophyll.

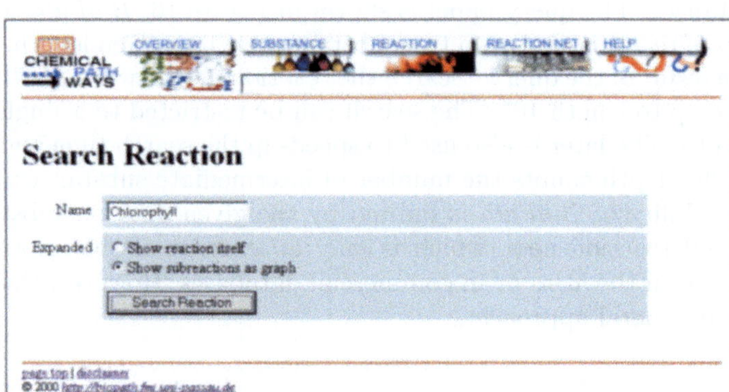

Fig. 15. Searching for the biosynthesis of the Side Chain of Chlorophyll.

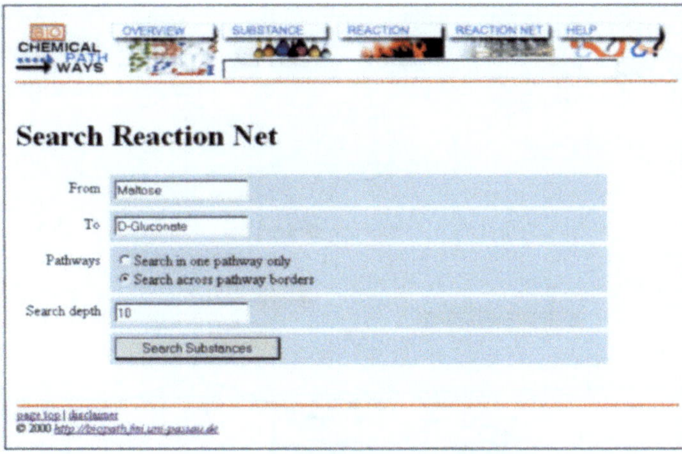

Fig. 16. Searching a reaction net.

References

1. Becker, M. Y., Rojas, I. (2001) A graph layout algorithm for drawing metabolic pathways. Bioinformatics **17** (5), 461–467
2. Brandenburg, F. J., Gruber, B., Himsolt, M., Schreiber, F. (1998) Automatische Visualisierung biochemischer Information. In: R. Hofestädt (ed.) Proceedings of the Workshop Molekulare Bioinformatik, GI Jahrestagung, Shaker Verlag, 24–38
3. Ellis, L. B., Hershberger, C. D., Wackett, L. P. (2000) The University of Minnesota Biocatalysis/Biodegradation Database: Microorganisms, Genomics and Prediction. Nucleic Acids Research **28** (1), 377–379
4. Forster, M., Pick, A., Raitner, M., Schreiber, F., Brandenburg, F. J. (2002) The System Architecture of the BioPath System. In Silico Biology **2** (3), 415–426
5. Fruchterman, T., Reingold, E. (1991) Graph Drawing by Force-directed Placement. Software – Practice and Experience **21** (11), 1129–1164
6. Garey, M. R., Johnson, D. S. (1979) Computers and Intractability: A Guide to the Theory of NP-Completeness. W. H. Freeman, New York
7. Himsolt, M. (2000) Graphlet: Design and Implementation of a Graph Editor. Software – Practice and Experience **30** (11), 1303–1324
8. Hofestädt, R., Thelen, S. (1998) Qualitative Modeling of Biochemical Networks. In Silico Biology **1**, 39–53
9. (1992) International Union of Biochemistry and Molecular Biology Nomenclature Commitee (1992) Enzyme Nomenclature. Academic Press
10. Kanehisa, M., Goto, S. (2000) KEGG: Kyoto Encyclopedia of Genes and Genomes. Nucleic Acid Research **28** (1), 27–30
11. Kanne, C.-C. (2000) BioPath database schema. Internal documentation
12. Kanne, C.-C., Schreiber, F., Trümbach, D. (1999) Electronic Biochemical Pathways. In: J. Kratochvil (ed.) Graph Drawing '99, Lecture Notes in Computer Science 1731, Springer-Verlag, 418–419

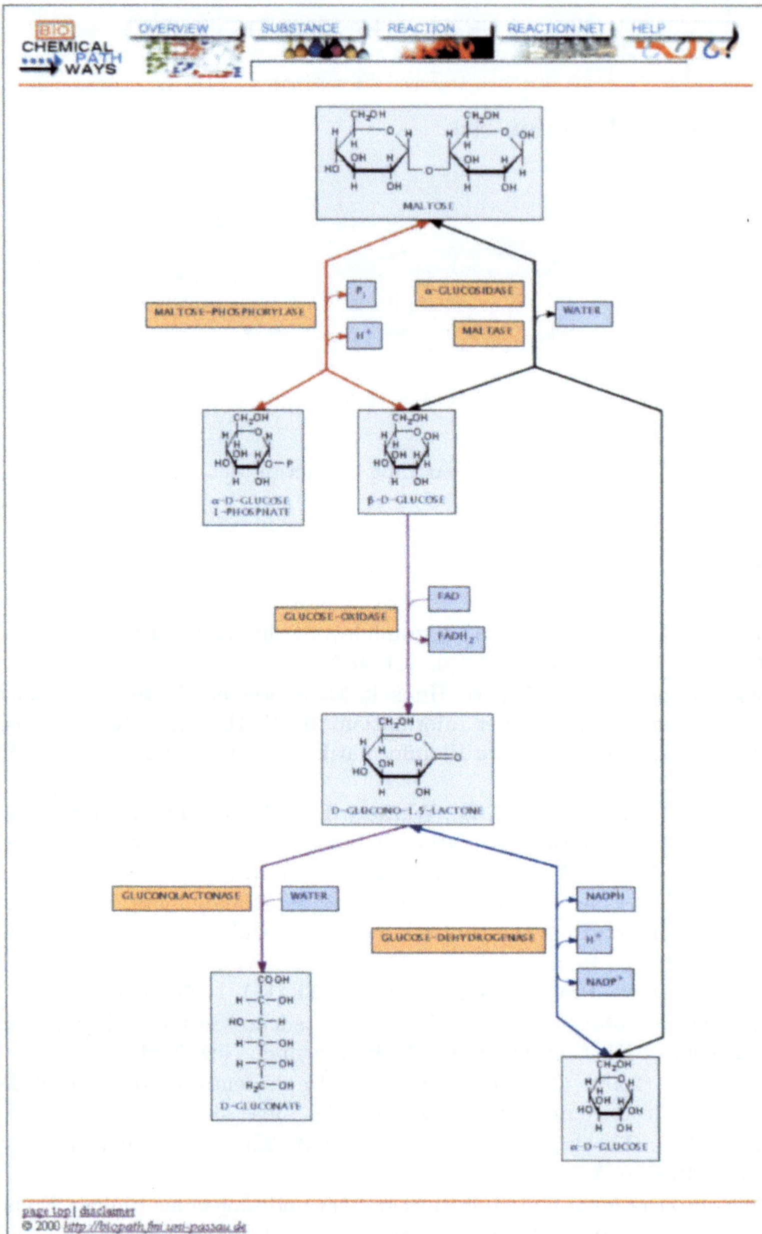

Fig. 17. A reaction net. This view contains structural formulas for substances. The image is automatically produced by the layout algorithm of *BioPath*.

13. Karp, P. D., Paley, S. M. (1994) Automated Drawing of Metabolic Pathways. In: H. Lim, C. Cantor, and R. Bobbins (eds.) Proceedings of the 3rd International Conference on Bioinformatics and Genome Research, 225–238
14. Karp, P. D., Riley, M., Saier, M., Paulsen, I. T., Paley, S. M., Pellegrini-Toole, A. (2000) The EcoCyc and MetaCyc database. Nucleid Acids Research **28**, 56–59
15. Mendes, P. (2000) Advanced Visualization of Metabolic Pathways in PathDB. In: Proceedings of the 8th Conference on Plant and Animal Genome
16. Michal, G. (1993) Biochemical Pathways (Poster). Boehringer Mannheim, Penzberg
17. Michal, G. (1999) Biochemical Pathways. Spektrum Akademischer Verlag, Heidelberg
18. Michal, G. (2000) Personal Communication.
19. Misue, K., Eades, P., Lai, W., Sugiyama, K. (1995) Layout Adjustment and the Mental Map. Journal of Visual Languages and Computing **6**, 183–210
20. `http://www.ebi.ac.uk/research/pfmp/`.
21. Reddy, V. N., Mavrovouniotis, M. L., Liebman, M. N. (1993) Petri Net Representations of Metabolic Pathways. In: L. Hunter, D. Searls, and J. Shavlik (eds.) Proceedings of the 1st International Conference on Intelligent Systems for Molecular Biology (ISMB'93), 328–336
22. Stryer, L. (1995) Biochemie. Spektrum Akademischer Verlag, Heidelberg
23. Sugiyama, K., Tagawa, S., Toda, M. (1981) Methods for Visual Understanding of Hierarchical System Structures. IEEE Transactions on Systems, Man and Cybernetics **SMC-11** (2), 109–125

DBdraw – Automatic Layout of Relational Database Schemas*

Giuseppe Di Battista[1], Walter Didimo[2], Maurizio Patrignani[1], and Maurizio Pizzonia[1]

[1] Università di Roma Tre, Dipartimento di Informatica e Automazione, Via della Vasca Navale 79, 00146 Roma, Italy
[2] Università di Perugia, Dipartimento di Ingegneria Elettronica e dell'Informazione, Via G. Duranti 93, 06125 Perugia, Italy

1 Introduction

DBdraw is a tool for the automatic layout of schemas coming from relational databases. The automatic production of high quality diagrams representing database schemas is a challenging task. In fact, such diagrams are strongly constrained (see Figure 1 for an example):

- each table of the database schema is usually represented as a box composed by a vertically ordered sequence of attributes, with the name of the table at the top
- edges, representing constraints or join paths between tables, link attributes of different tables
- edges may attach arbitrarily to the left side or to the right side of the boxes and should be incident on the box at the level of the corresponding attribute name.

Although many commercial tools provide some diagramming facility, generally such facilities rely on the user skills for producing readable and effective diagrams. However, drawing diagrams by hand is time consuming and the æsthetic results are often unsatisfactory. Further, a special attention is needed in order to keep the graphical documentation consistent with an evolving system.

DBdraw automatically produces such drawings, easing the task of maintaining up-to-date documentation, and helping the exploration of complex database schemas. While DBdraw is a tool interacting directly with the end-user through a friendly graphic interface, its drawing engine, available as an

* Work partially supported by European Commission - Fet Open project COSIN – COevolution and Self-organization In dynamical Networks – IST-2001-33555, by "Progetto ALINWEB: Algoritmica per Internet e per il Web", MIUR Programmi di Ricerca Scientifica di Rilevante Interesse Nazionale, and by "The Multichannel Adaptive Information Systems (MAIS) Project", MIUR Fondo per gli Investimenti della Ricerca di Base.

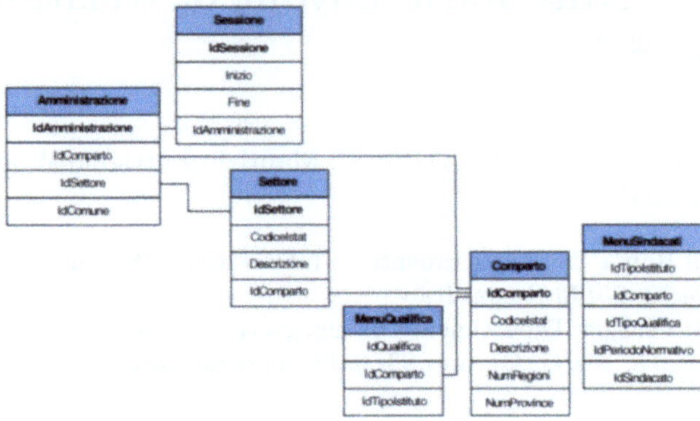

Fig. 1. An example of a diagram representing a small database schema.

independent library, may be accessed by other applications by means of an easy-to-use API.

The technique used by DBdraw in order to produce database schema drawings relies on the formulation of a constrained orthogonal graph drawing problem, which is addressed within the topology-shape-metrics approach described in Section 4.4 of the Technical Foundations. Such approach may be suitably tailored in order to take into account the complex constraints originated by this type of diagrams. Both the polynomial time algorithm for drawing diagrams of relational database schemas and the DBdraw architecture and user interface are described in the following sections.

2 Applications

2.1 The Application Domain

The *relational model*, due to Codd [5] and based on the intuitive concept of table, is the foundation of most current database management systems. In such a model a *table* with n columns is a set of ordered n-tuples, such that values in the same position of any two tuples have the same data type. Each table is identified by a unique name, and each column of the table is also identified by a name, called *attribute*, unique within that table. The name of the table with the ordered sequence of its attributes is called *table schema* while the set of tuples in a table is referred to as the *table instance*. A *database schema* is a set of table schemas with distinct table names, and a *database instance* is a set of table instances consistent with a certain database schema.

Each table schema is provided with a *key*, defined as a set of attributes of a table that unambiguously identifies its tuples (there are no two tuples of the table with the same values on the attributes of the key).

For a given application some database instances may represent meaningless information. To maintain the data consistency in commonly used database management systems several types of relationships and/or constraints between tables are defined (see [3] for a comprehensive survey). Each of them takes the form $(\langle T_1, A\rangle, \langle T_2, B\rangle)$, where T_1 and T_2 are table schemas and A and B are subsets of attributes of T_1 and T_2, respectively. Further, A and B have the same cardinality and have pairwise the same data type. The most used relationships, the *foreign keys* and the *join relationships*, are defined hereunder:

Foreign Key: given a table schema T, a set A of attributes of T, and a tuple t of an instance of T, denote by $t(A)$ the sub-tuple of t restricted to the attributes in A. A foreign key of the form $(\langle T_1, X\rangle, \langle T_2, K\rangle)$, where K is a key of table T_2, imposes that for each tuple t_1 in the instance of T_1, there exists a tuple t_2 in the instance of T_2 such that $t_1(X)$ is equal to $t_2(K)$.

Join Relationship: a join relationship of the form $(\langle T_1, A\rangle, \langle T_2, B\rangle)$ states that there is a frequently used join operation between T_1 and T_2, involving the subsets of attributes A and B. Database management systems allow also to specify the "behavior" of the join. For example, a user can say that the join should consider only the tuples that have the same values on the joined attributes (*natural join*). Otherwise, a user can say that the join should consider at least one tuple for each tuple of T_1, possibly with null values for the attributes of T_2, and only those tuples from T_2 that match at least one tuple in T_1 (*left outer join*). Refer to [3] for further details.

In the following both join relationships and foreign keys of the form $(\langle T_1, A\rangle, \langle T_2, B\rangle)$ are simply called *links*, and the pairs $\langle T_1, A\rangle$ and $\langle T_2, B\rangle$ are the *extremes* of the link. To simplify the terminology, we also say that a link $(\langle T_1, A\rangle, \langle T_2, B\rangle)$ is *incident* on all the attributes in the sets A and B.

In order to design, maintain, update, and query databases, users and administrators cope with the complexity of the database schemas describing the structure of the data. A graphical representation of such schemas greatly improves the friendliness of a database application and is essential for producing high-quality documentation. In the following section the drawing convention used by DBdraw to represent relational database schemas is described.

2.2 Drawing Conventions of the Application Domain

DBdraw's purpose is to visualize a database schema in terms of its table schemas and the links between them. The drawing convention adopted by DBdraw is mutated from the graphical representations found in commonly used systems for handling databases. Further, graphic constraints are enforced in order to improve the readability of the drawing. In particular, tables are not allowed to overlap and links are not allowed to traverse tables.

In the following such drawing convention is formally defined. For the sake of simplicity we only consider the case in which all links have the cardinality of A (and B) equal to one. It is not difficult to remove such restriction by adding suitable graphic attributes in a post-processing step.

Table schemas: each table schema is represented as a box and its attributes are sequentially listed in the box, with each attribute corresponding to a horizontal stripe. We suppose that the vertical order of the attributes of a table schema is given and that the drawing must preserve such an ordering. This feature allows the user to rank the attributes in order of "importance" or to put "related" attributes close together. The stripe at the top of each box is reserved for the table name. All the stripes have the same height. Two tables cannot overlap.

Links: each link $(\langle T_1, A\rangle, \langle T_2, B\rangle)$ is represented as a polygonal line p between the boxes of the two table schemas T_1 and T_2. The segments composing p are either horizontal or vertical (*orthogonal standard*); p is horizontally incident on the stripes associated with the attributes in A and B. A link cannot overlap any table. The only allowed overlaps between links are the crossings between a horizontal segment and a vertical segment belonging to distinct links.

We call DBS-DRAWING (*DataBase Schema-drawing*) a drawing of a database schema that respects the above conventions. An example of a DBS-DRAWING is depicted in Figure 1.

The algorithms used by DBdraw for computing DBS-DRAWINGS are described in the following section.

3 Algorithms

In this section we describe the algorithm used by DBdraw for computing DBS-DRAWINGS. First we give an overview of each basic step. Then each step is described in detail in a dedicated section. In [7] the overall process is shown to have a polynomial time complexity and its performance is measured by means of an experimental analysis.

For simplicity, we consider only the case in which for each link $(\langle T_1, A\rangle,$ $\langle T_2, B\rangle)$ the sets A and B have both cardinality equal to one. Otherwise, we just select one attribute for each of the two sets A and B. In fact, as mentioned in the section describing the drawing convention for database schema, suitable graphic attributes can be added to the drawing in a post-processing step in order to handle the general case.

3.1 Overview of the Drawing Process

Let S be a database schema. The *underlying* graph G_S of S is defined as follows:

- The vertices of G_S are the tables of S

- There is an edge in G_S between tables T_1 and T_2 if there is a link in S involving T_1 and T_2.

In what follows G_S is assumed to be connected. If G_S is not connected the algorithm described in the following is applied to every connected component, and the obtained drawing are subsequently arranged on the plane.

DBdraw uses a drawing process consisting of four main steps, informally described below:

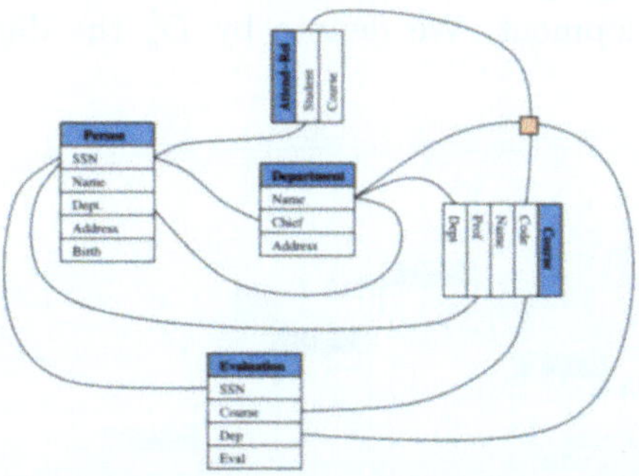

Fig. 2. The output of the Constrained Planarization step.

Constrained Planarization Given a database schema S, the purpose of this step is to obtain a planar embedding of G_S such that the circular order of the edges around each vertex v_T, representing a table T, is compatible with the specific sequence of attributes of T. The output is an embedded graph G'_S where dummy vertices of degree four are introduced to replace crossings (*cross-vertices*). Each link of S is represented in G'_S as an alternating chain of edges and cross-vertices (Figure 2).

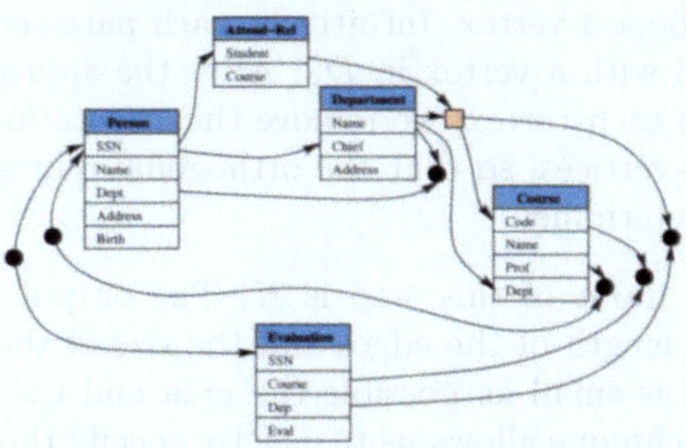

Fig. 3. The output of the Left-to-right Orientation step.

Left-to-right Orientation This step deals with the left-to-right development of the drawing. From this perspective the edges of the drawing are of two types: edges that monotonically follow the left-to-right direction and edges that perform one or more u-turns. A *u-turn* is a point where an edge changes its left-to-right orientation. A left-to-right shape is assigned to G'_s. A (possibly empty) sequence of u-turns is associated with each edge trying to minimize their total number. A u-turn is represented with a particular kind of dummy vertex (*u-vertex*) of degree two (Figure 3). The edges of the graph are made directed according to the computed left-to-right development. We denote by D'_s the digraph produced by this step.

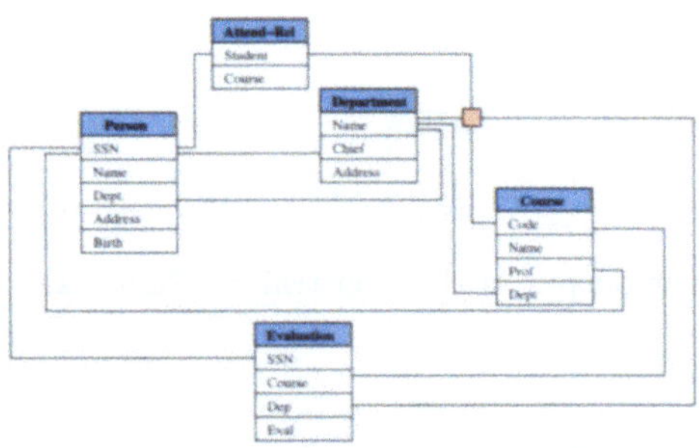

Fig. 4. The output of the Orthogonalization step.

Orthogonalization The result of this step is an orthogonal representation H of G'_S (Figure 4). H is obtained from D'_S by applying the transformation patterns depicted in Figure 9. For each vertex a pattern is selected according to its type. Each vertex may represent a table, may be a cross-vertex or may be a u-vertex. Intuitively, each pattern describes the part of H associated with a vertex in D'_S. After the appropriate pattern has been applied to each vertex, we remove the orientation of the edges and "absorb" the u-vertices, so that the orthogonal representation H of G'_S is completely determined.

Compaction The input of this step is H. The output is the final DBS-DRAWING. The length of the edges and the size of the vertices are computed, keeping as small as possible the area and the total edge length. The adopted technique allows us to exactly specify the incidence point of each link on the boxes representing the tables involved in the link. Cross-vertices introduced in the Constrained Planarization step are removed (Figure 5).

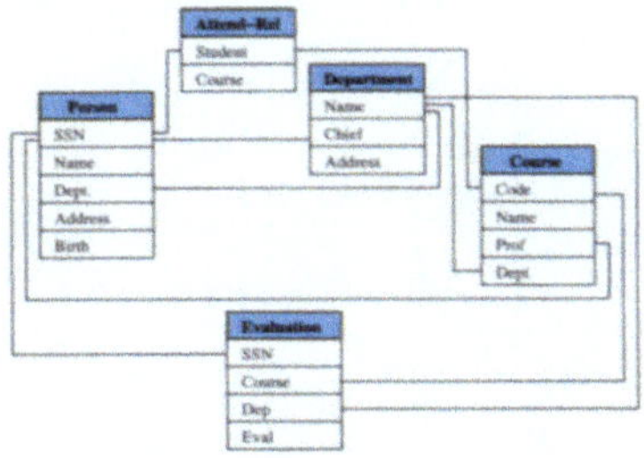

Fig. 5. The output of the Compaction step.

3.2 Constrained Planarization

In the Constrained Planarization step, a planarization is performed on G_S. The output of this step is an embedded graph G'_S that has the same vertices as G_S plus dummy vertices of degree four introduced to represent crossings (cross-vertices). Each link of S is represented in G'_S as an alternating chain of edges and cross-vertices. Furthermore, the embedding that we construct for G'_S is an *lr-embedding*. An lr-embedding is such that:

1. The edges incident on each vertex v_T representing a table T with attributes $a_1, \ldots, a_k$ are partitioned into $2k$ possibly empty sets $l_1, \ldots, l_k$, $r_1, \ldots, r_k$.
2. The edges of $l_i \cup r_i$ represent the links incident on attribute a_i.
3. The edges of l_i (r_i) are contiguous in the circular order around v_T.
4. Sets $l_1, \ldots, l_k, r_k, \ldots, r_1$ appear in this counter-clockwise order around v_T.

The edges of l_i (r_i) are called *left* (*right*) edges. Links represented by an edge of l_i (r_i) enter table T from the left (right) in the final drawing.

By using a standard planarization facility [8] in which some edges can be specified as non-crossable, the lr-embedding can be computed with the following procedure.

Chain-graph Construction A new graph C_{G_S}, called the *chain-graph of* G_S, is constructed from G_S. Namely, for each vertex v_T of G_S, associated with a table T with k attributes, a chain with $(k+2)$ vertices is introduced in C_{G_S}. Vertices and edges of the chain are called *attribute-vertices* and *attribute-edges*, respectively. The sequence of attribute-vertices composing the chain is $\{v_{\text{north}}, v_1, \ldots, v_k, v_{\text{south}}\}$, where v_i is associated with attribute a_i ($i = 1, \ldots, k$). The edges representing links incident on attribute a_i are made incident on v_i. Intuitively, attribute-vertices and attribute-edges represent the sequence of the attributes of the table, and vertices v_{north} and v_{south} represent the top and the bottom of the table, respectively (see Figure 6(a)).

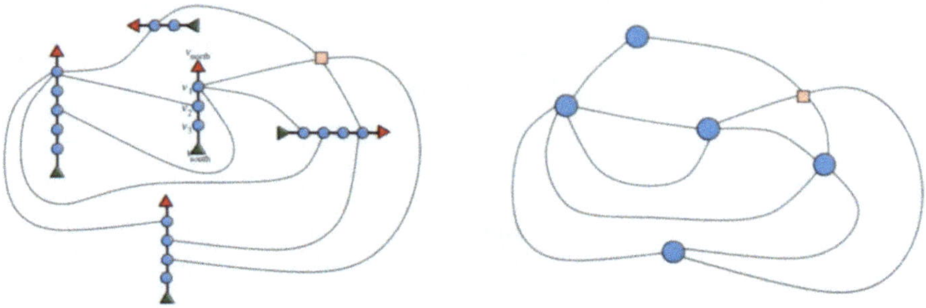

(a) (b)

Fig. 6. The chain-graph C_{G_S}, once planarized (a), corresponds to an embedding of the original graph G_S compatible with the order of tables' attributes. Such embedding can be obtained by contracting the chains (b). The square represents a cross-vertex while triangles represent the upper part or the lower part of a table.

Chain-graph Planarization A planarization is performed on C_{G_S} with the constraint that every attribute-edge of C_{G_S} is uncrossable. Since the subgraph of C_{G_S} induced by the uncrossable attribute-edges is a forest (in fact, it is a collection of paths) the constrained planarization is always possible. The embedded graph C'_{G_S} contains the same *attribute-vertices* and *attribute-edges* as C_{G_S}, while every other edge of C_{G_S} is represented in C'_{G_S} as an alternating chain of edges and cross-vertices. In Figure 6(a) the square represents a cross-vertex.

Chain Contraction The lr-embedding for G'_S is obtained from C'_{G_S} by contracting all the attribute-edges associated with the same table into a unique vertex. All the other edges and cross-vertices remain unchanged (see Figure 6(b)). More formally, the circular order of the edges around each vertex v_T is computed in the following way. For each table T consider the path of attribute-vertices $\{v_{\text{north}}, v_1, \ldots, v_k, v_{\text{south}}\}$ that represents T in C'_{G_S}. Each attribute-vertex v_i, with $i = 1 \ldots k$, is incident on two attribute-edges that we call the north attribute-edge and the south attribute-edge of v_i according to the north-south orientation of the path. For each attribute-vertex v_i we assign to l_i (r_i) the sequence of edges that is incident on v_i between the north (south) attribute-edge and the south (north) attribute-edge in counter-clockwise order. The circular sequence around v_T is obtained by concatenating $l_1, \ldots, l_k, r_k, \ldots, r_1$ in this order.

Observe that the above algorithm for finding an lr-embedding requires the capability of planarizing a graph in such a way that specific edges never intersect (uncrossable edges). This capability is available in existing graph drawing libraries (for example, GDToolkit [9]). We also observe that the above algorithm is correct. Its correctness is based on the following observations:

- The constrained planarization of C_{G_S} can always be performed since the graph induced by the uncrossable attribute-edges is a forest, and hence it is planar and acyclic. Its planarity guarantees that it can be used as a starting point for the Incremental Maximal Planar Subgraph algorithm of the Edge Removal step of the planarization technique described in Section 4.3 of the Technical Foundations, while its acyclicity allows the re-insertion of the remaining edges by computing a shortest path on the dual graph that does not make use of the edges of the dual graph corresponding to uncrossable edges of C_{G_S} (see Section 4.3 in the Technical Foundations for a detailed description of the Edge Re-Insertion step of planarization).
- An edge can be contracted only if the planarization step did not split it by inserting a cross-vertex. Since attribute-edges are uncrossable, they can always be contracted.
- The construction of the chain-graph performed in the first step makes it impossible, in the ordering of the edges around v_T, to have "mixings" of edges of l_i (r_i) with $l_j \cup r_j$ ($i \neq j$). This implies that the edges of l_i (r_i) appear consecutively around v_T.
- After the contraction of attribute-edges of table T, sets $l_1, \ldots, l_k, r_k, \ldots, r_1$ appear in this counter-clockwise order around v_T.

3.3 Left-to-right Orientation

In this step, which deals with the left-to-right development of the drawing, a (possibly empty) sequence of u-vertices is associated with each edge of G'_S. Informally, the purpose of u-vertices insertion is to obtain an orientation of the edges compatible with an upward drawing of the graph in which the edges incident on the left (right) side of a vertex corresponding to a table are incoming (outgoing) the vertex. Intuitively, when this upward drawing is positioned so that edges flow from left to right, all the tables are upright, that is, they have the title in the upper stripe. Each u-vertex has degree two and represents a u-turn in the final drawing, that is a left-to-right edge followed by a right-to-left edge or vice versa (see Figure 3).

U-vertices are introduced along with an orientation of the edges of G'_S, in such a way that the resulting digraph can be drawn upward planar in the left-right direction within the given embedding. The algorithm used by DBdraw for introducing u-vertices and assigning an orientation to the edges works in two steps, detailed below:

- **Bimodal Graph Construction:** a first suitable number of u-vertices is introduced and an orientation is given to all the edges of G'_S in order to obtain a digraph D'_S with a planar bimodal embedding (see Section 3.2 in the Technical Foundations for a definition of bimodal and bimodal embedding).
- **Upward Graph Construction:** a constrained version of the algorithm in [4] is applied on D'_S, in order to compute a minimum number of addi-

tional u-vertices that are needed to produce an upward planar drawing of the digraph in the left-right direction.

In the following we describe the two steps in detail.

Bimodal Graph Construction In the Bimodal Graph Construction step a digraph D'_S is computed in such a way that it has an associated bimodal planar embedding (see Section 3.2 in the Technical Foundations) that preserves the planar embedding of G'_S on the common vertices. In order to guarantee that a planar bimodal embedding of D'_S exists, we require the following properties to hold:

Property 1: all the left (right) edges incident on a vertex v of D'_S that represents a table are oriented incoming (outgoing) v.

Property 2: consider the two edges incident on a cross-vertex v of D'_S corresponding to the same link. Such edges are oriented one incoming and the other outgoing v.

Property 3: the two edges incident on an u-vertex v of D'_S are oriented either both incoming or both outgoing v.

The algorithm used by DBdraw for computing D'_S is based on the following strategy. At each step a different link of the graph is considered and all the edges that represent this link are oriented. During the orientation, it might be necessary to add one u-vertex on the link in order to satisfy Property 1. Since a link is taken into account exactly once, and since at most one new u-vertex is added for each link, D'_S can be computed in linear time in the number of edges of G'_S as follows.

For each link of G'_S, let $v_1, e_1, v_2, e_2, \dots, v_n, e_n, v_{n+1}$ $(n > 0)$ be the ordered sequence of vertices and edges that form the link. Vertices v_1 and v_{n+1} represent the extreme tables of the link, while the remaining vertices represent crossings. Two cases are possible:

Case (a): edge e_1 is a left edge of v_1.

1. Edge e_i is oriented incoming v_i, for any i in $1 \dots n-1$.
2. Edge e_n is oriented incoming v_n if e_n is a right edge of v_{n+1}. Otherwise, it is split into two new edges by adding a new u-vertex u and the two new edges are oriented both outgoing u.

Case (b): edge e_1 is a right edge of v_1.

1. Edge e_i is oriented outgoing from v_i, for any i in $1 \dots n-1$.
2. Edge e_n is oriented outgoing v_n if e_n is a left edge of v_{n+1}. Otherwise, it is split into two new edges by adding a new u-vertex u and the two new edges are oriented both incoming u.

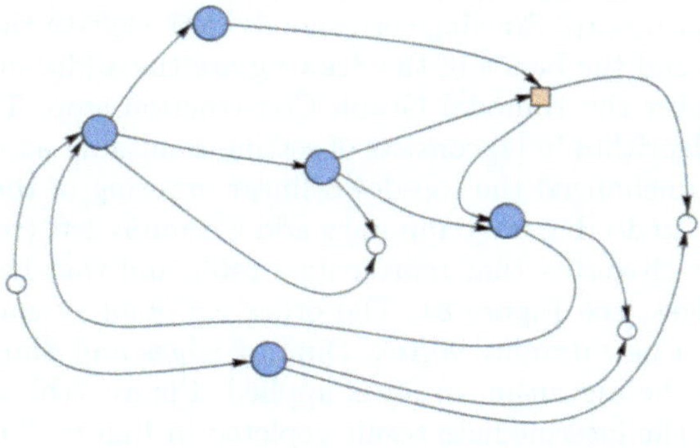

(a) Bimodal Graph Construction

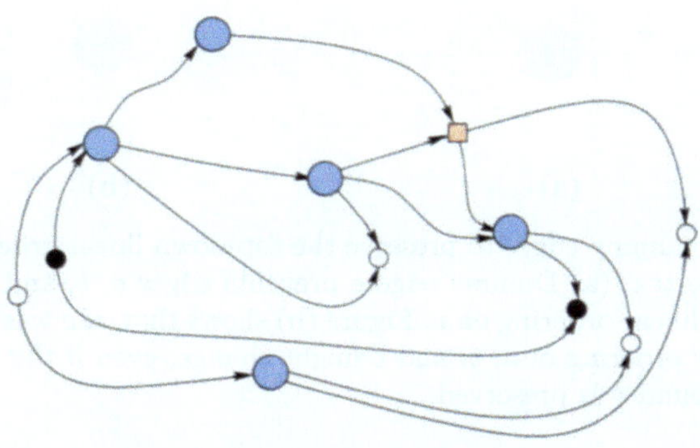

(b) Upward Graph Construction

Fig. 7. Left-to-right Orientation: (a) Assigning an orientation to the edges and adding u-turns to find a bimodal embedded digraph in the Bimodal Graph Construction step (u-vertices are represented as white circles). (b) Adding a minimum set of additional u-vertices to get an embedded upward planar digraph in the Upward Graph Construction step (the additional u-vertices are represented as black circles).

Observe that the split operation and the subsequent orientation of the produced edges are sufficient to keep Properties 1 and 3 always valid. Further, the orientations of the two edges representing the same link and incident on a cross-vertex are assigned in such a way that Property 2 also holds.

Figure 7(a) shows a digraph obtained by applying the above algorithm to the graph of Figure 6(b).

Upward Graph Construction This step is a simple variation of the algorithm presented in [4]. Namely, it computes a quasi-upward planar drawing of an embedded bimodal digraph with the minimum number of bends. The computed quasi-upward drawing corresponds to the left-to-right development of the schema and the bends of the drawing are the additional u-vertices we have to add after the Bimodal Graph Construction step. The variation we apply to the algorithm in [4] consists of setting a suitable set of constraints in order to keep unchanged the top-down linear ordering of the edges incident on each table. To do that we temporary add a dummy left (right) edge entering (leaving) each vertex that represents a table and that has only outgoing (incoming) edges (see Figure 8). The other endpoint of each dummy edge is attached to a new dummy vertex. Dummy edges and dummy vertices are removed after the algorithm in [4] is applied. Figure 7(b) shows a digraph obtained from the intermediate result depicted in Figure 7(a).

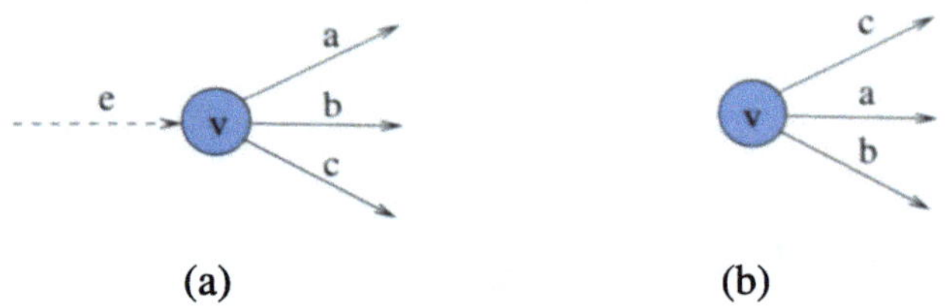

Fig. 8. Adding dummy edges to preserve the top-down linear ordering of the edges incident on a vertex. (a) Dummy edge e prevents edges a, b, and c from changing their top-down linear ordering on v. Figure (b) shows that, if e was not inserted, the top-down linear ordering of a, b, and c might change, even if the circular ordering of the edges around v is preserved.

3.4 Orthogonalization

This step yields an orthogonal representation H of G'_S preserving the left-to-right development of the drawing determined by the previous step. More formally, it is required that all the edges incoming a vertex v of H representing a table are incident on the left side of v, while all the edges outgoing v are incident on the right side of v. Also, the top-down ordering of the edges incident on v, computed in the u-turn assignment step, must not be changed.

We compute H from D'_S, by simply applying the transformation patterns shown in Figure 9. Namely, for each vertex v in D'_S three different cases are possible:

- If v represents a table then pattern (a) is applied.
- If v is a cross-vertex then pattern (b) is applied.
- If v is an u-vertex then pattern (c) or pattern (d) is applied depending on the direction of the two edges (incoming or outgoing) that incite on v.

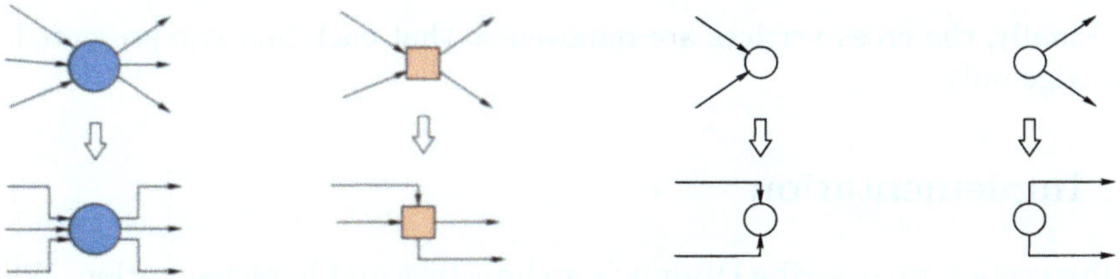

Fig. 9. Patterns for constructing an orthogonal representation after the left-to-right orientation. (a) Vertex representing a table; (b) Cross-vertex; (c,d) u-vertices.

Patterns (a) and (b) describe the angles between the edges that are incident on v plus part of the shape of such edges. Patterns (c) and (d) describe the shape of the edge in correspondence of a u-turn. Namely, we recall that in D'_S a u-turn is represented by a u-vertex, absorbed in H.

Hence, in H, we model a u-turn by adding two consecutive 90 degrees bends on the edge to which the u-turn belongs. After H is computed by applying the above defined procedure, the orientation of the edges of H is removed, that is, it is ignored from now on (see Figure 4).

Observe that the straightforward application of the above patterns may give rise to unnecessary bends on the edges. Namely, on some edges of H there may be sub-sequences of alternate left and right bends that can be removed. In [7] a simple post-processing algorithm for the removal of such avoidable bends is described.

3.5 Compaction

In this step the final DBS-DRAWING is computed from the orthogonal representation H by assigning coordinates to vertices and bends, and by giving the correct size to each vertex representing a table.

We essentially apply the compaction algorithm described in [6]: it computes a Kandinsky drawing (see Section 4.4 in the Technical Foundations) preserving the shape of H. The width we assign to each table is proportional to the length of the longest attribute of the table. The name of the table is also taken into account. The height we assign to each table is proportional to the number of attributes of the table itself.

We also have to guarantee that each link $(\langle T_1, A\rangle, \langle T_2, B\rangle)$, where A and B have cardinality equal to one, is incident on T_1 and T_2 at the heights of the attributes in A and B. The basic version of the algorithm described in [6] allows the edges to freely shift along the side they are incident on. However, it is possible to easily adapt such algorithm so that the point on which each edge is incident is pre-assigned.

Finally, the cross-vertices are removed so that each link is represented by one edge only.

4 Implementation

In this section we describe DBdraw's architecture and implementation. While DBdraw interacts directly with the end-user through a friendly interface, we devoted special attention to create modular and reusable code. This allows other database-related applications to use DBdraw's drawing engine. Thus, DBdraw architecture represents a carefully chosen tradeoff between use simplicity and flexibility. In the following we first introduce such an architecture and then describe it in detail. Our software system is composed by two main parts:

- The *DBdraw drawing engine*, a module that encapsulates the implementation of the `DBS-algorithm`. The drawing engine API allows to create the graph representing the database schema and to compute a drawing of it. The architecture of the drawing engine is further articulated into several parts, explained in detail afterwards.
- The *DBdraw main application* provides an interface for the end-user and communicates with the drawing engine by means of its API.

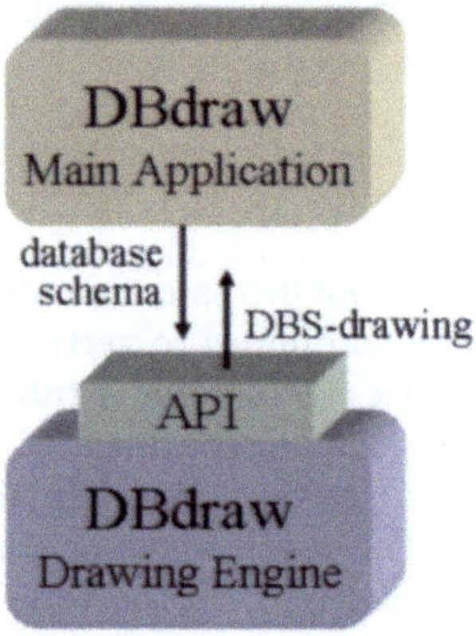

Fig. 10. The two main blocks of DBdraw architecture. We encapsulated the implementation of the `DBS-algorithm` into the *drawing engine*. The main application interacts with the drawing engine by means of a well defined API.

A schematic illustration of the architecture described above is depicted in Figure 10.

The two main parts into which the project is divided, the main application and the drawing engine, correspond to different skill levels needed for their development. Thus, in addition to facilitating the reuse of the core implementation of the algorithm in a multiplicity of systems, they follow naturally from the goal of efficiently employing the resources.

4.1 The Drawing Engine

An implementation "from scratch" of the `DBS-algorithm` would require several man-year of work. However, many graph drawing libraries, built for commercial or research purposes, may be effectively used in order to reduce the implementation and maintenance effort [1,9,12].

We chose to implement the `DBS-algorithm` in C++ using the GDToolkit[1] library. This library provides algorithms and data structures for graph drawing applications and supports both orthogonal and quasi-upward drawings within the topology-shape-metrics approach. Further, various constraints on the drawings are dealt with. GDToolkit is built on LEDA [11], using especially its basic data structures and the efficient planarity testing algorithm described in [10]. Figure 11 shows the drawing engine architecture. To have an idea of the relative weight of each layer we measured that GDToolkit consists of about 70,000 lines of code while the `DBS-algorithm` implementation consists of 3,000 lines of code. LEDA consists of about 200,000 lines of code, but only a small portion of it is used. The implementation of the `DBS-algorithm` with GDToolkit is described in detail in the next section.

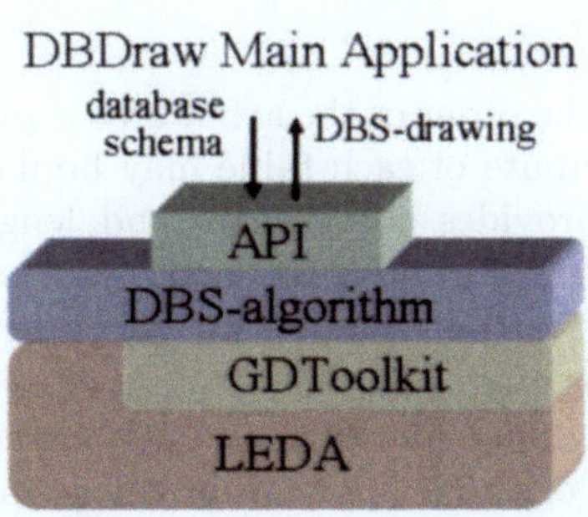

Fig. 11. The architecture of the drawing engine. The *DBS-algorithm* layer fills the gap between GDToolkit (a general graph drawing library) and the specific needs of the application.

Figure 12 shows the relevant methods of the API of the drawing engine. To improve the re-usability of the drawing engine, we especially studied the

[1] `http://www.dia.uniroma3.it/~gdt`

friendliness of its API. The interaction protocol with the drawing engine is quite simple and the standard usage consists of four steps:

1. Create an instance of the drawing engine.
2. Specify the schema using the input methods of the API that return identifiers for the tables, the attributes, and the created links.
3. Call the *compute* method, that validates the data and computes the drawing.
4. Retrieve the drawing by means of the output methods of the API.

The drawing engine API is written using the STL [2] data structures, so that it is not required to be familiar with specific GDToolkit or LEDA data structures in order to use it.

input	table	**new_table**()
	attribute	**new_attr**(table)
	link	**new_link**(attribute *src*, attribute *trg*)
	void	**set_table_width**(table t, unsigned int x)
commit and compute	void	**compute**()
output	point	**table_top_left**(table)
	list<point>	**link_polyline**(link)

Fig. 12. The most relevant methods of the API provided by the drawing engine: input methods allow to specify the schema, the *compute* method launches the computation, and output methods are used to retrieve graphic information.

Observe that, since the order of the attributes is preserved by the drawing algorithm, the first attribute of each table may be used to contain the table name. Also, the API provides coordinates and lengths in *grid units*. The developer may define all the graphic features, such as font sizes, colors, line styles, according to the freedom allowed by the chosen output device.

The DBdraw drawing engine may be thought of as an independent library. It was developed on a Linux platform and its testing was performed with a simple command-line oriented application whose input schemas were read from files written in XML-based format, and whose output was both shown on a window (using Tcl/Tk for graphic visualization) and saved in a postscript file. In order to make the drawing engine usable on a Microsoft Windows platform, it was wrapped into a Dynamically Linked Library (DLL).

4.2 The DBdraw Main Application and User Interface

The DBdraw main application is implemented in Visual Basic within the Microsoft Windows platform. Its main features are the following:

- It provides a graphical interface that allows the user to specify a Microsoft Access database (i.e., a `.mdb` file).
- It extracts the schema from the specified database.
- It allows the user to select the set of tables of the database schema to be visualized and to choose, for each table, one of the following visualization styles (see also Figure 13):

  Full all attributes of the table are shown.

  Partial only the attributes of the table that are linked to some other attributes are shown.

  Collapsed only the table name is shown (all links are attached to the name stripe).

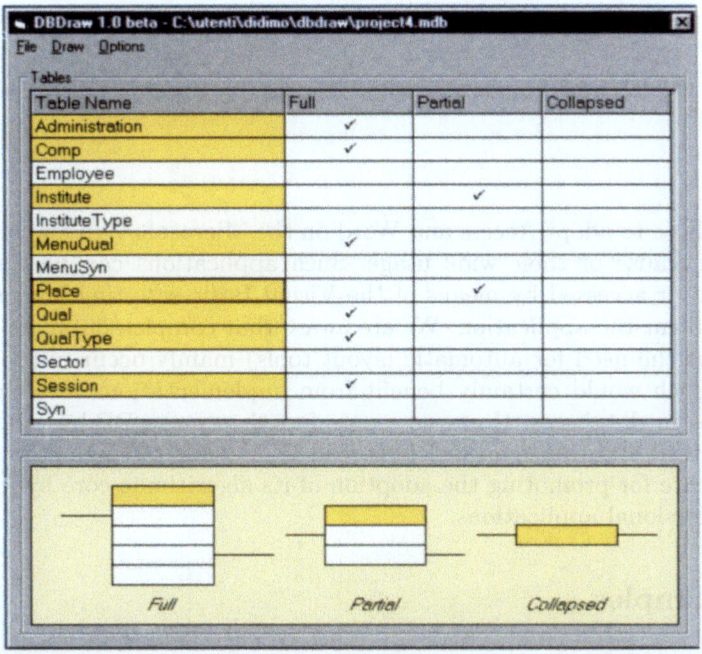

Fig. 13. The DBdraw interface allows the user to select the subset of the tables to be visualized and to choose, for each table, if it has to be visualized with all its attributes (i.e., `full`), only with the attributes that are linked to some other attributes (i.e., `partial`), or without attributes (i.e., `collapsed`).

- It allows the user to customize the graphic features of the drawing to be produced (see Figure 14).
- It computes the drawing, according to the given specifications, by using the drawing engine described above.
- It embeds the drawing in a Microsoft Word document whose name is specified by the user.

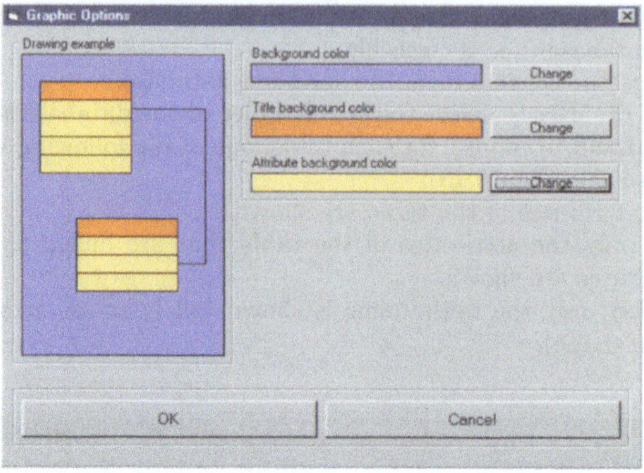

Fig. 14. The DBdraw window that allows the user to customize the drawing to be produced.

We chose to adopt Access and Word on the Microsoft Windows operating system because of their wide usage. Such applications can be easily programmed or accessed by means of the Visual Basic scripting language used to implement the application. We are aware that complex database schemas (and thus the need for automatic layout tools) mainly occur in professional areas, which would certainly benefit from implementations involving other platforms or databases. However, we preferred to make DBdraw easy to install, to test, and to use on widely spread PCs, while relying on its modular architecture for promoting the adoption of its algorithmic core by more specific professional applications.

5 Examples

Figures 15 and 16 provide some example of the DBdraw output within a Microsoft Word document. By selecting suitable subsets of the database tables, even big database schemas can be documented with a collection of drawings (DBdraw always inserts the pictures at the end of the selected Word file). Also, since the drawings are inserted as Microsoft Word Pictures into the document, they may be edited by hand if needed (DBdraw suitably groups the graphic objects in order to ease this refinement).

6 Software

The DBdraw system is available for download at
`http://www.dia.uniroma3.it/~dbdraw` or by contacting the authors.

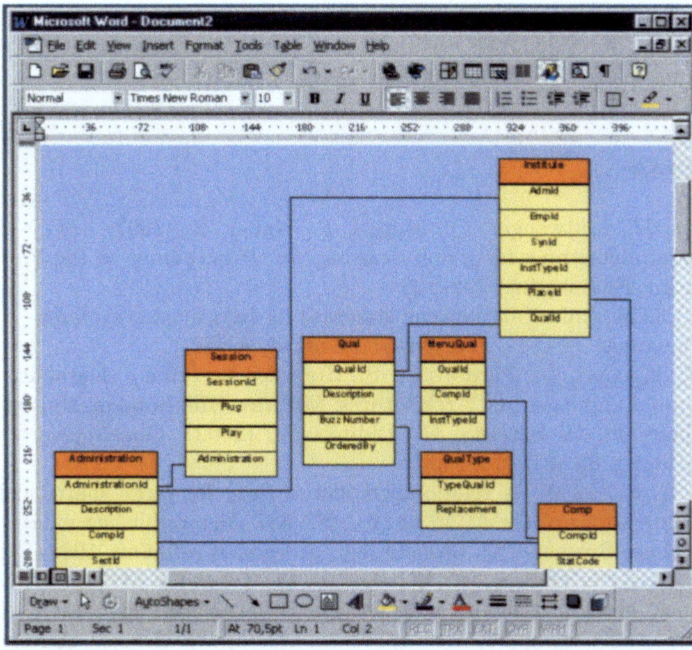

Fig. 15. An example of DBdraw output within a Microsoft® Word document.

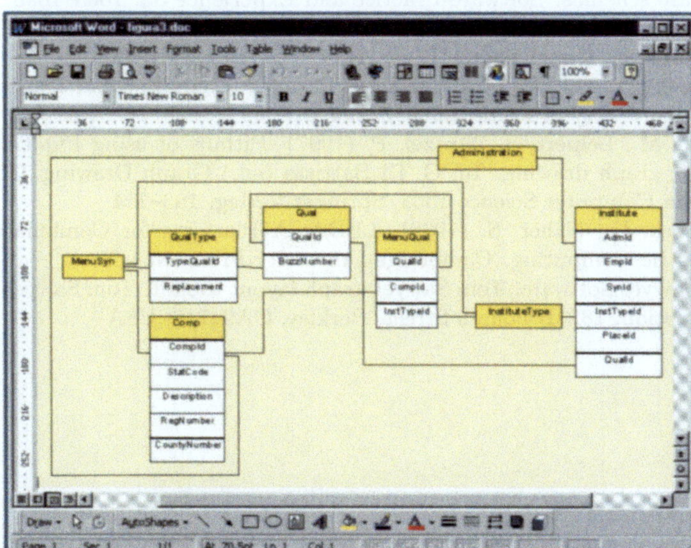

Fig. 16. An example of DBdraw output within a Microsoft® Word document.

Acknowledgment

Antonio Leonforte implemented part of the system.

References

1. Alberts, D., Gutwenger, C., Mutzel, P., Näher, S. (1997) AGD-Library: A library of algorithms for graph drawing. In: Proceedings of the Workshop on Algorithm Engineering, 112–123
2. ANSI X3J16. American national standard for information systems — programming language — C++. Approved standard, ANSI
3. Atzeni, P., Ceri, S., Paraboschi, S., Torlone, R. (1999) Database Systems: Concepts, Languages and Architetures. McGraw Hill, London, United Kingdom
4. Bertolazzi, P., Di Battista, G., Didimo, W. (2002) Quasi-upward planarity. Algorithmica **32** (3), 474–506
5. Codd, E. F. (1970) A relational model of data for large shared data banks. Communications of the ACM **13** (6), 377–387 Also published in/as: 'Readings in Database Systems', M. Stonebraker, Morgan-Kaufmann, 1988, 5–15
6. Di Battista, G., Didimo, W., Patrignani, M., Pizzonia, M. (1999) Orthogonal and quasi-upward drawings with vertices of prescribed size. In: J. Kratochvil (ed.) Graph Drawing '99, Lecture Notes in Computer Science, Springer-Verlag, 297–310
7. Di Battista, G., Didimo, W., Patrignani, M., Pizzonia, M. (2002) Drawing database schemas. Software-Practice and Experience **32**, 1065–1098
8. Di Battista, G., Eades, P., Tamassia, R., Tollis, I. G. (1999) Graph Drawing. Prentice Hall, Upper Saddle River, NJ
9. GDToolkit. (1999) An object-oriented library for handling and drawing graphs Third University of Rome, `http://www.dia.uniroma3.it/~gdt`
10. Jünger, M., Leipert, S., Mutzel, P. (1997) Pitfalls of using PQ-Trees in automatic graph drawing. In: G. Di Battista (ed.) Graph Drawing '97, Lecture Notes in Computer Science 1353, Springer-Verlag, 193–204
11. Mehlhorn, K., Näher, S. (1998) LEDA: A Platform for Combinatorial and Geometric Computing. Cambridge University Press, New York
12. Tom Sawyer Software. Tom Sawyer graph layout toolkit. Tom Sawyer Software Corporation, 1824B Fourth Street, Berkley, CA94710, USA

GoVisual

AUTOMATIC DIAGRAM LAYOUT

A Diagramming Software for UML Class Diagrams*

Carsten Gutwenger[1], Michael Jünger[2], Karsten Klein[1], Joachim Kupke[1], Sebastian Leipert[1], and Petra Mutzel[3]

[1] Research Center caesar, Ludwig-Erhard-Allee 2, D-53175 Bonn, Germany
[2] University of Cologne, Department of Computer Science, Pohligstraße 1, D-50969 Köln, Germany
[3] Vienna University of Technology, Institute of Computer Graphics and Algorithms, Favoritenstraße 9–11, A-1040 Wien, Austria

1 Introduction

UML diagrams have become increasingly important in the engineering and reengineering processes for software systems. Of particular interest are UML class diagrams whose purpose is to display class hierarchies (generalizations), associations, aggregations, and compositions in one picture. The combination of hierarchical and non-hierarchical relations poses a special challenge to a graph layout tool.

GoVisual is a graph drawing library that, in contrast to existing tools, treats the hierarchical and non-hierarchical relations neither alike nor as separate tasks in a two-phase process as in, e.g., Seemann [19]. Instead it provides unique techniques that visualize lucidly arranged, orthogonal diagrams featuring hierarchical and non-hierarchical elements in such a way that the directed edges of a component all follow the same direction. Transferred to UML-class diagrams, a layout is created which represents each inheritance hierarchy in an aligned fashion. A compact orthogonal layout (see Section 4.4 of the Technical Foundations) with a minimized number of crossings is calculated.

UML class diagrams consist of classes represented by rectangular regions containing the class name, attributes and operations of the class, and different kinds of relationships between classes that are represented as lines. We distinguish two kinds of relationships: *Generalizations* representing inheritance in class hierarchies and *associations* including *aggregations* and *compositions*. A UML class diagram can therefore be modeled as a graph $G = (V, A, E)$ consisting of two kinds of edges: arcs representing the generalizations in the set A, and edges representing the associations in the set E.

* This research was supported by Research Center caesar, Bonn, Germany

Figure 1 shows a small example of a UML class diagram taken from Purchase *et al.* [18]. Figure 1(a) shows the original layout by Purchase, Figure 1(b) shows an automatic layout computed by GoVisual. The diagram contains two hierarchies, clearly visible in the GoVisual layout in which the hierarchies have been colored blue and green, respectively.

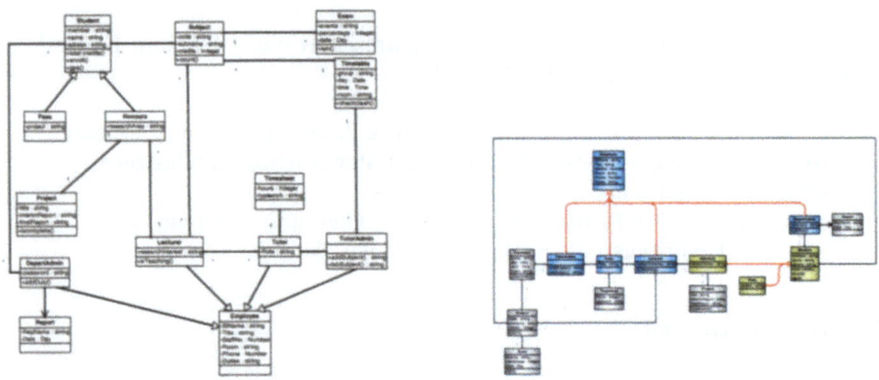

(a) Original Layout in [18].   (b) GoVisual UML Layout.

Fig. 1. UML class diagram for preference experiments assessing the effect of individual æsthetics [18].

Purchase *et al.* [18] have used this diagram to perform preference experiments for assessing the effect of individual æsthetics in the application domain of UML class diagrams. This study resulted in a priority listing of different æsthetics in this application domain. According to Purchase *et al.*, the most important aesthetic preferences for UML class diagrams are

- crossing minimization,
- bend minimization,
- horizontal labels,
- and joined inheritance arcs.

These æsthetic preferences are easily met in the automatic layout shown in Figure 1(b). Moreover, our new approach supports the visual perception of the human reader by

- drawing generalizations in the same class hierarchy always in the same direction,
- avoiding nesting of class hierarchies,
- highlighting the various class hierarchies by different colors,
- and highlighting the generalizations by color.

This approach allows a software engineer to visualize and analyze the hierarchical structure of the class hierarchies within a software project while using a clear orthogonal layout style. These hierarchies determine the layout of class diagrams and allow an easier access for the human reader to the structure of the project.

Complex class diagrams often use aggregation/composition hierarchies in addition to generalization hierarchies. These aggregations/compositions may describe a second hierarchical dimension that users wish to emphasize in a layout. In this chapter, we focus on generalization hierarchies, the same approach can be used to visualize hierarchies different from generalizations. This can be done for any kind of association. It is even possible to visualize all hierarchical dimensions within one diagram. However, such an approach does not reveal enough analytical information, since in this case the graph is usually fully directed, including directed cycles. Thus a layout based on such a directed graph does not emphasize any hierarchical dimensions.

1.1 State of the Art and Industrial Standard

The combination of hierarchical and non-hierarchical relations poses a special challenge to a graph layout tool. Commercial software typically uses Sugiyama-style methods, see, e.g., [4] and [5] that cannot properly distinguish between hierarchical and non-hierarchical relations.

Figures 2 and 3 show such typical industrial layouts. Both diagrams have been taken from different industrial model-driven CASE tools and show an object-oriented software project.

The examples in Figures 2 and 3 show clearly the disadvantages of a hierarchical layout style. While the example in Figure 2 shows technical problems such as unnecessary bends and edges passing through node areas, the example in Figure 3 provides some non hierarchical elements improving the layout. However, in both examples it is not possible to clearly identify for every edge the connected endpoints or to identify the hierarchies. We leave it to the reader to find out how many inheritance hierarchies are contained in both diagrams. In Section 5 the same diagrams are given with GoVisual layout clearly showing the number of inheritance hierarchies.

The next two Figures 4 and 5 demonstrate that any pure non-hierarchical visualization must fail in the automatic layout of class diagrams. Both Figures show the same graph that is used in Figure 2 and have been created by one of the leading CASE tool providers.

The layout given in Figure 4 is a typical symmetric layout that is the result of a low budget solution and leaves the human reader uninformed about the structure of the software project. The orthogonal layout of the same diagram demonstrates, apart from the obvious technical weaknesses, that the missing hierarchical information still does not reveal any information on the project.

The weakness of strictly hierarchical or strictly non hierarchical layout algorithms for mixed hierarchical graphs has been recognized early by See-

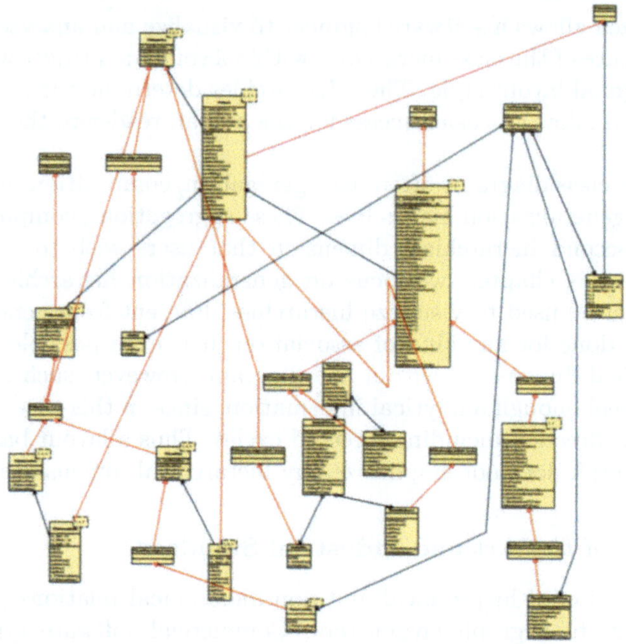

Fig. 2. Industrial layout in Sugiyama style.

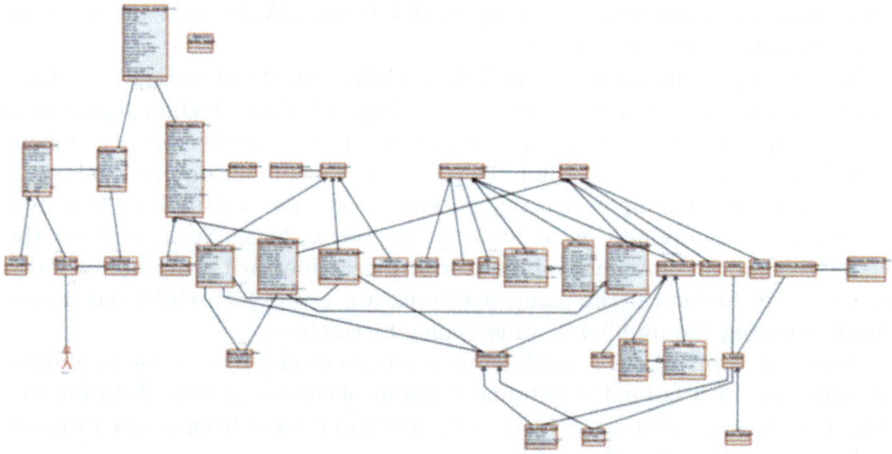

Fig. 3. Industrial layout in Sugiyama style.

mann [19], who presented a two phase method combining Sugiyama layout for the inheritance hierarchies and a routing method for the undirected edges. Figure 6 shows a layout of a diagram that has been drawn using the SugiBib system.

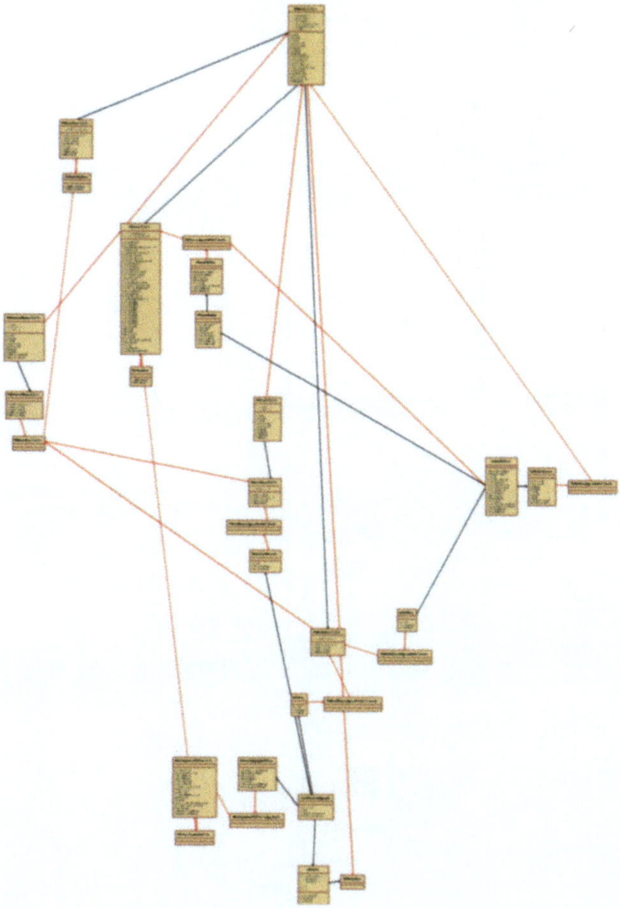

Fig. 4. Industrial layout in symmetric style. Same diagram as in Figure 2.

The drawback of this method is at hand: routing edges within a given drawing results in severe combinatorial problems that end in local optimization methods giving difficult to read results with a rising number of undirected edges. The approach by Seemann [19] was the first to be reported on this special issue and has been enhanced by Eichelberger [8]. Up to now, only very few other approaches have been reported to solve this problem. Recently, Eiglsperger and Kaufmann [9] have enhanced this method and included an implementation into their software system *yFiles*, as presented in the yFiles chapter in this book.

Figure 7 shows a layout that is a result of a semiautomatic approach used by a large variety of layout software tools. The objects and the generalizations are drawn by hand while the associations have been placed automatically, using some routing algorithms.

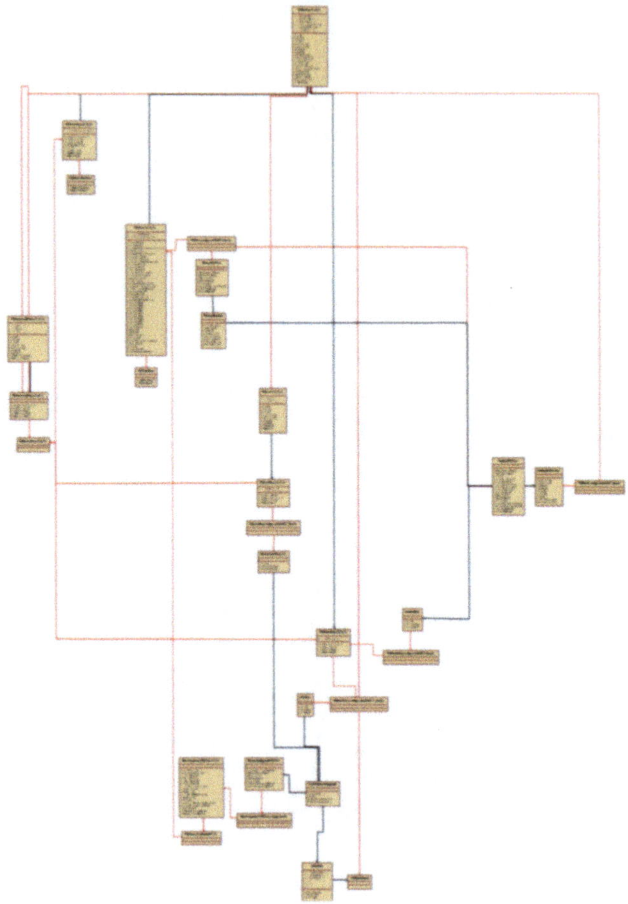

Fig. 5. Industrial Layout in orthogonal style. Same diagram as in Figure 2.

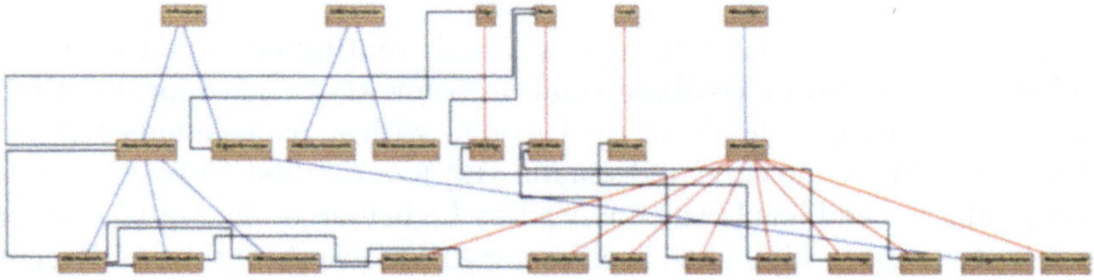

Fig. 6. SugiBib style layout.

1.2 The GoVisual Approach

Several aspects are important when drawing class diagrams: The generalizations induce hierarchical components (*hierarchies*) of the graph, thus each

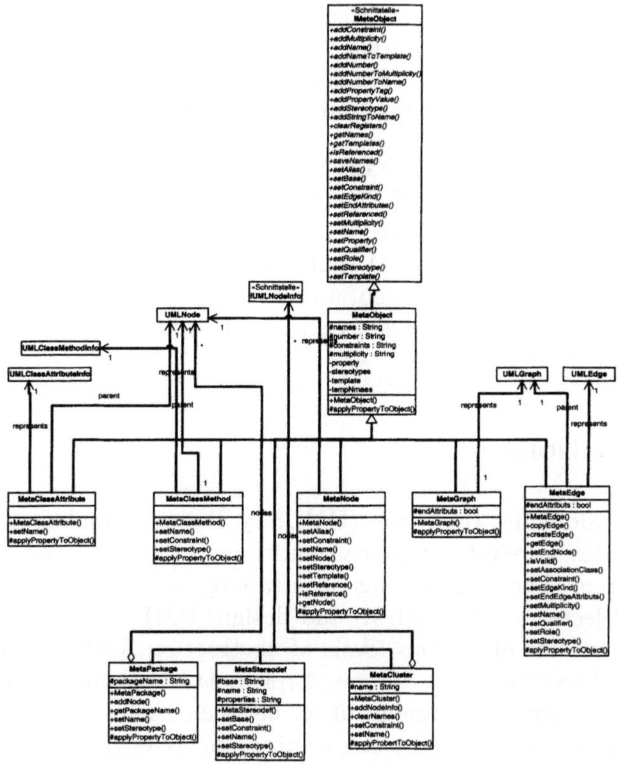

Fig. 7. Layout made by hand using auto routing for edges.

hierarchy must be drawn such that all arcs run in the same direction; there are no restrictions on how the edges in the set E must be drawn. We call a drawing of G that satisfies these requirements a *mixed-upward* drawing. Moreover, the number of crossings between relationships should be small, generalizations belonging to different inheritance hierarchies should never cross, one hierarchy should not enclose another hierarchy, and the area covered by the drawing should be small.

For a clear visualization of the specific combination of hierarchical and non-hierarchical components in UML class diagrams, we put special emphasis on meeting a balanced mixture of the following æsthetic criteria:

- *Crossing minimization*
- *Bend minimization*
- *Orthogonal layout*
- *Uniform direction within each class hierarchy*: Arcs of a class hierarchy should point in a consistent direction.
- *No nesting of one class hierarchy within another*: A class hierarchy is not enclosed by a circle (in the undirected sense) of arcs of a different hierarchy.

- *Merging of multiple inheritance edges*: inheritance lines join prior to reaching the super class, rather than being presented as separate arcs.
- *Good edge labelling*: Labels are placed at predefined positions (beginning, end or midpoint of an edge) minimizing the overlap area.

Following these guidelines, the GoVisual approach consists of two steps. In the first step, a *mixed-upward planarized representation* is computed that is a planar representation P_G of G in which edge crossings are replaced by dummy vertices of degree 4, and that admits a planar drawing that is also mixed-upward. In the second step, a mixed-upward planar drawing of P_G is constructed, and the dummy vertices are replaced by edge crossings in order to obtain a drawing of G.

2 Applications

The Unified Modeling Language (UML) by Booch, Rumbaugh and Jacobson [3] provides a mainly graphical notation to represent the artifacts of a software system. The notation has been rapidly adopted as the accepted notation for object-oriented analysis and design. UML incorporates notations to describe systems at various levels of abstraction. UML diagrams can be used to model requirements, designs, implementations and tests. Since these diagrams are means of communication between customers, developers and others involved in the software engineering and re-engineering process, it is critical that the diagrams present information clearly. Appropriate layout of these diagrams can assist in achieving this goal (see [18]).

Of particular interest are UML class diagrams whose purpose is to display class hierarchies (generalizations), associations, aggregations, and compositions in one picture.

3 Algorithms

A mixed-hierarchical graph G is a graph $G = (V, A, E)$ consisting of an arc set A of *generalizations* and an edge set E of *associations*, such that the digraph $G_A = (V, A)$ induced by the generalizations of G is acyclic.

We generalize the notion of planarity, upward planarity and planarization to mixed-hierarchical graphs as follows: Let $G = (V, A, E)$ be a mixed-hierarchical graph. A *mixed-upward planar* drawing of G is a planar drawing of G in which the implied drawing of each connected component of G_A has the property that all arcs are drawn following the same direction. The components of G_A are called the *hierarchies* of G. An arc $(w, v) \in A$ is directed from w to v. In UML-notation, the node v is said to be the *super class* of w and w is the *child* of v that *inherits* from v. Let $v_1, v_2, \ldots, v_k \in V$, $k \geq 2$, be super classes of a node w. Then w *multiply inherits* from $v_1, v_2, \ldots, v_k$ and such a constellation is called *multiple inheritance*. A hierarchy that does not contain multiple inheritance is called an *inheritance tree*.

G is called *mixed-upward* planar if it admits a mixed-upward planar drawing. An *embedding* of G is a combinatorial embedding of G with a fixed external face. Notice that, in contrast to simple planarity, it is not possible to choose an arbitrary face as external face. An embedding that is realized by a mixed-upward planar drawing is called *mixed-upward*. A planarized representation of G (seen as an undirected graph) which is also mixed-upward planar is called a *mixed-upward planarized representation* of G.

Our drawing model for generalizations is shown in Figure 8. Consider a node v in an inheritance hierarchy with children $w_1, \ldots, w_k$, $k \geq 2$. All arcs leading to v are joined in a single point from which a line with an arrow head leads to v. Altogether, only two bends per edge are required. The UML specifications allow to use this model of representation in UML class diagrams and many users prefer it.

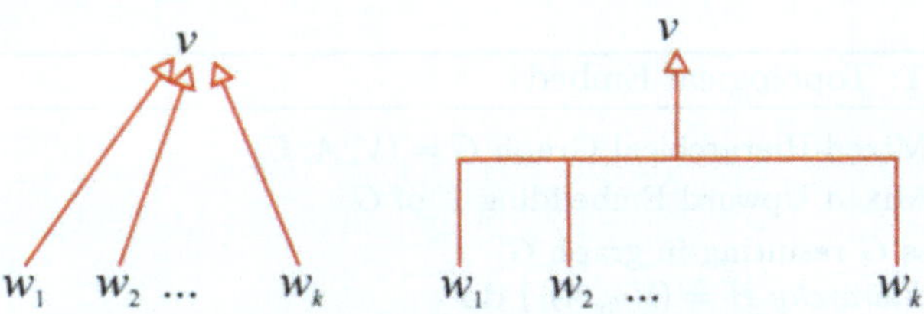

Fig. 8. The drawing model for generalizations.

Let $v_1, v_2, \ldots, v_k \in V$, $k \geq 2$, be super classes of a node w. Then different to the previous case the edges entering node w do not join before entering w but are kept separate. Figure 9 illustrates this situation.

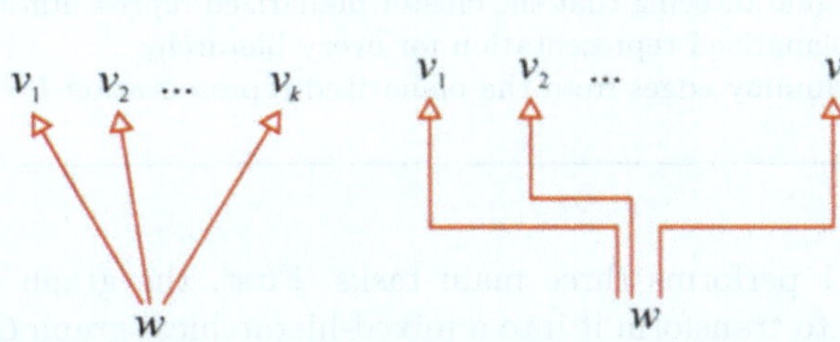

Fig. 9. The drawing model for multiple inheritance generalizations.

Two hierarchies H_1 and H_2 in an embedding Γ of a planarized representation P_G of G might be nested in the following sense. Let $\tilde{H}_1$ denote the subgraph of P_G induced by all arcs and edges in P_G whose corresponding arc in G is incident only to vertices in H_1, and define $\tilde{H}_2$ analogously for H_2. We say that H_2 is *nested* in H_1 in Γ if there is an undirected cycle c formed by arcs of $\tilde{H}_1$ such that $\tilde{H}_2$ is in the interior of c in Γ.

3.1 GoVisual Orthogonal UML Drawing Framework

In this section, we first give an overview on the strategy of the layout algorithm for UML-class diagrams. Consider a mixed-hierarchical graph $G = (V, A, E)$ that represents a UML-class diagram. The GoVisual drawing framework follows a strategy as it is described in Section 4.4 of the Technical Foundations: It first planarizes a graph G, computing a mixed-upward planarized representation and then in a second step computes the orthogonal layout of the mixed hierarchical graph G.

The computation of the mixed-upward planarized representation is the more interesting part of the layout algorithm. The second step performing the computation of the orthogonal layout is more tedious due to complex implementational details, and we therefore give more room to the first part. The computation of the mixed-upward planarized representation is sketched in Algorithm 1.

Algorithm 1: Topological Embed

Input : Mixed-Hierarchical Graph $G = (V, A, E)$
Output: Mixed Upward Embedding Γ of G
Pre-process G resulting in graph G'
for *every hierarchy* $H = (V_H, A_H)$ **do**
  Compute an upward planarized representation P_H of H
  Construct *st*-graph P_H^{st} from P_H
  Add all remaining associations between vertices of V_H to P_H^{st}, constructing the final upward planarized representation of H
end
Compute a cluster planarized representation Γ of G' using P_H^{st} for every hierarchy H guaranteeing that the cluster planarized representation induces an upward planarized representation for every hierarchy
Remove all dummy edges from the planarized representation Γ of G'
Return Γ

Algorithm 1 performs three main tasks. First, the graph G is preprocessed in order to transform it into a mixed-hierarchical graph G' that meets our requirements for the drawing model. This step is described in detail in Section 3.2. In the second and third main steps of Topological Embed, a mixed-upward planarized representation of G' is computed. Apart from the minimization of the edge crossings, this computation must meet two requirements: The hierarchies need to be directed in uniform direction and nesting of hierarchies is not allowed. Thus GoVisual subdivides the planarization of the graph G' into two steps. First, GoVisual computes for every hierarchy an upward planarized embedding to ensure a uniform direction. Second, the graph is clustered, gathering every hierarchy in its own cluster, in order to ensure that there will be no nesting of hierarchies in the subsequent planarization step. Each of the two steps is described in detail in Sections 3.3 and 3.4.

3.2 Preprocessing

The drawing model presented at the beginning of this section alters the graph that has to be drawn. We can easily find an example, where its application leads to a crossing although the embedding of the graph is mixed-upward planar (see Figure 10(a)). This means that the mixed-upward planarized representation produced in the planarization step does not define the number of crossings in the final drawing, further crossings might occur.

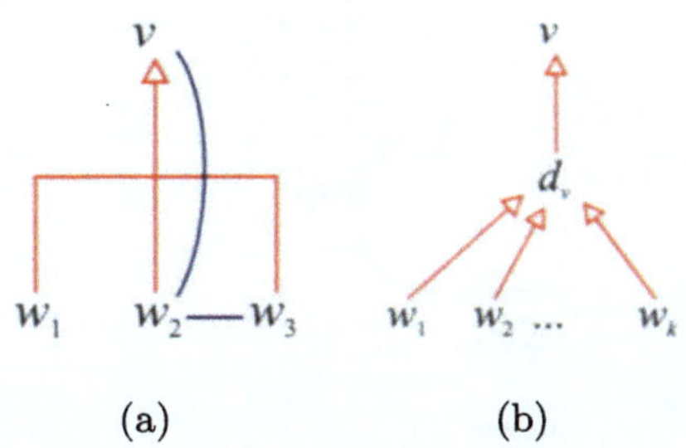

Fig. 10. Drawbacks of the drawing model for generalizations and the modifications made in the preprocessing step.

Therefore, we also alter the graph accordingly in a preprocessing step such that the number of crossing vertices in the planarized representation is in fact the number of crossings in the final drawing (compare Figure 10(b)). For each vertex v in a class hierarchy with at least 2 children $w_1, \ldots, w_k$, we introduce a new vertex d_v representing the point where the edges from the children to v are joined. Each edge (w_i, v) is replaced by a new edge (w_i, d_v), and a new edge (d_v, v) is added. We call the inserted vertices d_v *generalization mergers* and the graph resulting from the preprocessing step $G' = (V', A', E)$.

3.3 Upward Planarization

Upward planarization is performed by Topological Embed on every hierarchy to ensure a uniform direction for this hierarchy. Each hierarchy $H = (V_H, A_H)$ of G represents a directed graph. In order to compute an upward planarized representation P_H of H, several techniques can be applied.

If H has only a single sink (base class), the upward planarity test for directed acyclic graphs by [2] can be applied. If H is upward planar, the algorithm also computes an upward planar embedding of H in time $O(|V_H|)$. In this case, no crossings are necessary at all. A straight-forward extension of the test for graphs with several sinks is to introduce a super-sink t and to add arcs from all sinks of H to t. This is equivalent to demand that all sinks have to be on the external face, which makes sense for UML class diagrams. On the other hand, the general problem of upward planarity testing is $\mathcal{NP}$-complete (see [12]). Figure 11 shows a hierarchy H represented by red edges. The hierarchy H has a single sink and is obviously upward planar, thus H and P_H are identical.

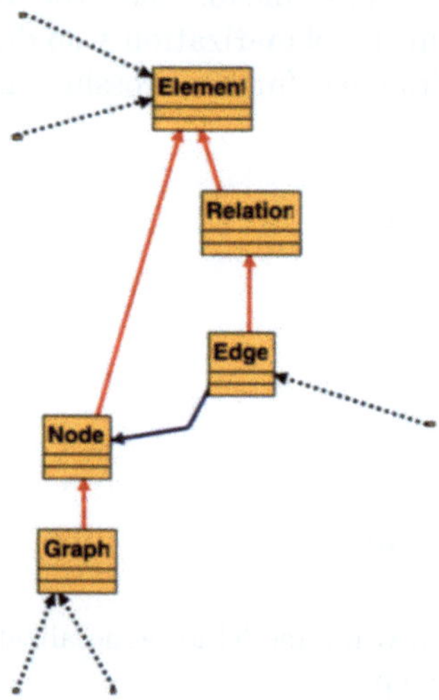

Fig. 11. The hierarchy H is shown by red edges, associations between nodes of V_H are blue. Associations between V_H and $V \setminus V_H$ are shown as dotted black lines. H and P_H are identical.

If the upward planarity test fails, techniques have to be applied that replace edge crossings with dummy vertices. Possible approaches are to adapt the crossing minimization step of the Sugiyama algorithm [20,7,11,15], or to use the technique described in [9].

Since every upward planar embedding is subgraph of a planar st-digraph, we can augment the resulting upward planarized representation P_H to a planar st-digraph P_H^{st}. Finally, we reinsert the remaining associations between vertices in V_H using a standard technique as described in [1] or the SPQR-tree based optimal algorithm in [13].

Figure 12 shows P_H^{st} of the example from Figure 11. The st-graph P_H^{st} is presented by the green and the blue edges. The green edges are the original edges from H. To construct the st-graph we use either existing associations between nodes of V_H or add extra edges. Here we use one association shown as blue edge between the nodes "Node" and"Edge", and add an extra edge between "Element" and "Graph". Until the computation of the mixed upward

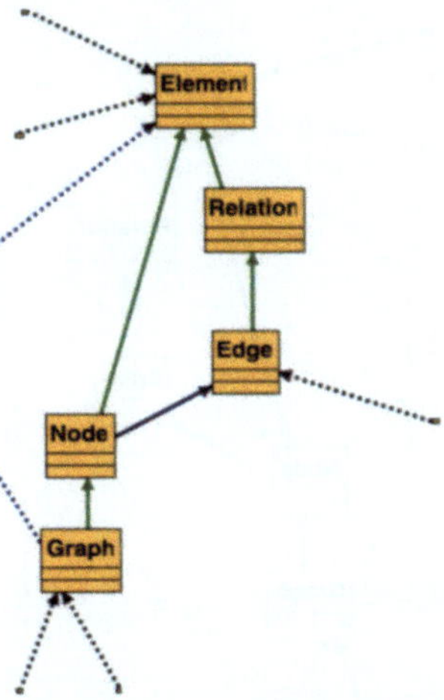

Fig. 12. P_H^{st} of the example from Figure 11. P_H^{st} is shown by green and blue edges.

planar embedding is finished, the association ("Node","Edge") is considered to be directed.

3.4 Computation of Cluster Planarized Representations

In order to avoid nesting of hierarchies, we place each hierarchy into a cluster and apply the cluster planarization algorithm. By the previous step described in Section 3.3 every cluster is already planar. Figure 13 shows the example of Figure 12 with P_H^{st} defining a cluster.

For each cluster, we compute the planar embedding of the corresponding P_H^{st} and construct the wheel graph which represents all possible permutations of the vertices on the external face of a cluster (see [10]). We make sure that this wheel graph corresponds to an upward planar embedding of P_H^{st}. These wheel graphs are connected with the remaining edges between vertices of different clusters, and a planar subgraph of the resulting graph is computed which contains all edges in the wheel graphs and a set F of edges connecting vertices in different clusters. Since it is essential to have all wheel graph edges in the planar subgraph, we cannot apply the PQ-based algorithm (see [14]). Instead, we use the algorithm based on iterative planarity testing. In the next step, we construct a cluster planar embedding of the graph consisting of all the graphs C_i and the edges in F.

Finally, we re-insert the edges between vertices in different clusters that are not contained in F. This can be done as described in [6]. The resulting cluster planarized graph has been constructed such that all hierarchies are embedded upward planarized and nesting of hierarchies is avoided. It remains to remove the dummy edges that do not correspond to associations and generalizations which have been introduced to construct st-graphs of the upward planarized hierarchies.

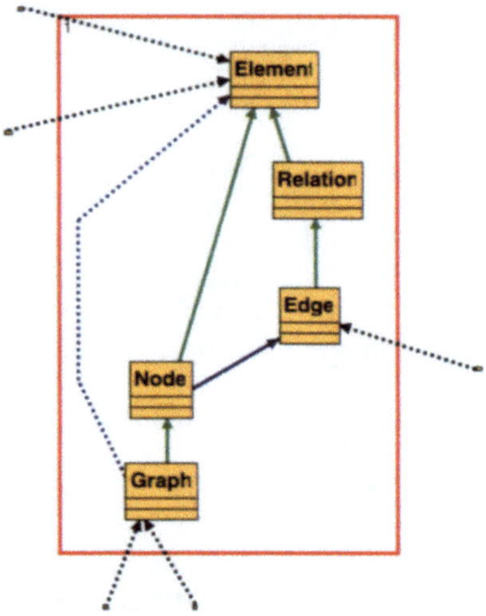

Fig. 13. P_H^{st} induces a cluster.

3.5 The Orthogonal Drawing Step

For simplicity, we restrict ourselves to single-inheritance hierarchies. We apply the *topology-shape-metrics* approach as proposed in [22] and explained in Section 4.4 of the Technical Foundations. The previous steps described in Sections 3.1–3.4 give us the topology of the drawing, i.e., an embedded mixed-upward planarized representation Γ of graph G'. Since each hierarchy is a tree, no two generalizations cross and all the generalizations from a super class v to its children $w_1, \ldots, w_k$ can be drawn with at most two bends as shown in Figure 8.

The shape of the drawing is determined as follows. First, Γ is transformed into a 4-graph Γ' by replacing each high-degree vertex v with a face f (called *cage*) such that $\deg(v) = \deg(f)$ as described in [17]. Then we apply the bend-minimization algorithm of Tamassia [21] as described in [17] or the Giotto algorithm as described in [22] with certain degree and bend constraints. These constraints guarantee that generalizations are always drawn as in the model described at the beginning of this Section and that cages have rectangular shape.

The compaction phase computes the metrics of the drawing, i.e., the final coordinates. Constructive flow-based compaction (see [16]) is used to get a first drawing of the expanded graph Γ'. In this step, we have to make sure that each cage is large enough so that the real vertex can be placed into it. Then, Γ' is re-transformed into Γ by placing each high-degree vertex into its cage and routing the adjacent edges in an orthogonal fashion within the cage. Finally, flow-based improvement compaction is applied, in order to reduce the size of the drawing and to remove unnecessary bends introduced during the edge routing step.

4 Implementation

The orthogonal UML layout algorithm presented in this chapter is integrated into a large framework of layout algorithms and data structures for the automatic layout of diagrams, called GoVisual. GoVisual is an object-oriented C++ class library.

The GoVisual C++ class library is an independent library based on its own fast and efficient data structures and combinatorial algorithms. It currently provides the layout and labelling styles as listed below. All layout styles provide a set of drawing and optimization algorithms that can be combined to a layout algorithm that provides the best results for the user within the chosen style. Furthermore a variety of parameters can be manipulated within each style.

- Orthogonal Layout for UML Class Diagrams.
- Orthogonal Cluster Layout providing an orthogonal layout for cluster graphs that focuses on the crossing minimization between edges and the minimization of the number of bends of the edges (see e.g. [6]).
- Orthogonal Layout having a focus on the minimization of crossings between edges and the minimization of the number of bends of the edges (see Section 4.4 of the Technical Foundations).
- Tree Layout for the visualization of non-circular structures (see Section 4.1 of the Technical Foundations).
- Layered Layout visualizing data that is meant to reflect the existence of a prioritized ranking system (see Section 4.2 of the Technical Foundations).
- Force-directed Layout for displaying hidden symmetries within a diagram (see Section 4.5 of the Technical Foundations).
- Circular Layout for network visualization.
- Advanced Labelling offering a method to automatically place labels of edges, respecting the size and the type of the labels as well as the desired position at the edge and maximizing the overlap-free area.
- Labelling placing labels of connectors either at one of the two ends of the connector or at its midpoint.

4.1 API

The API enables users to access the layout algorithms within a C++, .NET, or Java (using Java Native Interface JNI) JNI) environment and to integrate them into their own applications. To access a layout algorithm, the user only needs to create a data structure that contains information on the relationships of the diagram. After successfully applying a layout algorithm, the layout information of the diagram is stored in this data structure.

The software is currently available for Windows® platforms 95, 98, ME, NT, 2000, XP; versions for Unix and Linux systems are in preparation.

Programming Language C++. The API supplies C++ header files (.h-files), a dynamic link library govisual.dll, and the corresponding import library govisual.lib. The import library is either meant to be used with Microsoft® Visual Studio® 6.0 or Borland® C++ Builder 6.0.

Programming Language Java. The API supplies C++ header files and the libraries govisual.dll and govisual.lib as described for the programming language C++. Furthermore, the API provides an extra dynamic library govisual_JNI.dll that implements the native functions for accessing the layout methods. The libraries govisual_JNI.dll and govisual.dll are loaded at run time by the Java interpreter. Both libraries are only suited for Windows and must be replaced accordingly on other operating systems. The Java class library that accesses the two C++ libraries via the native interface is contained in the Java archive file govisual.jar. This class library represents the actual interface for the user.

Microsoft .NET Framework. The API supplies an assembly prepared for the Microsoft .NET framework. Via the Common Language Runtime (CLR) the library can be used for C#, Visual Basic, JScript, J#, C++.NET, and any other language where a compiler that supports the CLR is available.

4.2 Plug-Ins: Microsoft Visio, Borland Together ControlCenter, Gentleware Poseidon for UML

GoVisual is also available as a Plug-In for Microsoft Visio 2000/2002 on Windows NT/2000/98/Me/XP. This provides the tools for producing layouts of IT-diagrams, network device and topology diagrams, business diagrams, and UML class diagrams from within a Microsoft Visio environment. Microsoft Visio itself allows to create and visualize a diagram using many different shapes and connectors.

GoVisual is also available as Plug-In for Borland Together ControlCenter and for Gentleware Poseidon for UML. Both, the ControlCenter and Poseidon are model-driven development tools for object oriented software projects.

After installation of the Plug-In in either Poseidon, Together ControlCenter, or Visio, a GoVisual menu entry appears on the toolbar, allowing to choose an appropriate layout algorithm for the diagram. As in the API, the user is able to combine drawing and optimization algorithms in order to achieve the best results. We decided to use sliders that allow to choose between different optimization goals since users tend to ignore complex explanations on advantages and drawbacks on the different methods.

Figure 14 shows the layout menu as well as the options menu with a typical user friendly slide bar to choose between different optimization algorithms.

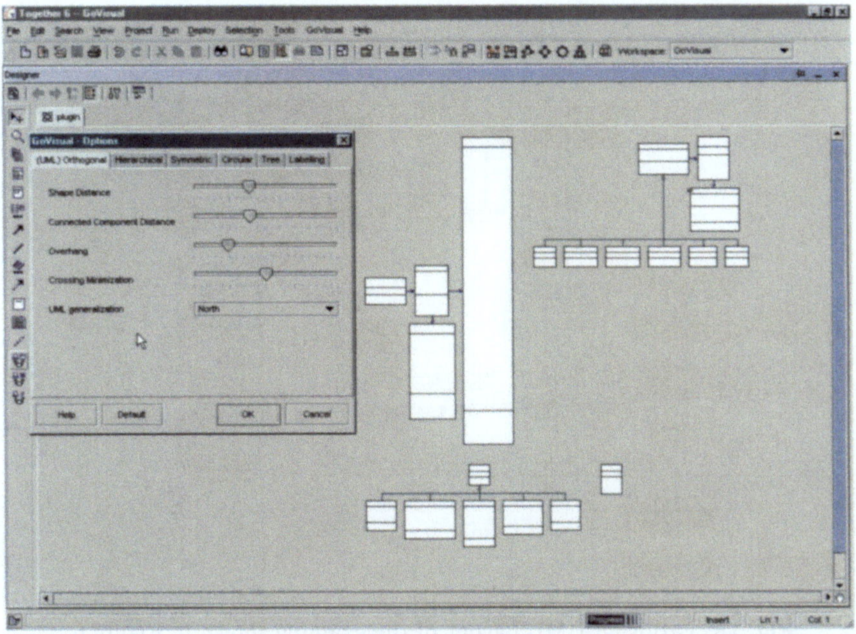

Fig. 14. GoVisual within Borland Together Control Center.

5 Examples

This section shows different UML diagrams that have been laid out using GoVisual. Figure 15 gives a GoVisual layout of the diagram that was presented in Figure 6 to demonstrate the state of the art layout by [19]. The new layout contains no crossings at all (compared to 59 crossings in Figure 6) and seven bends in association (compared to 46 bends in associations in Figure 6).

Figures 16 and 17 give similar layouts for the semiautomatically produced UML layout as shown in Figure 7. Figure 16 gives the GoVisual layout without coloring of the generalization edges and the nodes belonging to the only hierarchy in this graph. The new layout contains no crossings at all (compared to eight crossings in Figure 7) and one bend in an association (compared to 14 bends in associations in Figure 7). Moreover, the inheritance hierarchy is clearly visible. In Figure 17 we present the same graph with the nodes of the inheritance hierarchy being colored, enhancing the visual perception of the human reader even more.

Figure 18 gives a GoVisual Layout of a UML class diagram that we already showed in Figures 2, 4, and 5. While it was impossible to understand the structure of the software project presented by the diagram in any of the industrial layouts, it becomes immediately clear in the new layout. In particular, the human reader immediately recognizes three inheritance hier-

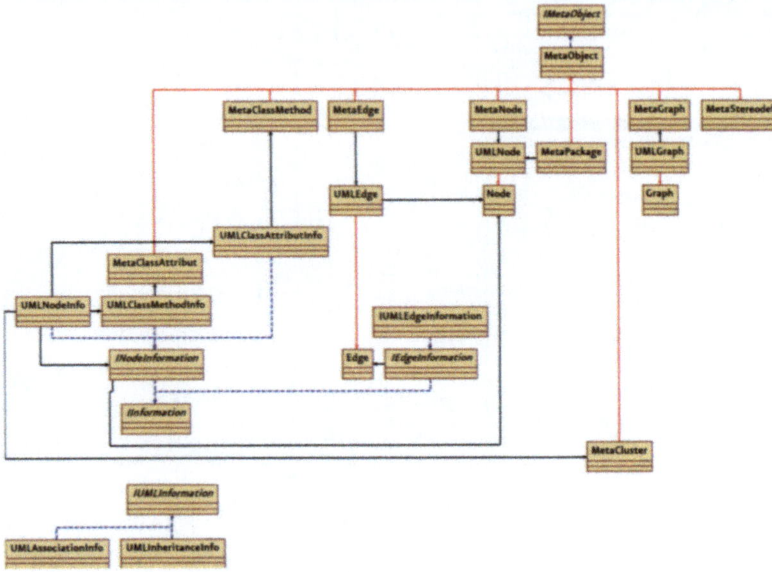

Fig. 15. GoVisual UML Layout of the example shown in Figure 6.

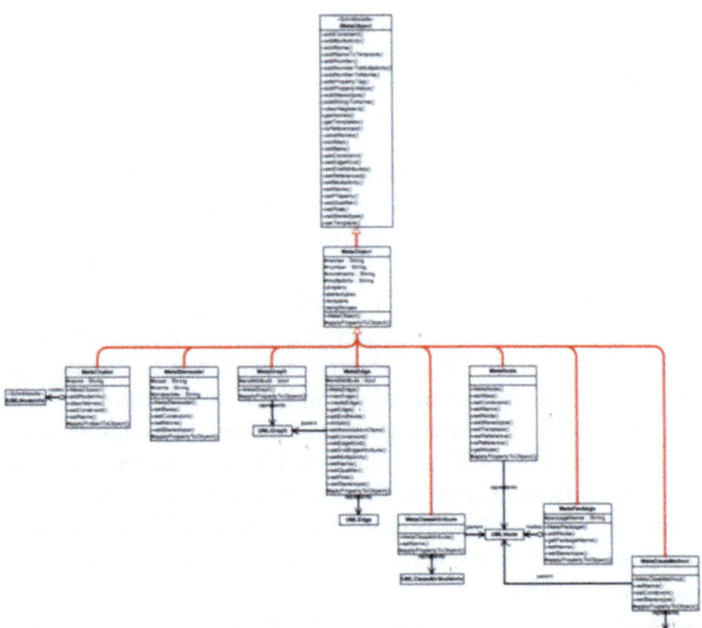

Fig. 16. GoVisual UML Layout of the example shown in Figure 7.

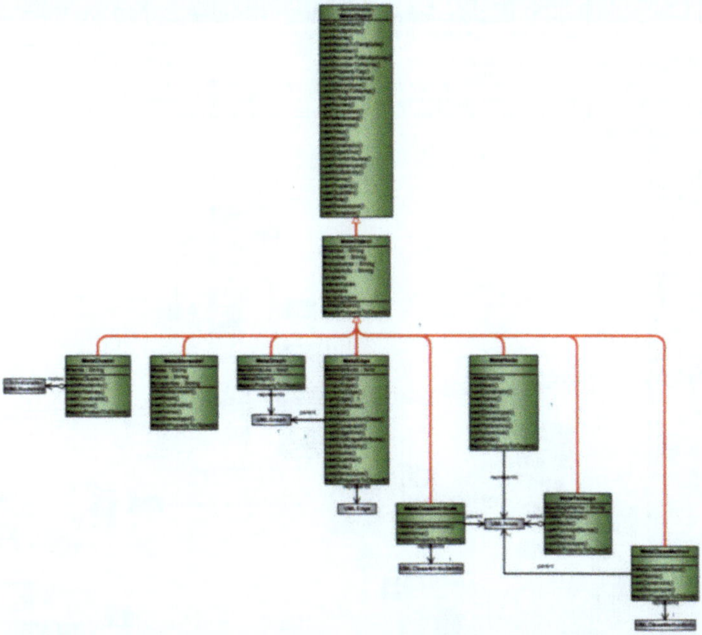

Fig. 17. GoVisual UML Layout of the example shown in Figure 7 including coloring of the hierarchy.

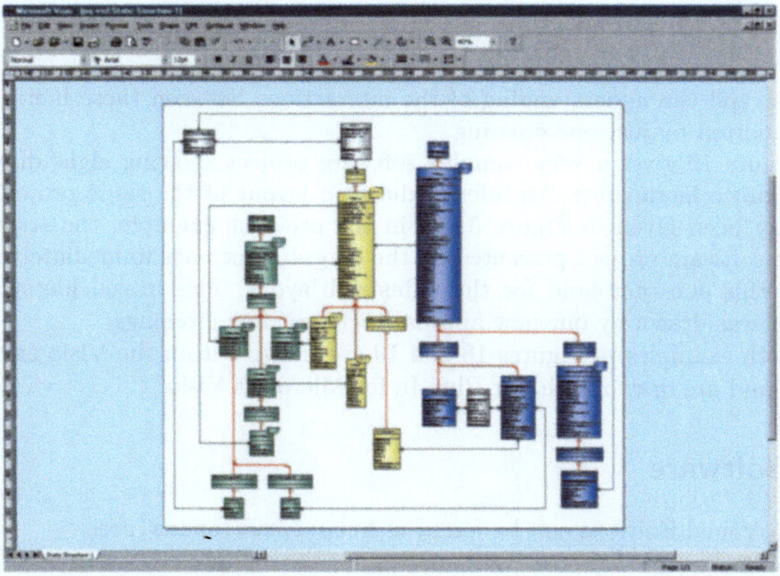

Fig. 18. GoVisual UML Layout of the example shown in Figure 2, 4, and 5.

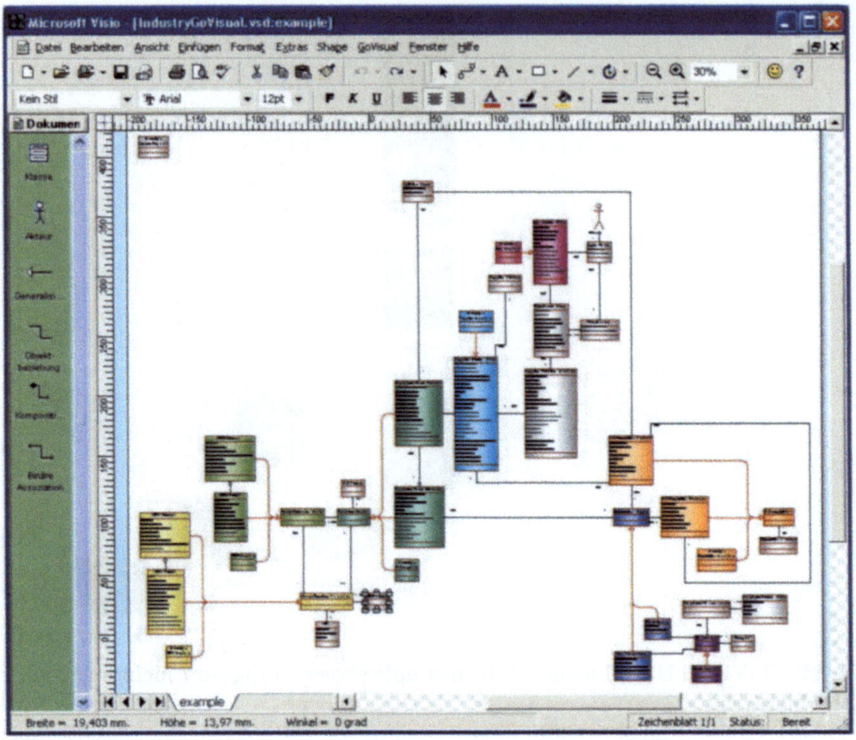

Fig. 19. GoVisual UML Layout of the example shown in Figure 3.

archies and the understanding of the interactions between these hierarchies is supported by just one crossing.

Figure 19 gives a very complex software project showing eight different inheritance hierarchies. An inferior diagram layout of the same project has already been given in Figure 3. As in the previous example, the structure of the software project presented by the diagram becomes immediately clear while this does not hold for the industrial layout. This mixed hierarchical layout was drawn by our new approach without any crossings.

Both examples in Figures 18 and 19 are shown within the Visio environment and are drawn with our Plug-In for Microsoft Visio.

6 Software

All GoVisual Editions can be found at `http://www.oreas.com`.

6.1 API

The API UML layout package provides techniques for the visualization of mixed-hierarchical structures. Orthogonal cluster layout algorithms are also available as API. Standard techniques such as circular layout, symmetric layout, tree layout, hierarchical layout, and orthogonal layout are also available.

6.2 PlugIn for Borland Together ControlCenter

GoVisual is available as Plug-In for Borland® Together® ControlCenter™ featuring the UML layout software. The software comes along with orthogonal layout, symmetric layout, and hierarchical layout providing users a full range of layout algorithms that can be applied to the different UML diagram types.

6.3 PlugIn for Gentleware Poseidon for UML

GoVisual is available as Plug-In for Gentleware® Poseidon® for UML featuring the UML layout software. The software comes along with orthogonal layout, symmetric layout, and hierarchical layout providing users a full range of layout algorithms that can be applied to the different UML diagram types.

6.4 PlugIn for Microsoft Visio

GoVisual is also available in three different editions as Plug-In for Microsoft® Visio 2000/2002 on Windows NT/2000/98/Me/XP. The Network Edition features three established techniques: circular layout, symmetric layout, and tree layout. The Professional Edition includes all functionality of the Network Edition and features two professional techniques: hierarchical layout and orthogonal layout. The UML Edition includes all functionality of the Professional Edition and features the UML layout.

References

1. Di Battista, G., Eades, P., Tamassia, R., Tollis, I. G. (1999) Graph Drawing. Prentice Hall
2. Bertolazzi, P., Di Battista, G., Mannino, C., Tamassia, R. (1998) Optimal upward planarity testing of single-source digraphs. SIAM Journal on Computing **27** (1), 132–169
3. Booch, G., Rumbaugh, J., Jacobson, I. (1999) Unified Modeling Language User Guide. Addison Wesley Longman
4. Rational Software Corporation. (2002) Rational Rose, Rational XDE
5. TogetherSoft Corporation. (2002) Together ControlCenter
6. Di Battista, G., Didimo, W., Marcandalli, A. (2002) Planarization of clustered graphs. In: P. Mutzel, M. Jünger, and S. Leipert (eds.) Graph Drawing '01, Lecture Notes in Computer Science 2265, Springer-Verlag, 60–74
7. Eades, P., Kelly, D. (1986) Heuristics for reducing crossings in 2-layered networks. Ars Combinatoria **21** (A), 89–98
8. Eichelberger, H. (2002) SugiBib. In: P. Mutzel, M. Jünger, and S. Leipert (eds.) Graph Drawing '01, Lecture Notes in Computer Science 2265, Springer-Verlag, 467–468

9. Eiglsperger, M., Kaufmann, M. (2001) An approach for mixed upward planarization. In: Proc. 7th International Workshop on Algorithms and Data Structures (WADS'01), Lecture Notes in Computer Science 2125, Springer-Verlag, 352–364
10. Feng, Q.-W., Cohen, R. F., Eades, P. (1995) Planarity for clustered graphs. In P. Spirakis (ed.) Algorithms – ESA '95, Lecture Notes in Computer Science 979, Springer-Verlag, 213–226
11. Gansner, E. R., Koutsofios, E., North, S. C., Vo, K. P. (1993) A technique for drawing directed graphs. IEEE Transactions on Software Engineering **19** (3), 214–230
12. Garg, A., Tamassia, R. (1995) On the computational complexity of upward and rectilinear planarity testing. In: R. Tamassia and I. G. Tollis (eds.) Graph Drawing '94, Lecture Notes in Computer Science 894, Springer-Verlag, 286–297
13. Gutwenger, C., Mutzel, P., Weiskircher, R. (2001) Inserting an edge into a planar graph. In: Proceedings of the Twelwth Annual ACM-SIAM Symposium on Discrete Algorithms (SODA '01), ACM Press, 246–255
14. Jünger, M., Leipert, S., Mutzel, P. (1998) A note on computing a maximal planar subgraph using PQ-trees. IEEE Transactions on Computer-Aided Design **17** (7), 609–612
15. Jünger, M., Mutzel, P. (1996) 2-layer straightline crossing minimization: Performance of exact and heuristic algorithms. Journal of Graph Algorithms and Applications (JGAA) **1** (1), 1–25, `http://www.cs.brown.edu/publications/jgaa/`
16. Klau, G. W., Klein, K., Mutzel, P. (2000) An experimental comparison of orthogonal compaction algorithms. Technical report, Technische Universität Wien
17. Klau, G. W., Mutzel, P. (1998) Quasi-orthogonal drawing of planar graphs. Technical Report MPI-I-98-1-013, Max–Planck–Institut für Informatik, Saarbrücken
18. Purchase, H., Allder, J.-A., Carrington, D. (2001) User preference of graph layout aesthetics: A UML study. In: J. Marks (ed.) Graph Drawing '00, Lecture Notes in Computer Science 1984, Springer-Verlag, 5–18
19. Seemann, J. (1997) Extending the sugiyama algorithm for drawing UML class diagrams. In: G. Di Battista (ed.) Graph Drawing '97, Lecture Notes in Computer Science 1353, Springer-Verlag, 415–424
20. Sugiyama, K., Tagawa, S., Toda, M. (1981) Methods for visual understanding of hierarchical systems. IEEE Transactions on System, Man, and Cybernetics **SMC-11** (2), 109–125
21. Tamassia, R. (1988) On embedding a graph in the grid with the minimum number of bends. SIAM Journal on Computing **16** (3), 421–444
22. Tamassia, R., Di Battista, G., Batini, C. (1988) Automatic graph drawing and readability of diagrams. IEEE Transactions on System, Man, and Cybernetics **SMC-18** (1), 61–79

CrocoCosmos – 3D Visualization of Large Object-Oriented Programs

Claus Lewerentz and Andreas Noack

Brandenburg Technical University at Cottbus, Computer Science Department,
Software Systems Engineering Research Group, Postbox 10 13 44,
D-03013 Cottbus, Germany

1 Introduction

Software belongs to the most complex human-made artifacts. The size and complexity of programs has constantly grown over the last years. Today in many application domains (e.g., e-business, switching systems) software systems with millions of lines of code are constructed. They consist of many thousands of components and subsystems. Prefabricated frameworks and component technology make it possible to quickly build very large programs which typically go through a long lasting evolution process with adaptations and extensions of the existing code. Such reengineering and maintenance activities require good support for program analysis and understanding. In the context of program comprehension typical questions are "How good is the quality of the program with respect to maintainability?", "Where are the most critical parts?", "What is the overall structure of the system?", "How are particular parts interdependent?" (cf. [19], [21]).

One way to support program comprehension is software visualization based on automatically extracted information about the internal program structure and on derived software metrics data [14]. Typical examples are inheritance or call graphs depicting program entities like subsystems, classes, or functions, and inheritance or call relations between them. There are many other approaches visualizing different aspects of software systems (cf. [12]).

For an effective use of software visualizations in the context of program comprehension and reengineering of real-world systems they have to fulfill some important requirements:

1. Geometric properties of a system's visualization have to allow for a valid interpretation with respect to the system properties. The size and geometric distance of graphical entities representing particular program elements, for instance, has to have sound correlation with the underlying program structure and thus an interpretation in the problem domain. This provides a basis for producing visual patterns that are clearly related to structural patterns of intended or undesired constructions.
2. The visualizations should be well suited to represent large software structures, i.e., high resulting data volumes. Typical software in industrial development projects nowadays consists of 10^5–10^7 lines of source code

organized in 10^4-10^5 functions in 10^3-10^4 classes or files, contained in 10^2-10^3 packages or subsystems. Thus, the visualization approach has to scale well and to support hierarchical visual structures with robust transitions between different hierarchy levels.

3. The visualization technique has to be flexible and adaptable in order to provide means for the creation and exploration of different views which appropriately support specific analysis and comprehension tasks.

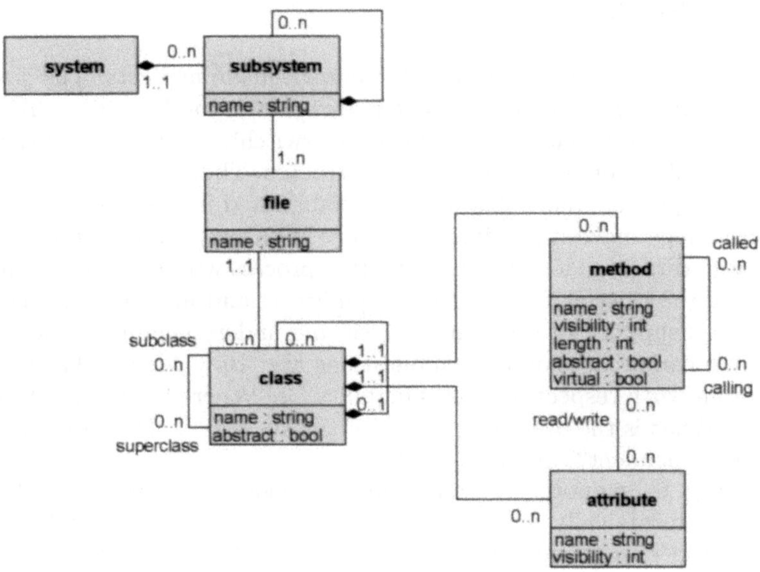

Fig. 1. Schema for the representation of object-oriented programs.

In our metrics-based software analysis approach [21,13] we use a product abstraction of object-oriented programs that results in large attributed graph structures with several thousand vertices and tens of thousands of edges representing different logical views on a software system. Figure 1 shows a simplified schema for the internal representation of object-oriented programs on the level of subsystems and classes with the relations for class nesting, method call, attribute access, and inheritance. On this level we abstract from the code structure within methods and represent particular instruction level information (e.g., the number of lines of code for a method or a class) by metrics values which are part of the schema as attributes. Views on this schema correspond to hierarchical call, use, or inheritance graphs.

The CrocoCosmos tool creates three-dimensional visual representations of the graph structures resulting from the instantiation of this schema for large

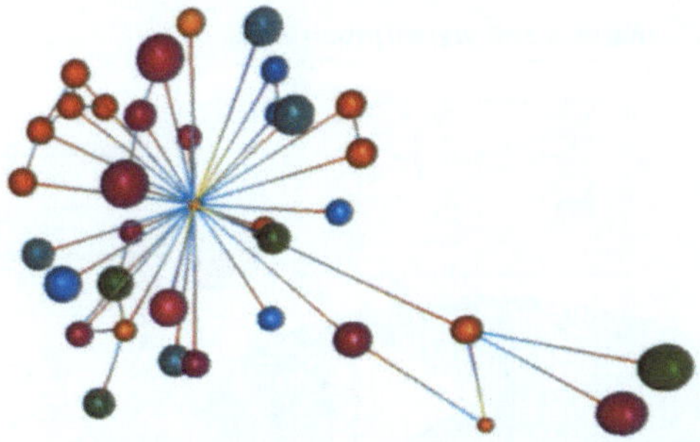

Fig. 2. Example visualization.

programs. As illustrated in Figure 2, vertices represent program entities and colored edges represent relations of different types. Particular properties of the individual entities are encoded by geometrical vertex properties and edge directions are encoded by color transitions. The positions of the vertices in 3D space reflect the relational structure of the visualized program. The use of 3D space instead of 2D space is motivated by the experience that the additional degree of freedom in many cases drastically enhances the spatial unfolding of large graph structures. Section 3 explains and discusses our layout approach in detail.

2 Applications

CrocoCosmos is part of a comprehensive experimental software analysis tool set to support analysis, comprehension, and quality assessment of large object-oriented programs. Based on parsing, structure extraction and transformation, and metrics calculation, different analysis views of programs are created and used for interactive exploration (cf. Figure 3). The 3D-graph view is one particular view which mainly supports overall structure recognition and the visual detection of potentially anomalous program constructions like overly complex inheritance structures or repetitive structures caused by code clones.

The visualizations were used in several industrial case studies for software quality assessment, review preparation and reengineering support (cf. [21,15]). The experiences show that the visualizations complement other analysis data, tabular views and browsing structures in a very useful way. Their particular strength is that the 3D-graphs provide overall pictures as well as detailed structural insights, that are difficult to derive from the other views. In several cases the 3D-visualizations showed very directly unexpected structures which were clearly related to complex and cumbersome internal structures of the analyzed software (cf. Section 5.2 for examples). It is, however, necessary to learn to interpret the visual structures and to relate visual patterns to desired or problematic program structures. There is still substantial empirical work to be done.

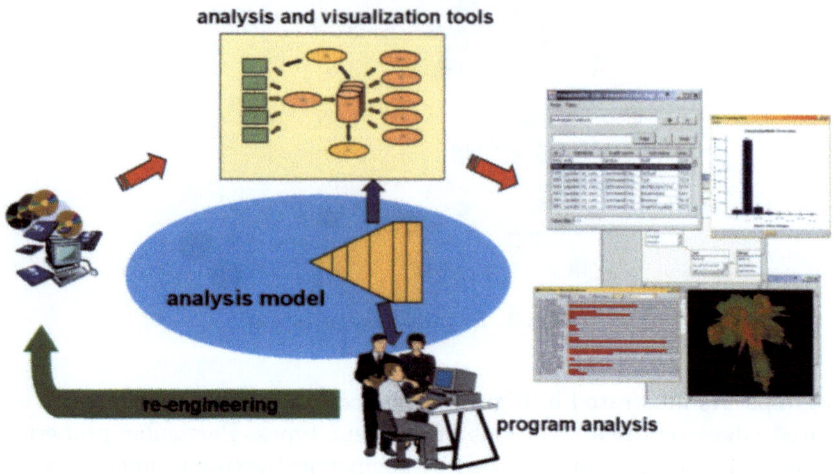

Fig. 3. Analysis and visualization of software systems.

3 Algorithms

CrocoCosmos uses force-directed methods to draw graph models of programs. This choice is motivated by the requirements for effective software visualizations listed in Section 1. Consider the third requirement, adaptability to different views on software systems. This means drawing graphs with different graph-theoretic properties. Inheritance graphs, for instance, are acyclic and very sparse, while call graphs often have large strongly connected components and many times more edges.

Force-directed methods are easily adaptable to different kinds of graphs. In general, they have two parts: an energy model, and an algorithm for finding a state of minimum total energy. (Alternatively, the model may be defined as force system and the algorithm searches for an equilibrium configuration where the total force on each vertex is zero.) The drawing criteria are explicitly specified in the energy model and can be changed without modification of the algorithm.

Section 4.5 in the Technical Foundations gives an introduction to force-directed methods and lists some popular force and energy models. However, these models are not well suited for some important graphs of software systems. In this section we develop an energy model for the drawing of reference graphs, which include call, attribute access, and inheritance relations. Therefore we state some graph-theoretic properties of reference graphs, derive criteria for their drawings, discuss existing energy models with respect to these criteria, and formalize the criteria to obtain a new energy model. Finally we address the first requirement of Section 1 by proving the interpretability of distances in the drawings of this energy model.

3.1 Properties of Reference Graphs

In general, the vertices of a *reference graph* are structural entities of a software system like methods, classes or subsystems. There is a directed edge from a vertex u to another vertex v if and only if a method of entity u calls a method of entity v, or a method of u uses an attribute of v, or a class of u directly inherits from a class of v. Including inheritance and attribute usage adds relatively few edges, so most of the following also applies to call graphs.

For clarity of presentation, we simplify the notion of a reference graph in two respects: Firstly, we consider the edges as undirected. In our visualizations, the direction and the type of the edges is only indicated by their coloring (cf. Section 4), and does not affect the positions of the vertices. Secondly, we treat the components of the reference graph separately. So in the following, reference graphs are undirected, connected, simple graphs.

Table 1 shows some properties of reference graphs of four software systems. For a graph $G = (V, E)$ and using the notations of the Technical Foundations Chapter, these properties are defined as follows:

- Average degree: $\frac{1}{|V|} \sum_{v \in V} \deg(v) = \frac{2|E|}{|V|}$.
- Density: $\frac{2|E|}{|V|(|V|-1)}$, the fraction of the possible edges that actually exist.
- Average graph-theoretic distance: $\frac{1}{|V|(|V|-1)} \sum_{u,v \in V,\, u \neq v} \mathrm{dist}(u, v)$.
- Diameter: $\mathrm{diam}(G) = \max\{\mathrm{dist}(u, v) \mid u, v \in V\}$, the maximum graph-theoretic distance.
- Clustering coefficient $\gamma(u)$ of a vertex u with $\deg(u) \geq 2$ [22]:

$$\frac{2}{\deg(u)(\deg(u)-1)} \left|\{\{v, w\} \in E \mid v, w \in \mathrm{adj}(u)\}\right|,$$

  the fraction of those possible edges between neighbors of u which actually exist in the graph.
- Clustering coefficient of a graph: $\frac{1}{|\{v \in V | \deg(v) \geq 2\}|} \sum_{v \in V,\, \deg(v) \geq 2} \gamma(v)$, the average clustering coefficient of all vertices with at least two neighbors. In all four reference graphs of Table 1 more than 90 percent of the vertices have at least two neighbors.

Number of Vertices	Number of Edges	Average Degree	Density	Average Distance	Diameter	Clustering Coefficient
170	691	8.13	0.0481	2.71	5	0.247
539	2239	8.31	0.0154	3.39	8	0.382
662	3690	11.15	0.0169	2.88	11	0.334
1508	9759	12.94	0.0086	2.74	10	0.275

Table 1. Properties of the reference graphs of four software systems.

Three observations are of particular importance for the drawing of reference graphs:

1. The average distance of vertices and the diameter are very small compared to the number of vertices. This raises the problem of how to avoid drawing many vertices and edges in very small areas or volumes.
2. The clustering coefficients are high. While in random graphs (i.e., graphs where every pair of different vertices is connected with equal probability) the clustering coefficient is approximately equal to the density, it is much higher in the four reference graphs. So reference graphs probably have natural clusters, i.e., subsets of vertices with many internal edges (high cohesion) and few edges to outside vertices (low coupling). These natural clusters should be apparent in the visualization.
3. The average degree is high. Drawings of graphs with that many edges often appear cluttered. So ideally the viewer would know where edges are without actually seeing them. This can be partially achieved by indicating the number of edges connecting two subgraphs by the closeness of the subgraphs.

3.2 Discussion of Existing Energy Models

This section explains why most popular force and energy models, in particular those mentioned in Section 4.5 of the Technical Foundations, are not well suited to drawing reference graphs. For a more detailed discussion see [17].

An energy model specifies what is considered a good drawing. More precisely, for a given graph, a drawing with high total energy is considered worse than a drawing with lower total energy. Force and energy are just two different perspectives on the same problem: Force is the negative gradient of energy, thus an equilibrium state of a force model is a *local* minimum of energy. We prefer the perspective of energy minimization because *local* minima can have high energies and therefore give bad drawings compared to the *global* minimum.

Section 4.5 in the Technical Foundations introduces the models of Eades [6], Fruchterman and Reingold [9], Frick *et al.* [8], and Davidson and Harel [5], which are sums of a term for the spring energy and a term for the repulsion energy. (The model of Davidson and Harel has two additional terms.) These terms formalize a popular criterion for good drawings: Adjacent vertices should generally be closer than non-adjacent vertices. This conforms to our goal to make dense subgraphs visually apparent, and thus our energy model (introduced in Section 3.4) has the same form.

But the particular terms differ, because the energy models from the Technical Foundations enforce an additional property of the drawing: uniform edge lengths. Strong forces act between adjacent vertices towards some fixed desired edge length (which is a parameter of the models), while the repulsive forces between vertices decay rapidly with growing distance. This results in distances between adjacent vertices which are almost independent of global properties of the graph.

Uniform edge lengths are not desirable in drawings of reference graphs. Table 1 shows that the average graph-theoretic distance of two vertices is only about 3. The result of drawing such graphs with uniform edge lengths are hundreds of edges of length 1 in a circle or sphere of diameter 3 – a clutter that does not reveal much about the structure of the software system (except its small diameter). Section 5.1 illustrates this with a comparison of drawings of the Fruchterman-Reingold model and our energy model. The same argument rules out the energy model of Kamada and Kawai [11] (also introduced in Section 4.5 of the Technical Foundations) which aims at Euclidean distances of the vertices being proportional to their graph-theoretic distances.

All mentioned force and energy models easily generalize to different desired edge lengths for each edge, i.e., to the drawing of graphs with weighted edges so that the desired length of every edge depends on its weight. Further energy models serving this purpose were proposed in the literature on information visualization [4,7] and multidimensional scaling (e.g. [2]). So our first approach was to apply a similarity measure to determine the desired distance of every pair of vertices, and to compute drawings that preserve these distances at least on an ordinal scale [14,20]. One requirement for the desired distances is that vertices of the same cluster of the graph should be closer to each other than vertices of different clusters. So specifying desired distances requires knowledge of the clusters of the graph, but most variants of the graph clustering problem are $\mathcal{NP}$-hard. (See [1,18] for surveys on graph clustering.)

In the following, we introduce an energy model that does not take desired edge lengths as input parameter. Instead, it is only the interplay of attractive and repulsive forces which reveals the global structure of the graph. In this respect our approach is similar to that of Hendley *et al.* [10] who, however, did not publish their force model and an analysis of its properties. The main advantages over energy models which aim at preserving given desired distances are:

1. Knowledge about the clusters of the graph is not required as input, but provided as output.
2. Instead of hoping that the given desired distances are preserved in the drawing, it can be proved that the distances in the minimum energy drawing are interpretable.

3.3 The Cut Ratio as a Measure of Coupling

In this subsection we define the cut ratio of two clusters and explain why its inverse is an appropriate distance of these clusters in the drawing. In the next subsection an energy function is introduced whose minimization produces a drawing in which clusters have this distance – without taking any explicit information about clusters as input.

Let V_1 and V_2 be two nonempty, disjoint subsets of the set of vertices V. Then the *cut* that separates V_1 and V_2 is the set of edges connecting both subsets:

$$\mathrm{cut}(V_1, V_2) = E[V_1 \cup V_2] \setminus (E[V_1] \cup E[V_2])$$

The *ratio* of this cut is the fraction of the possible edges between V_1 and V_2 which actually occur:

$$\mathrm{ratio}(V_1, V_2) = \frac{|\mathrm{cut}(V_1, V_2)|}{|V_1| \cdot |V_2|}$$

The ratio of a cut was introduced as quality metric for partitions of circuits by Wei and Cheng [23], and was more recently applied as a metric for coupling in the clustering of call graphs [16]. Because it is normalized with respect to the number of possible edges, its interpretation is independent of the size of V_1 and V_2. If, for example, $|V_1| = |V_2| = 2$, then a cut size of 4 means maximum coupling. If $|V_1| = |V_2| = 10$, the same cut size means loose coupling. This is reflected by the ratio of the cuts which takes the maximum possible value 1 in the first case and the near-minimum value 0.04 in the second case. Wei and Cheng [23] present the same idea from the opposite perspective: For all cuts of a random graph the expected value of the *ratio* is equal, while the expected *size* of the cuts strongly depends on the sizes of the separated sets of vertices.

Suppose $\mathrm{ratio}(V_{11}, V_{12}) \gg \mathrm{ratio}(V_1, V_2)$ and $\mathrm{ratio}(V_{21}, V_{22}) \gg \mathrm{ratio}(V_1, V_2)$ for all partitions of V_1 into non-empty sets V_{11} and V_{12} and all partitions of V_2 into non-empty sets V_{21} and V_{22}, i.e., V_1 and V_2 are clusters with high cohesion and low coupling. Then the intra-cluster distances in the drawing should be small, and the distance between V_1 and V_2 should be much greater and depend on the coupling of V_1 and V_2. Since $\mathrm{ratio}(V_1, V_2)$ measures the coupling, $\frac{1}{\mathrm{ratio}(V_1, V_2)}$ is an appropriate distance of V_1 and V_2:

- Higher couplings imply lower distances. More precisely, doubling the number of edges between V_1 and V_2 halves their distance.
- If no edge connects V_1 and V_2, their distance is infinite. This causes no problems when different components of a graph are treated separately.
- The minimum distance is 1, so even strongly coupled subgraphs are not drawn at the same position.

At the same time, using the inverse ratio of the cut as distance also ensures small intra-cluster distances, because the ratios of the cuts that separate a cluster are high.

3.4 The LinLog Energy Model

In the *LinLog energy model*, the total energy of a drawing is

$$U = \sum_{\{u,v\} \in E} \|p_u - p_v\| - \sum_{\{u,v\} \in V^{(2)}} \ln \|p_u - p_v\|$$

where $V^{(2)}$ denotes the set $\{\{u,v\} \mid u,v \in V, u \neq v\}$ of all subsets of V with exactly two elements, and p_v denotes the position of vertex v. To avoid infinite energies we always assume that different vertices have different positions.

We now analyze the distances in a *one-dimensional* minimum LinLog energy drawing of a graph $G = (V, E)$ where each vertex v has the position x_v. The set of vertices V is partitioned into two sets V_1 and V_2 such that:

1. $V = V_1 \cup V_2, V_1 \cap V_2 = \emptyset$, $V_1 \neq \emptyset$, $V_2 \neq \emptyset$, and
2. the vertices in V_1 have smaller coordinates than the vertices in V_2: $\forall v_1 \in V_1\ \forall v_2 \in V_2 : x_{v_1} < x_{v_2}$.

Let us examine drawings where some $d \in \mathbb{R}$ is added to the coordinates of all vertices in V_1, and which do not violate the second condition, i.e., $d < \min\{x_v \mid v \in V_2\} - \max\{x_v \mid v \in V_1\}$. The total energy of these drawings is the sum of the energy *within* each of the two subgraphs $G[V_1]$ and $G[V_2]$, and the energy *between* these two subgraphs:

$$U(d) = \sum_{\{u,v\} \in E[V_1] \cup E[V_2]} |x_u - x_v| - \sum_{\{u,v\} \in V_1^{(2)} \cup V_2^{(2)}} \ln |x_u - x_v|$$

$$+ \sum_{\{u,v\} \in E \setminus (E[V_1] \cup E[V_2])} (|x_u - x_v| + d) - \sum_{\{u,v\} \in V^{(2)} \setminus (V_1^{(2)} \cup V_2^{(2)})} \ln(|x_u - x_v| + d)$$

By definition of the x_v, this function has a global minimum at $d = 0$, so $U'(0) = 0$.

$$U'(d) = \left|E \setminus (E[V_1] \cup E[V_2])\right| - \sum_{\{u,v\} \in V^{(2)} \setminus (V_1^{(2)} \cup V_2^{(2)})} \frac{1}{|x_u - x_v| + d}$$

$$0 = |\operatorname{cut}(V_1, V_2)| - \sum_{\{u,v\} \in V^{(2)} \setminus (V_1^{(2)} \cup V_2^{(2)})} \frac{1}{|x_u - x_v|}$$

Inserting the harmonic mean of the distances between V_1 and V_2

$$\operatorname{harm}(V_1, V_2) = \frac{|V_1| \cdot |V_2|}{\sum_{\{u,v\} \in V^{(2)} \setminus (V_1^{(2)} \cup V_2^{(2)})} \frac{1}{|x_u - x_v|}}$$

we get

$$0 = |\operatorname{cut}(V_1, V_2)| - \frac{|V_1| \cdot |V_2|}{\operatorname{harm}(V_1, V_2)}$$

$$\operatorname{harm}(V_1, V_2) = \frac{|V_1| \cdot |V_2|}{|\operatorname{cut}(V_1, V_2)|} = \frac{1}{\operatorname{ratio}(V_1, V_2)}$$

So we have shown that wherever one cuts a one-dimensional minimum LinLog energy drawing of a connected graph into two non-empty subgraphs, the harmonic mean of the inter-subgraph distances equals the inverse ratio of the cut. Thus valid (and useful, see Section 3.1) inferences about the structure of the graph can be made from the positions of the vertices.

The harmonic mean of the inter-subgraph distances is more appropriate than the arithmetic or geometric mean here because it weights small distances higher than large distances. This corresponds well to our intuitive notion of the distance of two subgraphs. If the intra-subgraph distances are much smaller than the inter-subgraph distances, the three means are roughly equal.

Unfortunately, the result does not generalize to two- or higher-dimensional minimum energy drawings. However, we have neither theoretical nor empirical reasons to believe that it is seriously violated in practice. In particular, the one-dimensional case is a good approximation when the intra-subgraph distances are much smaller than the inter-subgraph distances.

A more detailed analysis of the LinLog energy model and additional energy models for reference graphs can be found in [17].

4 Implementation

In the reference model of information visualization developed by Card *et al.* [3, Chapter 1], visualizations are considered as series of adjustable mappings from raw data to views of visual structures. This section describes the mappings of CrocoCosmos.

4.1 Data Extraction

The raw data of CrocoCosmos is the source code of an object-oriented program. The source code is mapped to an attributed nested graph (see Section 2.6 of the Technical Foundations for the definition of nested graphs) which is an instance of the schema depicted in Figure 1:

- Program entities, like methods, attributes, classes, files, and subsystems, are mapped to vertices of the graph.
- The containment hierarchy of the program is mapped to the inclusion tree of the nested graph. The containment hierarchy includes the relations of methods and attributes to their containing class, of classes to their containing file, and of files and subsystems to their containing subsystem.
- Other relations of program entities, mainly the "uses" relation between methods and attributes, the "calls" relation between methods, and the "inherits from" relation between classes, are mapped to directed edges.
- The vertices of the graph are attributed with the values of metrics. Metrics map properties of program entities, like the size or the number of incoming and outgoing relations, to numbers. A particular set of metrics can be defined for the entities of each level of the hierarchy, i.e., methods, classes, files, subsystems and the whole system.

4.2 Level of Detail and Filtering

By choosing the level of detail and applying filtering mechanisms, the user defines a mapping from the nested graph to a graph without hierarchy. The level of detail can be set globally, and modified for each vertex individually by replacing it by its children and vice versa. For example, first showing the whole system at class level and then replacing a class by its methods and attributes results in a detailed view of this class in global context.

Because the inclusion tree of the nested graph is not represented in the main visualization, CrocoCosmos provides an additional window that shows the containment hierarchy of the software system. This hierarchy window is closely linked to the main view. For example, clicking on a vertex in the hierarchy window focuses this vertex in the main view.

The user also controls which vertices and edges of the chosen level of detail are included in the hierarchy-free graph and which are elided. This makes it possible to examine parts of a program in isolation, or to start with a few methods and explore how they are used by the remaining system.

4.3 Graph Layout

Force-directed layout algorithms attribute each vertex of the graph with a position in three-dimensional space. To adapt the drawing criteria to the properties of the graph and the purpose of the visualization, the user can choose between different energy models. For example, the Fruchterman-Reingold model produces readable layouts of inheritance graphs, while the LinLog model can reveal the structure of denser graphs like reference graphs. Section 3 discusses energy models in more detail.

4.4 Visual Mapping

The attributed graph is mapped to a visual structure as follows:

- Vertices are mapped to volumes.
- The shape, size and color of a volume represent the type and metric values of the corresponding vertex. For example, all methods can be displayed as stars, classes as spheres, files as cubes, and subsystems as pyramids. The diameter of the sphere representing a class can be defined by its number of methods, and all classes of the same subsystem might have the same color. All these mappings are controlled by the user.
- Edges are mapped to straight lines.
- The type and direction of an edge is shown by the color transition of the corresponding line. For example, a blue-yellow line indicates an inheritance relation from the entity at the blue end to the entity at the yellow end.

4.5 View Transformation

The user controls the point and direction of view by moving freely through the three-dimensional space. Viewpoints can be saved to return to them later. An additional way to change the view is focusing on a particular vertex by clicking on it in the hierarchy window, as mentioned in Section 4.2.

When the mouse cursor is moved on a volume the name of the corresponding program entity is shown. Clicking on a volume opens a details-on-demand window with metric values or the source code of the corresponding entity.

5 Examples

The first subsection shows the ability of the LinLog energy model to reveal the structure of graphs for some pseudo-random graph with expected clusters. The second subsection sketches an analysis of a real-world software system with CrocoCosmos.

5.1 Random Graphs

The Figures 4, 5 and 6 show drawings of pseudo-random graphs with clusters for our LinLog energy model (introduced in Section 3) and the well-known Fruchterman-Reingold model (discussed in Section 3.2).[1] In all figures, the LinLog model (left drawings) reveals the clusters more clearly than the Fruchterman-Reingold model (right drawings).

The graph of Figure 4 is a pseudo-random graph with eight clusters of 50 vertices each. The probability of an edge $\{u, v\}$ is 0.2 if u and v belong to the same cluster and 0.01 otherwise. The eight clusters are clearly separated in the drawing for the LinLog model, but the borders of the clusters look fuzzy and some vertices do not seem to belong to any cluster. This is to be expected of a random graph: Some vertices have a small degree, and hence drift to the border of the drawing. Other vertices are equally connected to two clusters, and are drawn between these clusters.

To illustrate this point, Figure 5 shows another graph with eight clusters of 50 vertices each. The clusters are cliques (complete graphs, edge probability 1), while the inter-cluster edge probability is 0.2. The drawing of the LinLog model looks more orderly than in Figure 4, because every vertex is guaranteed to be adjacent to all other vertices of its cluster. Nevertheless, separating clusters is difficult: every vertex is adjacent to 49 vertices of its own cluster, but on average to 70 vertices of other clusters.

The graph of Figure 6 is a pseudo-random graph with one central cluster of 200 vertices and three "satellite" clusters of 100 vertices each, called cluster A, B and C. The probability of an edge $\{u, v\}$ is

[1] The examples in this section are two-dimensional because three-dimensional visualizations are not adequately represented by printouts.

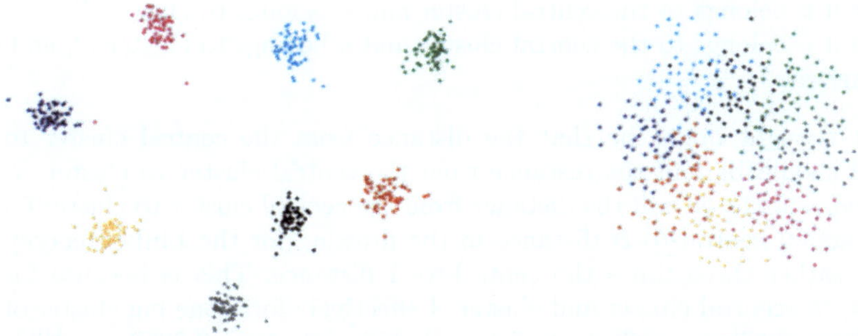

Fig. 4. Pseudo-random graph with intra-cluster edge probability 0.20, inter-cluster edge probability 0.01; left: LinLog model, right: Fruchterman-Reingold model.

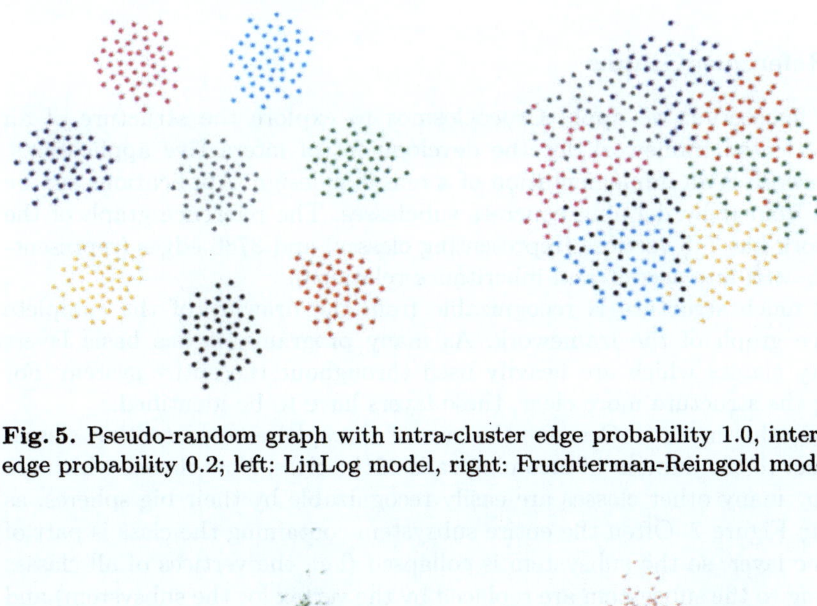

Fig. 5. Pseudo-random graph with intra-cluster edge probability 1.0, inter-cluster edge probability 0.2; left: LinLog model, right: Fruchterman-Reingold model.

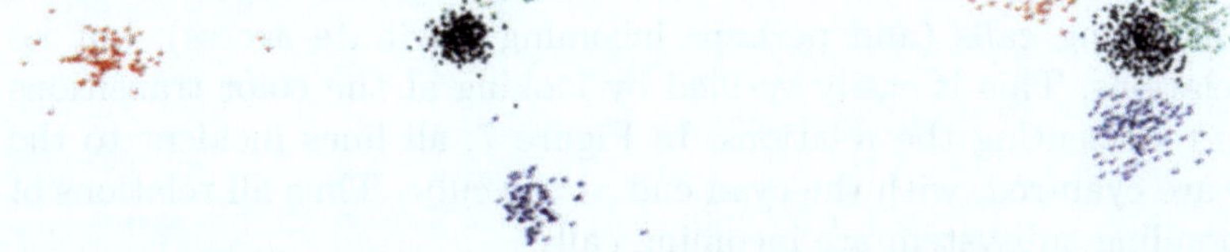

Fig. 6. Pseudo-random "satellite" graph; left: LinLog model, right: Fruchterman-Reingold model.

- 0.064 if u and v belong to the same cluster,
- 0.016 if u belongs to the central cluster and v belongs to cluster A,
- 0.008 if u belongs to the central cluster and v belongs to cluster B,
- 0.004 if u belongs to the central cluster and v belongs to cluster C, and
- 0 otherwise.

The first thought might be that the distance from the central cluster to cluster A should be half the distance from the central cluster to cluster B, which again should be half the distance from the central cluster to cluster C. But the actual central-to-B distance in the drawing for the LinLog energy model is rather three times the central-to-A distance. This is because for cluster B, the central cluster and cluster A effectively form one big cluster of 300 vertices, yielding an effective edge probability of about $0.0053 = \frac{0.016}{3}$. On the other hand, cluster B has little influence on the central-to-A distance because it is relatively far away from both. So the LinLog model did not only separate different clusters, it also produced interpretable distances between the clusters.

5.2 Reference Graphs

In this subsection we apply CrocoCosmos to explore the structure of an object-oriented framework for the development of interactive applications. A framework is an implementation of a reusable design. Applications can be derived from it by defining concrete subclasses. The reference graph of the framework has 745 vertices (representing classes) and 3786 edges (representing call, attribute access, and inheritance relations).

Not much structure is recognizable from the drawing of the complete reference graph of the framework. As many programs, it has basic layers of utility classes which are heavily used throughout the entire system. For making the structure more clear, these layers have to be identified.

To do this in CrocoCosmos, the size of the spheres representing classes can be set to the number of incoming calls of the class. Now classes which are called by many other classes are easily recognizable by their big spheres, as shown in Figure 7. Often the entire subsystem containing the class is part of the basic layer, so the subsystem is collapsed (i.e., the vertices of all classes belonging to the subsystem are replaced by the vertex for the subsystem) and all relations of the subsystem are shown. The basic layer of a system should have only incoming calls (and perhaps incoming attribute access), but no outgoing relations. This is easily verified by looking at the color transitions of the lines representing the relations. In Figure 7, all lines incident to the green cube are cyan-red, with the cyan end at the cube. Thus all relations of the corresponding subsystem are incoming calls.

In this way the layer structure can be discovered, and it can be verified that lower layers do not use upper layers. Classes and subsystems of basic layers can be easily understood and reused, because they do not use

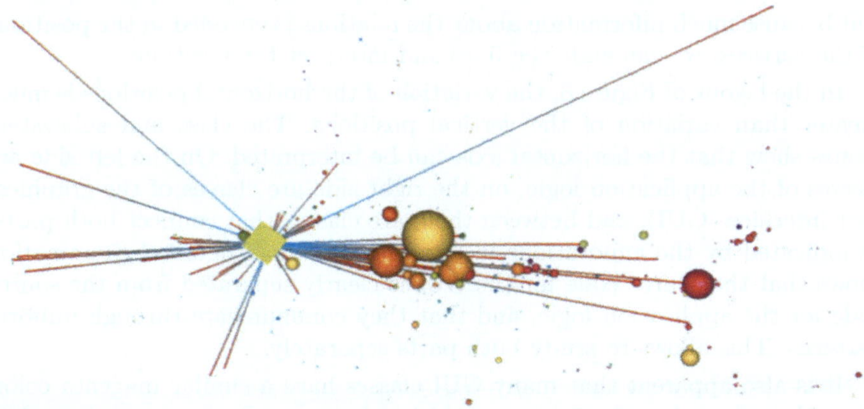

Fig. 7. Reference graph of a framework. The diameter of each sphere is proportional to the number of incoming calls of the corresponding class. One subsystem is collapsed and its relations are shown.

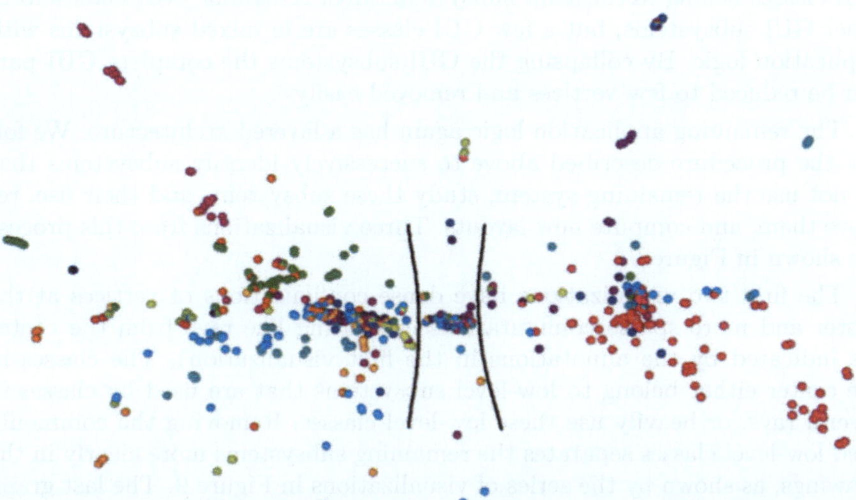

Fig. 8. Reference graph after the removal of the basic layer.

the remaining system. Often the basic layer has to be removed to make the structure of the remaining system more clear. Which low-level utilities (e.g., exceptions, console output, pre- and postconditions) a high-level class uses is not relevant for understanding its relations to other high-level classes.

Figure 8 shows a layout of the reference graph after the classes of the basic layer are removed. In contrast to Figure 7, all classes are drawn with equal size, independent of metric values. There are still so many relations that the drawing appears cluttered when all corresponding lines are shown.

But because much information about the relations is encoded in the positions of the vertices, we can elide the lines and interpret the positions.

In the layout of Figure 8, the variation of the horizontal positions is much greater than variation of the vertical positions. The class and subsystem names show that the horizontal axis can be interpreted: On the left side are classes of the application logic, on the right side are classes of the graphical user interface (GUI), and between them are classes that connect both parts, as indicated by the annotations in the figure. A more detailed examination shows that the source code for the GUI is clearly separated from the source code for the application logic, and that they communicate through uniform patterns. This allows to study both parts separately.

It is also apparent that many GUI classes have a similar magenta color. The color of a sphere indicates to which subsystem the corresponding class belongs: All classes of the same subsystem have the same color. However, large systems have so many subsystems that different subsystems sometimes have very similar colors. In Figure 8, the colors correctly indicate that most GUI classes belong to the same subsystem. Most remaining GUI classes form other GUI subsystems, but a few GUI classes are in mixed subsystems with application logic. By collapsing the GUI subsystems the complete GUI part can be reduced to few vertices and removed easily.

The remaining application logic again has a layered architecture. We follow the procedure described above to successively identify subsystems that do not use the remaining system, study these subsystems and their use, remove them, and compute new layouts. Three visualizations from this process are shown in Figure 9.

The first two visualizations have dense configurations of vertices at the center and more sparse configurations emanating like rays from the center (as indicated by the annotations in the first visualization). The classes in the center either belong to low-level subsystems that are used by classes in several rays, or heavily use these low-level classes. Removing the commonly used low-level classes separates the remaining subsystems more clearly in the drawings, as shown by the series of visualizations in Figure 9. The last graph has such a clear structure that we produced the layout with the Fruchterman-Reingold model instead of the LinLog energy model.

The rays represent high-level parts of the system which are related to the low-level classes in the center, but only loosely related to each other. Sometimes the removal of a low-level class even disconnects a ray from the rest of the system. These disconnected parts are not shown in the figure to save space (which explains the decrease of the number of vertices from the top to the bottom drawing). In each ray and each disconnected component, the spheres have the same or only few different colors, which indicates that the corresponding classes belong to the same or only few different subsystems. Thus the subsystems are cohesive and loosely coupled, which conforms to a fundamental software design rule.

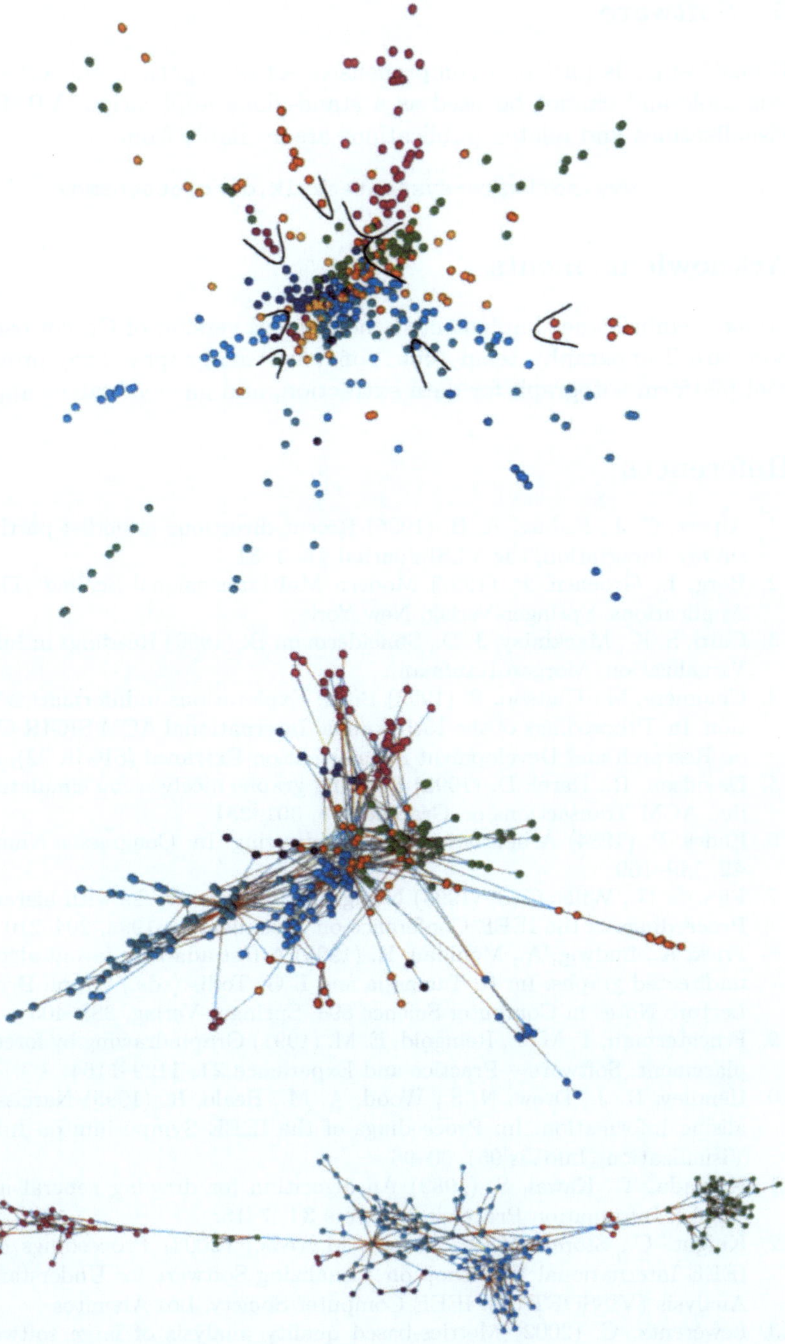

Fig. 9. Reference graphs of the application logic after successive removal of low layers (from top to bottom).

6 Software

CrocoCosmos is part of a comprehensive set of experimental software analysis tools and cannot be used as a stand-alone application. VRML files of visualizations and related publications are available from

`www.software-systemtechnik.de/crococosmos.`

Acknowledgements

Frank Steinbrückner implemented the original version of CrocoCosmos. The Software Tomography team (`www.softwaretomography.com`) provided the tool platform sotograph for data extraction, and gave valuable support.

References

1. Alpert, C. J., Kahng, A. B. (1995) Recent directions in netlist partitioning: a survey. Integration, the VLSI Journal **19**, 1–81
2. Borg, I., Groenen, P. (1997) Modern Multidimensional Scaling: Theory and Applications. Springer-Verlag, New York
3. Card, S. K., Mackinlay, J. D., Shneiderman, B. (1999) Readings in Information Visualization, Morgan Kaufmann
4. Chalmers, M., Chitson, P. (1992) Bead: Explorations in information visualization. In: Proceedings of the 15th Annual International ACM SIGIR Conference on Research and Development in Information Retrieval (SIGIR'92), 330–337
5. Davidson, R., Harel, D. (1996) Drawing graphs nicely using simulated annealing. ACM Transactions on Graphics **15**, 301–331
6. Eades, P. (1984) A heuristic for graph drawing. In: Congressus Numerantium **42**, 149–160
7. Eick, S. G., Wills, G. J. (1993) Navigating large networks with hierarchies. In: Proceedings of the IEEE Conference on Visualization 1993, 204–210
8. Frick, A., Ludwig, A., Mehldau, H. (1995) A fast adaptive layout algorithm for undirected graphs. In: R. Tamassia and I. G. Tollis (eds.) Graph Drawing '94, Lecture Notes in Computer Science 894, Springer-Verlag, 388–403
9. Fruchterman, T. M. J., Reingold, E. M. (1991) Graph drawing by force-directed placement. Software – Practice and Experience **21**, 1129–1164
10. Hendley, R. J., Drew, N. S., Wood, A. M., Beale, R. (1995) Narcissus: Visualising information. In: Proceedings of the IEEE Symposium on Information Visualization (InfoVis'95), 90–96
11. Kamada, T., Kawai, S. (1989) An algorithm for drawing general undirected graphs. Information Processing Letters **31**, 7–15.
12. Knight, C., Storey, M.-A., Munro, M. (eds.) (2002) Proceedings of the 1st IEEE International Workshop on Visualizing Software for Understanding and Analysis (VISSOFT'02). IEEE Computer Society, Los Alamitos
13. Lewerentz, C. (2002) Metrics-based quality analysis of large software products. In: R. R. Dumke and M. Bundschuh (eds.) Software-Metriken in der Praxis. Tagungsband des DASMA Software Metrik Kongresses METRIKON 2001, Shaker Verlag, 133–146

14. Lewerentz, C., Simon, F. (2002) Metrics-based 3D visualization of large object-oriented programs. In [12], 70–77
15. Lewerentz, C., Simon, F., Steinbrückner, F., Breitling, H., Lilienthal, C., Lippert, M. (2002) External validation of a metrics-based quality assessment of the JWAM framework. In: R. Dumke and D. Rombach (eds.) Software-Messung und -Bewertung, Deutscher Universittsverlag, 32–49
16. Mancoridis, S., Mitchell, B. S., Chen, Y., Gansner, E. R. (1999) Bunch: A clustering tool for the recovery and maintenance of software system structures. In: Proceedings of the International Conference on Software Maintenance (ICSM'99), 50–59
17. Noack, A. (2003) Energy models for drawing clustered small-world graphs. Technical Report 07/03, Computer Science Reports, Brandenburg University of Technology at Cottbus
18. Pothen, A. (1997) Graph partitioning algorithms with applications to scientific computing. In: D. E. Keyes, A. Sameh, V. Venkatakrishnan (eds.) Parallel Numerical Algorithms, Kluwer Academic Publishers, 323–368
19. Proceedings of the 10th International Workshop on Program Comprehension (IWPC'02), IEEE Computer Society, Los Alamitos 2002
20. Simon, F. (2001) Meßwertbasierte Qualitätssicherung. Dissertation, Fakultät für Mathematik, Naturwissenschaften und Informatik, Brandenburgische Technische Universität Cottbus
21. Simon, F., Lewerentz, C., Bischofberger, W. (2002) Software quality assessments for system, architecture, design and code. In: D. Meyerhoff, B. Laibarra, R. van der Pouw Kraan, A. Wallet (eds.), Software Quality and Software Testing in Internet Times, Springer-Verlag, 230–249
22. Watts, D. J., Strogatz, S. H. (1998) Collective dynamics of 'small-world' networks. Nature **393**, 440–442
23. Wei, Y.-C., Cheng, C.-K. (1991) Ratio cut partitioning for hierarchical design. IEEE Transactions on Computer-Aided Design **10**, 911–921

ViSta – Visualizing Statecharts*

Rodolfo Castelló[1], Rym Mili[2], and Ioannis G. Tollis[2]

[1] Institute of Technology at Monterrey, School of Engineering and Computer Science, H. Colegio Militar 4700, Chihuahua, Chih, 31300, México
[2] The University of Texas at Dallas, Department of Computer Science, Box 830688, Richardson, TX 75083-0688, USA

1 Introduction

Statecharts are widely used for the requirements specification of reactive systems. This notation captures the requirements attributes that are concerned with the behavioral features of a system, and models these features in terms of a hierarchy of diagrams and states. The usefulness of statecharts depends primarily on their readability, that is the capability of the drawing to convey the meaning quickly and clearly. Several visualization tools for the specification of reactive systems are available in the market [15,26,24,1]. Even though these tools are helpful in organizing designers' thoughts, they are mostly sophisticated small scale graphical editors, and therefore are inadequate for the modeling of complex reactive systems. Specifically, hand made diagrams quickly become unreadable when the specification complexity and size increase. Therefore computer assistance is of paramount importance for the graphical representation of complex reactive systems.

In this chapter we present a tool suite for the static and interactive visualization of statechart diagrams. We proceed in two steps: we manually extract behavioral information from a textual description, and store it into interactive templates; then we automatically generate graphs that model statecharts in a hierarchical fashion. The resulting drawings enjoy several properties: they have a low number of arc crossings; they emphasize the natural hierarchical decomposition of states into sub-states; and they have a good aspect ratio.

The automatically produced graphical representation is an effective requirements assessment tool since it allows the specifier to shift focus from organizing the mental or physical structure of the requirements to its analysis. In addition, the interdependence between the textual, template and graphical representations ensures consistency between the different documents and therefore facilitates the verification and validation effort.

1.1 Related Work

Statemate [15] is a graphical tool used to represent reactive system requirements from three perspectives: *structural*, *functional* and *behavioral*. The

* Research supported in part by Sandia National Labs and by the Texas Advanced Research Program under grant number 009741-040.

structural view provides a hierarchical decomposition of the system into its components; the functional view describes the functions and processes of the system; the behavioral view uses statecharts to represent state change. The user of Statemate draws statecharts manually, using a graphical editor. No automatic layout feature is offered by the tool. *Rational Rose* [28] offers a feature to layout UML statechart diagrams. This feature assigns high level objects to horizontal layers. Sub-objects are drawn randomly and are not laid out by the tool. In addition, labels are automatically placed in the middle of edges, and no attempt is made to avoid overlaps between labels and other graphical elements of the diagram. *ObjectTime* [26] is a graphical tool used to visualize requirements written in the *Room* formal specification language. It uses graphics to describe the structure and behavior of reactive systems. *Telelogic* [24] is a tool suite used to visualize, develop, implement and test distributed real time systems. It is based on formal languages such as SDL, and graphical notations such as statecharts and UML. *Artisan Real-Time Studio* [1] uses a UML based notation to model the functionality and design of real-time systems. However, the graphical representations offered by the tools discussed above are all hand made through a graphical editor.

The statechart layouts produced by our tool are based on several techniques that include layered drawing, labeling, and floor-planning. We also provide algorithms for interactive operations (such as insertions and deletions) that preserve the mental map of the drawings. Our algorithm for layered drawings is a variant of the algorithm by Sugiyama *et al.* [33] described in Section 4.2 of the Technical Foundations that is tailored to statecharts. A comprehensive approach to layered drawings of directed graphs is described in Sugiyama *et al.* [33]. Several extensions and variations of this approach have been introduced in the literature. A comprehensive survey is given in [2]. A first extension that takes into consideration cycles and dummy nodes for large edges (i.e., edges that span more that one level) was introduced by Rowe *et al.* [29]. Gansner *et al.* [12,13] provide a technique to draw directed graphs using a simplex-based algorithm that assigns vertices to layers; at the same time, they provide an extension to the basic algorithm of Sugiyama *et al.* by drawing edge-bends as curves. A divide-and conquer approach is described by Messinger *et al.* [21] to improve the layout-time performance for large graphs consisting of several hundred vertices. More recently, a combination of the algorithm of [33] with incremental-orthogonal drawing techniques was proposed by Seemann [31] to automatically generate a layout of UML class diagrams. In [16], Harel and Yashchin discuss an algorithm for drawing edge-less high-graph-like structures. The problem of drawing clustered graphs without crossings was studied in [10,11]. Most of the research on the *Edge Labeling Problem* (ELP) has been done on labeling graphs with fixed geometry, such as geographical and technical maps. Kakoulis and Tollis [17,18] present an algorithm for the ELP problem that can be applied to layered drawings with fixed geometry. Gansner *et al.* [13] use a simple approach to solve the ELP problem for layered drawings: they assign labels to the middle position of edge lines. However, they assume that edge labels are small and do not consider the possibility of overlap with other drawing components. In our work, we address the problem of graph drawings with flexible geometry. Finally, in order to reduce the area and improve the aspect ratio of the statechart drawings we apply floor-planning techniques inspired by the ones used for the area minimization of VLSI layouts [20,32]. This chapter is based on work originally published in [7,8].

In our approach, the layered, labeling, and floor-planning techniques are designed to work in a cooperative environment to aid in the preservation of the mental map. Misue *et al.* [22] present three models for mental map maintenance, based on the position of the nodes in the diagram: the orthogonal ordering; the proximity relations; and the topology. They provide two layout adjustment techniques that preserve the mental map. The first technique aims at making nodes disjoint during the modification of the original diagram. The second technique is oriented towards displaying certain parts of the diagram like a view.

North [23] presents a heuristic for layered layouts of directed graphs that incorporates position and order node stability. This heuristic moves nodes between adjacent ranks based on median sort. Seemann [31] combines layered with orthogonal techniques for the incremental layout of UML class diagrams. Ryall *et al.* [30] present a constraint-based approach to layout small graphs. These constraints are enforced by a generalized spring algorithm. Several techniques for the preservation of the mental map in orthogonal drawings have been proposed [4,5,25]. Papakostas and Tollis [25] discuss a systematic approach that applies to interactive orthogonal graph drawings of vertices of degree at most 4.

2 Applications

Statecharts [14] are extended finite state machines used to describe control aspects of reactive systems. They provide mechanisms to describe synchronization and concurrency, and manage exponential explosion of states by using state decomposition. In the statechart notation, a state is denoted by a box labeled in the upper left corner. Directed arcs are used to denote transitions between states. A transition label has the form $E[C]/A$, where E is a boolean combination of external stimuli; C is a boolean combination of conditions; and A is an action that is executed when the transition is active, E occurs, and C is true. In Figure 1, the transition between states S_a and S_b occurs when stimuli e is received and condition c is true; this will result in the execution of action a.

In the statechart notation, a state can be repeatedly decomposed into sub-states in two ways, through the *OR* or the *AND* decomposition. The *OR* decomposition reflects the hierarchical structure of a state machine and is

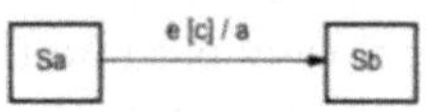

Fig. 1. Transitions in statecharts.

represented by encapsulation (see Figure 2). The *AND* decomposition reflects concurrency of independent state machines and is represented by splitting a box with lines (see Figure 3).

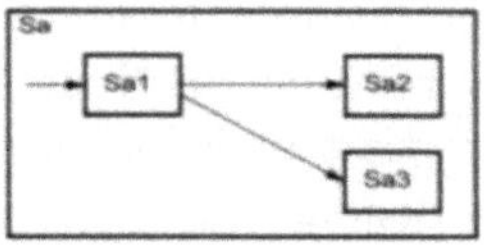

Fig. 2. OR Decomposition.

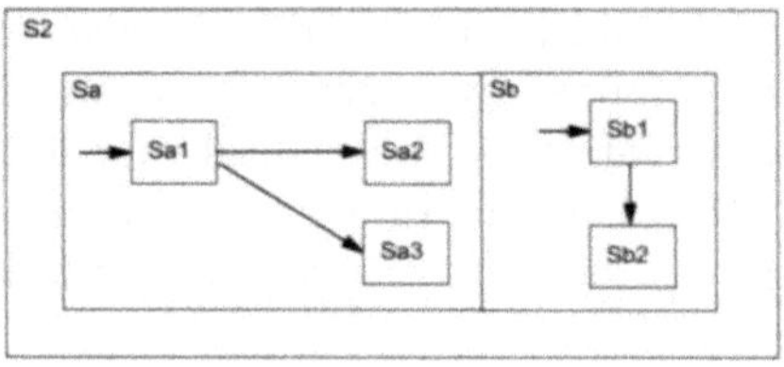

Fig. 3. AND Decomposition.

The underlying structure of a statechart is an *AND*/*OR* tree where the leaves are called *basic* states. We call this structure a *decomposition tree*. The root of a decomposition tree corresponds to the system state; leaves correspond to atomic states. Each object in the tree can be decomposed through the *AND* or *OR* decomposition. Figure 4 shows the decomposition tree that corresponds to the statechart depicted in Figure 3.

3 Algorithms

The foundation of our framework for the visualization of statecharts is the following Algorithm 1.

The procedure that draws leaves is trivial: Each leaf is drawn as a rectangle that is wide enough to accommodate its label. The algorithms for drawing the *AND* and *OR* nodes are more complicated and one can choose among

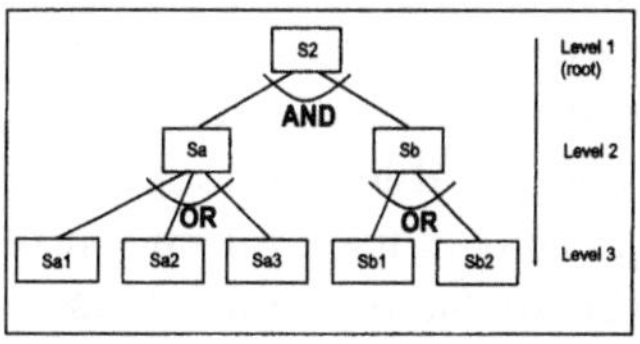

Fig. 4. Decomposition tree of a statechart.

Algorithm 1: Visualization of statecharts.

Input : Decomposition Tree T
Output: Statechart Drawing of T

1. The decomposition tree T is traversed in order to determine the dimensions and point of origin of the drawing of every node, in a recursive manner.
2. If a node v is a leaf then a simple drawing procedure is called that produces a labeled rectangle. It returns the point of origin and the dimensions of the rectangle.
3. If v is an *AND* node then a recursive algorithm constructs the drawings of every child node of v and places the drawings next to each other.
4. If v is an *OR* node then a recursive algorithm
   - first constructs the drawings of every child of v,
   - then, it assigns each child to a specific layer. For the sake of simplicity, we generate our drawings horizontally, from left to right. A similar approach can be used to generate vertical drawings.

---

many approaches. We have chosen to draw *AND* nodes using techniques similar to floor-plans [19,32,34] or inclusion drawings [9], and *OR* nodes using a modified version of Sugiyama's algorithm [33] decribed in Section 4.2 of the Technical Foundations. Our framework will still be operational if the user decides to use other algorithms.

3.1 Drawing *AND* Nodes

An *AND* node reflects concurrency of independent state machines. The simplest way to draw an *AND* node is to place the drawings of its children vertically next to each other. The height of the *AND* node is equal to the maximum height of its children's rectangles and its width is equal to the sum of the widths of its children's rectangles. This approach is very simple and thus very desirable. However, it is not very efficient in terms of area. The size of each node depends on the recursive drawings of the sub-state nodes that are nested in it. Hence, it is possible that certain *AND* nodes of the decomposition tree are very large in one dimension or the other. This implies that an unfortunate combination of two sub-node rectangles, one with large height and one with large width, will result in a drawing of the *AND* node that occupies a very large area (which is mostly empty). This is clearly undesirable. Additionally, the aspect ratio of the drawing, another important æsthetic criterion, is not controllable. We tackle this problem by applying (a) the *floor-planning* concept that is used for the minimization of area of VLSI chip [19,32,34], and (b) the *inclusion* concept used to minimize the drawing area of trees in [9].

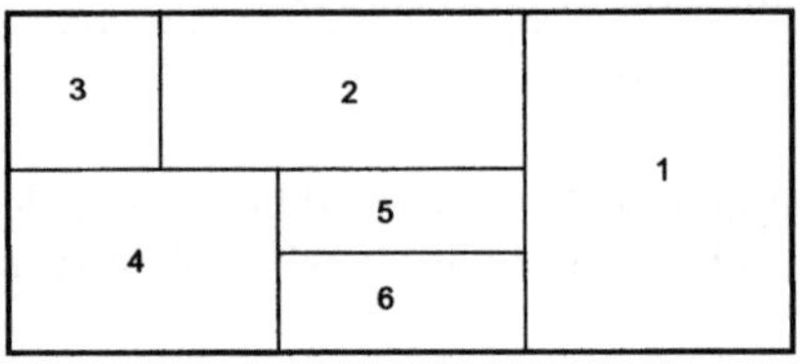

Fig. 5. A slicing floor-plan.

Floor-planning partitions a floor rectangle into *floor-plans* using line segments called *slices*. Each slice is either vertical or horizontal. Floor-plans are combined in such a way that the enclosing rectangle covers a minimum area (see Figure 5). A floor-plan is *slicing floorplan* whenever the floor-plan is an atomic rectangle[1] or there exists a slice that divides the rectangle into two. The floor-planning problem has an efficient solution when the floor-plan is slicing [20,32]. However, the slices in our problem are not fixed as either vertical or horizontal. This has to be decided by some algorithm. From this point of view, our problem is also similar to the tree drawing problem mentioned above. For the inclusion convention each non-leaf node is a rectangle that contains the rectangles of its subtrees. The problem of optimizing the area by choosing vertical and horizontal slices is $\mathcal{NP}$-hard in general, see for example [9]. If the tree is binary and the sizes of the leaf nodes are restricted, then a dynamic programming algorithm can minimize the area of an inclusion drawing in about quadratic time [9]. Unfortunately, our trees are general and the size of the subtrees depends on the structure of the statechart.

Although one could apply either (a) the general slicing floor-planning technique for drawing the *AND* nodes [32], or (b) a modification of an inclusion drawing algorithm, none of them can guarantee optimal results. Also, due to the structure of statecharts, and the fact that the size of any *OR* node can be arbitrarily large we have decided to use some simple heuristics that can be applied to statecharts. To this effect, we define the following drawing criteria for statecharts:

[1] one that cannot be further decomposed.

- Leaves are used to represent atomic states whose size depends solely on their labels. Since labels are usually written horizontally (for readability purposes), we will draw leaves horizontally.
- The AND decomposition reflects concurrency, and is represented by splitting an AND-state rectangle into a number of concurrent sub-states. One of the most important æsthetic criteria in graph drawing is *symmetry* [27]. As discussed before, due to the recursive nature of each (sub)state, the dimensions of the various sub-states could be incompatible if placed next to each other. Thus we choose to slice AND-state rectangles either horizontally or vertically, in order to reduce the total area and control the aspect ratio.
- OR states can be drawn in a layered fashion using either a horizontal or a vertical layering depending on the slicing type of the parent node (i.e., horizontal / vertical slicing). This is discussed in the next subsection.

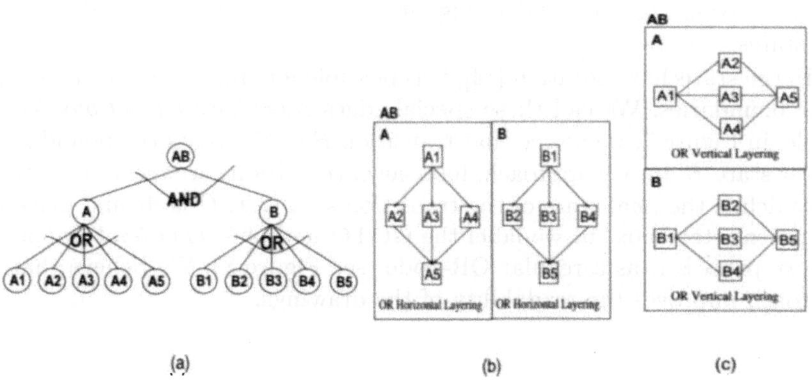

Fig. 6. AND-OR combination: (a) AND/OR decomposition tree, (b) AND vertical slicing with OR horizontal layering, (c) AND horizontal slicing with OR vertical layering.

Our goal is to generate drawings that use the horizontal and vertical dimensions in a uniform way, in order to obtain drawings with small area and good aspect ratio. To this effect we define several heuristics: The AND/OR heuristic applies to the case where the parent is an AND node and the children are OR nodes (see Figure 6(a)). There are two cases:

1. The parent node (AND) is sliced vertically. Then the children nodes (OR) will be drawn on horizontal layers (see Figure 6(b)). In this case, the height of the parent object is the height of the highest child node; and the total width of the parent is the sum of the children's widths.

2. The parent node (AND) is sliced horizontally. Then the children nodes (OR) are drawn on vertical layers (see Figure 6(c)). In this case the height of the parent node is the sum of children's heights; and the width of the parent node is the width of the widest child.

Clearly, the above algorithm for drawing *AND* nodes (excluding the drawing of *OR* nodes) has linear time-complexity with respect to the number of sub-states in such a node. Heuristics that handle the other cases (OR/AND, AND/AND, and OR/OR) are defined similarly. For a complete description see [6,7].

3.2 Drawing *OR* Nodes

An *OR* node reflects the decomposition of states into sub-states. The sub-states of an *OR* node are drawn as rectangles. The drawing (and hence the dimensions of the enclosing rectangle) of an OR node is obtained by recursively performing a layered drawing algorithm [3] on the node and each of its sub-states.

In the statechart notation [14], it is possible for transitions to cross super-state boundaries. We call these special edges *inter-level transitions*. For example, in Figure 7, we notice that transition *B3-C2* crosses the boundaries of parent state *B*. In our approach, inter-level transitions are treated as follows: a) we define the final state of the transition as a *GOTO* node and place it in the parent state box; b) we label the GOTO node "*GOTO final-statename*" and we process it as a regular OR-node (see Figure 8). We believe that this approach improves the readability of the drawings.

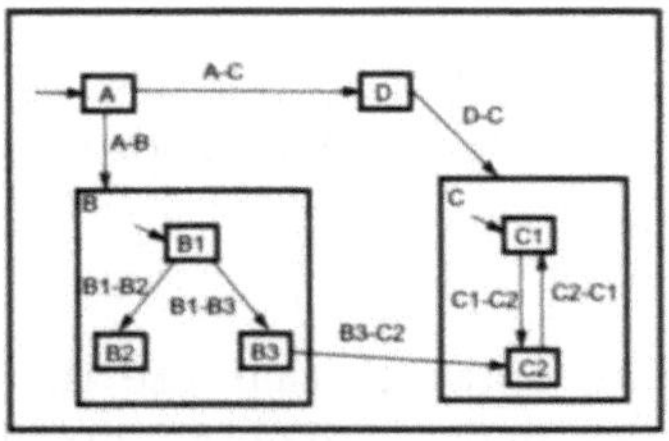

Fig. 7. Inter-level transitions.

The algorithm that constructs the drawing of an OR node has the following steps: (i) sub-states are drawn recursively; and (ii) sub-states are assigned to layers by using a modified version of Sugiyama's algorithm [33] described in Section 4.2 of the Technical Foundations (see Algorithm 2). Sub-states are assigned to layers by applying the following two steps:

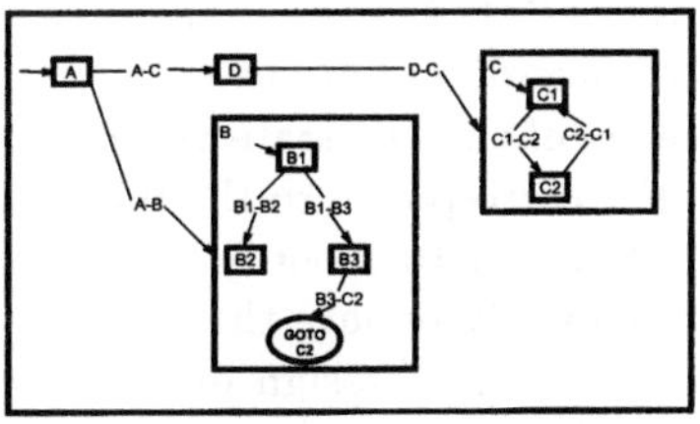

Fig. 8. Goto State.

Algorithm 2: Generation of an OR state final drawing

Input : Set A of sub-states of an OR state
Output: Layered drawing of the OR state with real dimensions
layeredDrawing(A)
Set *hierarchy.height* $= 0$
Set *hierarchy.width* $= 0$
for i = *1 to depth(layeredDrawing of* A*)* **do**
  Set *layer[i].largestWidth* = largest width among the objects in *layer[i]*
  if *layer[i+1]* $\leq$ *depth(layeredDrawing of* A*)* **then**
    add *layer[i].largestWidth* as an offset to the *origin_x* of every object in *layer[i+1]*
  end
  Set *layer[i].height* = summation of each object's height at *layer[i]*
  if *hierarchy.height* $<$ *layer[i].height* **then**
    Set *hierarchy.height* = *layer[i].height*
  end
  Set *hierarchy.width* = *hierarchy.width* + *layer[i].largestWidth*
  Increase the *origin_y* of each object in *layer[i]* in order to deal with the height of each object and avoid overlapping
end

---

1. We construct a hierarchy of sub-states by treating each sub-state as a point by calling Algorithm 3.
2. We incorporate into the hierarchy the dimensions (i.e., height and width) of each node in the drawing. The resulting hierarchy is used to determine the height and width of the parent object/state, as well as the coordinates of the origin of the object's rectangle.

It is easy to modify the above algorithm in order to produce drawings that are directed from left to right and their nodes are placed on vertical layers. Most of the steps of the algorithm have linear time-complexity with respect to the number of edges of the graph. The last step of procedure *hierarchyDrawing* attempts to beautify the obtained drawing by reducing the number of edge crossings, see Section 4.2 in the Technical Foundations.

Algorithm 3: Layered drawing of an OR state

Input : Set A of sub-states of an OR state
Output: Layered drawing of the OR state without dimensions

1. Assign the node that corresponds to the initial state to the first layer.
2. Apply a *depth-first* search to identify those edges that form graph-cycles; then we temporarily remove them.
3. Once the cycles are removed, assign every node v to a specific layer which is determined by the length of a longest path from the start node to v. At this stage, every node is assigned an x coordinate.
4. Add dummy vertices to deal with edges whose initial and final states are not in adjacent layers.
5. Apply a node ordering procedure whose purpose is to minimize edge crossings (see Section 4.2 in the Technical Foundations) within each layer. This ordering provides the y coordinate for each node.

Our approach is based on the general *layer by layer sweep* paradigm [3]. The time-complexity of this step of the algorithm depends on the number of vertices that exist on each layer. If layer L contains $|L|$ nodes, then the time required by the algorithm is $O(|L|^2)$. Clearly, the total time for this step depends upon the distribution of nodes into layers.

3.3 Final Drawing

The final drawing of the statechart represented by the decomposition tree is computed by performing the following steps:

1. Each non-leaf node of the decomposition tree is equipped with two (*width, height*) pairs as follows:
   OR node: (vertical_layering_width, vertical_layering_height), and (horizontal_layering_width, horizontal_layering_height).
   AND node: (vertical_slicing_width, vertical_slicing_height), and (horizontal_slicing_width, horizontal_slicing_height)
2. The horizontal/vertical drawing dimensions are computed in a recursive manner, by traversing the decomposition tree in a top-down fashion as described by Algorithm 4.
3. The root node of the decomposition tree will decide which is the best width/height pair, as described by Algorithm 5.
4. We generate the drawing by traversing the decomposition tree top-down once more, assigning the correct layering/slicing option to every node.

As described above, when the drawing of the children nodes is completed, it takes a time proportional to the number of children to determine the horizontal and vertical drawings of the parent node. Of course, at the expense of extra computation time one can allow a higher number of drawings (or

Algorithm 4: Computation of horizontal and vertical drawing dimensions

Input : Decomposition tree T
Output: Dimension of both horizontal and vertical drawings
for *all* $node_i \in T$ **do**
  if $node_i$*.decompositionType =AND or* $node_i$*.decompositionType =OR* **then**
    Determine the dimensions for both the vertical drawing and the horizontal drawing.
  end
  else
    Determine the dimensions as a LEAF.
  end
end

Algorithm 5: Computation of best width/height

Input : Root node n of decomposition tree T
Output: Best width/height
if *root.horizontal_width * root.horizontal_height* $<$ *root.vertical_width * root.vertical_height* **then**
  Generate drawing with root as horizontal_layering (slicing)
end
else
  Generate drawing with root as vertical_layering (slicing)
end

combinations) to be computed for each internal node. However, this may lead to an exponential number of combinations. Recall that for the inclusion drawings of trees, the optimization of the area is an $\mathcal{NP}$-hard problem, in general [9].

3.4 Interactive Operations in Statecharts

The framework presented in this chapter describes algorithms that produce drawings of static statecharts. The techniques try to optimize various æsthetics, such as bends, crossings, area, etc. This implies that even when a minor modification is performed on a drawing (e.g., addition of a node or a transition), the layout algorithms will re-order the nodes in such a way that these æsthetic criteria are met. Hence, the structure of the resulting drawing could be very different from the original one. In this section, we discuss a technique that we comprehensively presented in [7] and can be used to preserve the *mental map* (i.e., the structure) of statecharts. This is important since the designer/specifier may find mistakes/omissions and hence may need to delete and/or insert states and/or transitions without loosing the mental map. Our approach is based on the *relative coordinate* and *no-change* scenarios:

- The *delete* operation allows deletion of nodes and edges. The simplest way to implement the delete operation is to follow the no-change scenario. In other words, the node and/or edge are simply removed from the drawing without changing the coordinates of the rest of the nodes and edges.
- The *insert* operation allows insertion of nodes and edges. Here we use the relative-coordinates scenario. We apply a layout algorithm that preserves the relative position of the selected states (nodes). The main drawing features of the algorithm that are affected by the insert operation are: (1) the placement on layers of the sub-states of an OR decomposition, and (2) the position of these sub-states inside the layers.

Let us consider the first feature, i.e., the placement of OR-sub-states on layers. When a new transition (edge) is added to the drawing, the insert operation works as follows:

1. Verify that the layout algorithm has been applied.
2. Select the set of states that need to preserve their mental map.
3. Add a new transition to the diagram.
4. Keep the direction of the transitions.
5. Do not identify new cycles, that is, disable the depth-first search algorithm.
6. Determine the direction of the new transition using the current layer assignments of its initial and final states.
7. If the transition is between two states in the same layer, then stop the interactive insert operation and apply the normal layout algorithm.

When a new state (node) is added to the drawing, insert operation for the placement of sub-states on layers works as follows:

1. Verify that the layout algorithm has been applied.
2. Select the set of states that need to preserve their mental map.
3. Add a new state:
4. Keep the direction of the transitions.
5. Do not identify new cycles, that is, disable the depth-first search algorithm.
6. Determine the new layers by applying the following criteria:
   (a) If the new state shifts the position of one selected state, then shift the position of the entire selected group.
   (b) If the new state is positioned in between selected states of the group, then keep the new state in its position, and shift the selected states positioned on subsequent layers to the right.

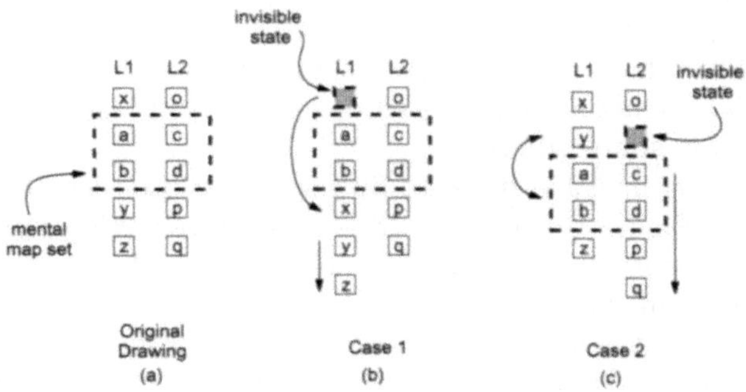

Fig. 9. Edge crossing reduction for mental map preservation: cases 1 and 2.

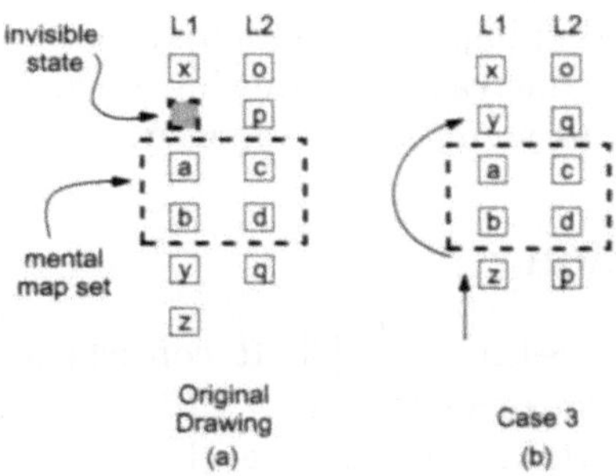

Fig. 10. Edge crossing reduction for mental map preservation: case 3.

The second feature that is affected by the preservation of the mental map, is the placement of states on the same layers. Specifically, our *edge crossing reduction* algorithm (see [6] for details) is modified as follows: the selected group of states on a specific layer is treated as a single state; the edge crossing reduction algorithm shifts the complete group as needed, and inserts invisible nodes when necessary.

We consider three cases that we illustrate through Figures 9 and 10.

1. *Case 1.* If the edge crossing reduction algorithm determines that state x is best placed below b (Figure 9(b)):
   (a) Insert an *invisible state* in x's position.
   (b) Shift down all states below state b, e.g., states y and z.
   (c) Place x below b.
2. *Case 2.* If the edge crossing reduction algorithm determines that state y is best placed above a (see Figure 9(c)):
   (a) In layer $L1$ shift down the position of the selected states, e.g., a and b.
   (b) Place y above a.

   (c) For all the states in other layers that include part of the selection (e.g., layer $L2$):
      i. Shift down the position of the states in such a way that the original structure of the selection is preserved (e.g., states c, d, p, and q are shifted down).
      ii. Insert invisible states to fill the empty positions (e.g., above c).
3. *Case 3.* In Figure 10(a), if the edge crossing reduction algorithm determines that state y is best placed above a and the position above a is occupied by an *invisible!state*:
   (a) Move y to the position occupied by the invisible state.
   (b) Shift up the position of every state below the original position of y (e.g., z).
   (c) Delete the *invisible!state* (see Figure 10(b)).

The preservation of the mental map has disadvantages: some edge crossings may not be removed; improper edges may be inserted; and the insertion of invisible states may increase the drawing area. Hence, the mental map feature is offered only as an option to the user.

4 Implementation

ViSta was originally presented in [8]. It consists of four components: the *template wizard*, the *statechart!graphical editor*, the *statechart!visualization tool*, and the *central database* (see Figure 11).

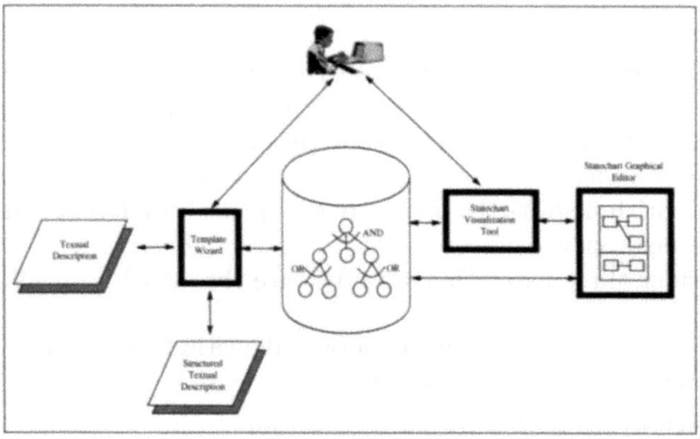

Fig. 11. System overview.

The tool's graphical user interface is shown in Figure 12. It offers four frames. The *text* frame (shown in the top-left part of Figure 12) is used to input a textual description of requirements. The *template!wizard* frame (shown in the top-right part of Figure 12) is used to extract and store information into a set of templates. The *structured text* frame (shown in the bottom-right part of Figure 12) displays the structured textual description that is derived from the information stored in the database. Finally, the *graphical editor* (shown in the bottom-left part of Figure 12) displays the statechart drawings.

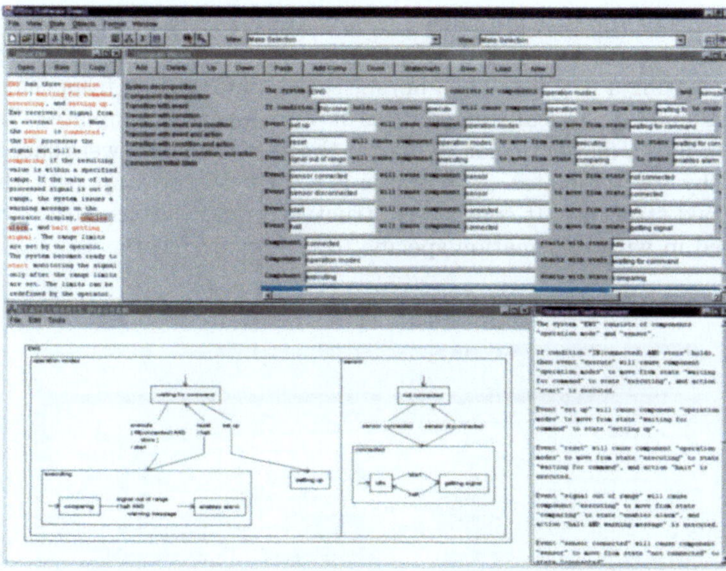

Fig. 12. Tool's GUI.

The user has the choice of entering the information either through the template wizard or directly through the graphical editor.

The data stored in the central database is summarized in a *decomposition tree*. As discussed in Section 2, this structure reflects the decomposition of super-states into sub-states. A node in the decomposition tree includes the following information: its name; its width and height; the coordinates of its origin point; a pointer to its parent; the list of its children; its decomposition type (e.g., *AND*, *OR* or *leaf*); the list of incoming arcs; the list of outgoing arcs; a list of attributes; and finally its aliases. The root of a decomposition tree corresponds to the system super-state; leaves correspond to atomic states. Each non-leaf node in the tree can be decomposed through the *AND* or *OR* decomposition.

The information is entered in the central database either through the template wizard or the statechart graphical editor. ViSta uses this information to automatically update the graphical, textual and template representations.

Template Wizard and Graphical Editor. The template wizard guides the user through the steps necessary for the construction of statechart drawings. It is used when a textual description of requirements exists, and the user wants ViSta to generate the drawings. The template wizard forces the user to provide specific behavioral information based on the original requirements document; it stores this information in the central database, and generates a fixed-format structured document. The wizard's elaborate user interface allows the user to view the textual file, input data into templates, and view the output structured requirements document at the same time.

The user inputs a textual description by either opening an existing document or creating a new file. Then he/she selects information from the textual document and dynamically introduces it into a set of templates. Selected parts turn into a distinct color to inform the user that they were successfully accepted by the templates. A template is a form-based component that has a predefined structure. It consists of structured propositions with text fields to be filled in with information specific to the requirements.

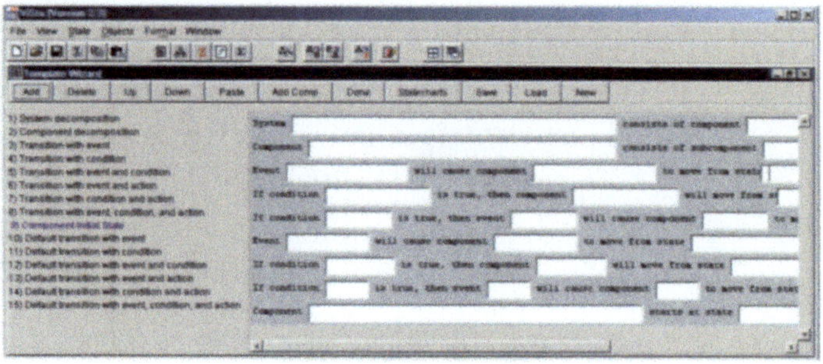

Fig. 13. Template Representation.

As shown in Figure 13, the template wizard offers various types of templates. These include **System Decomposition**, **Component decomposition**, **Transition with event**, **Transition with event and condition**, **Transition with event and action**, **Transition with condition and action**, **Transition with event, condition and action**, **Component initial state**.

The template descriptors can be easily expanded or modified as needed. They are not hard-coded, but are stored in an external configuration file. The user adds necessary templates by clicking on the template type on the left of the template view. This action highlights the chosen type and, after the user clicks the **Add** button on the template view tool-bar, the corresponding template form appears on the right hand side of the template view. It is possible to view all the templates shown on the right hand side by using the scrollbar in case they are larger then the available screen space. In addition, the user can delete or rearrange template forms in the template view by highlighting the necessary template and clicking on the **Delete**, **Up**, or **Down** buttons on the tool-bar. Such features as *saving* a template view, *clearing data* from it, *loading* existing template, or *generating the statechart representation* of the templates are also provided.

As the user selects information in the textual description and fills it in the corresponding input fields of the templates, a structured requirement document is generated. The structured output is constructed by tracing the user's input actions in the template view. Hence, as the user adds on to the templates, the structured document is dynamically updated with changes. The data collected from the templates is also stored in a central database, which is used to generate and update the graphical and structured textual representations.

The user may decide to directly draw statecharts using the graphical editor. In the graphical editor, statechart elements are described using *item-forms* (e.g., state-form, transition-form). When the user selects a graphical icon (e.g., state, transition, or default state) and clicks in the drawing area, an item-form pops up. Figure 14 and 15 show a state-form and a transition-form. The user fills in the empty fields.

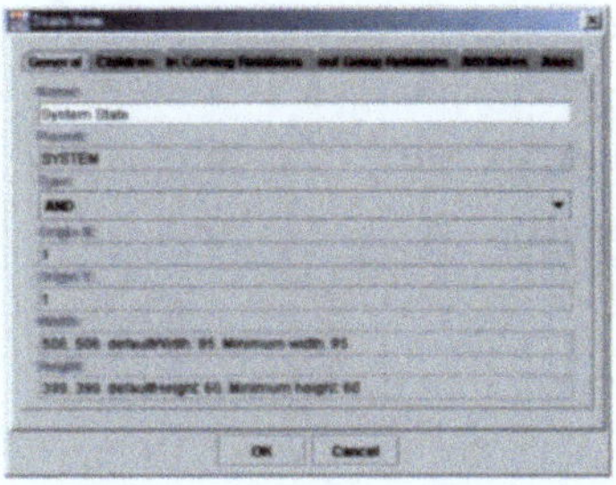

Fig. 14. A Sample StateForm.

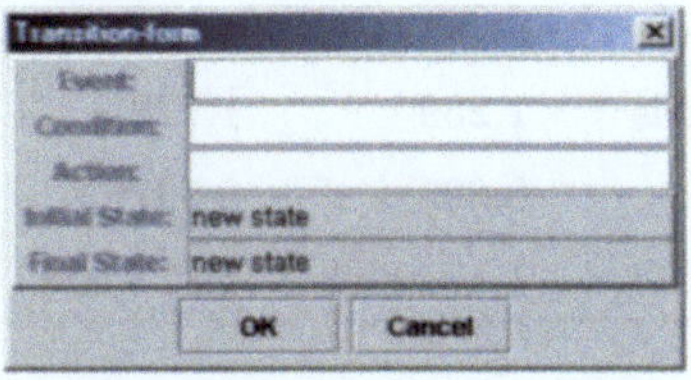

Fig. 15. Transition-Form.

The information captured in the item-forms is immediately stored in the central database, and is used by *ViSta* to generate (or update) the graphical, template and structured descriptions.

5 Examples

In Figures 16–19 we present two statechart examples that were used with Rational Rose 1999 and ViSta.

Our results are summarized in Table 1. Also, Table 2 shows the statistics of three more statecharts produced by ViSta[2]. These drawings cannot be produced automatically by Rational Rose 1999. We notice that, after running ViSta, the drawings have: (1) fewer edge-crossings; (2) a lower number of edge bends; (3) a smaller area; and (4) a good aspect ratio.

Table 1. Comparison of statecharts drawn by our algorithms.

Aesthetic	Example 1		Example 2	
Criteria	Rational	ViSta	Rational	ViSta
Edge Crossings	2	0	6	0
Edge Bends	2	5	7	3
Edge Label Overlap	10	0	10	0
State-Edge Overlap	4	0	0	0

Table 2. Comparison of statecharts drawn by our algorithms.

Aesthetic Criteria	Example 3	Example 4	Example 5
Edge Crossings	0	0	0
Edge Bends	19	18	18
Width in pixels	875	1,029	861
Height in pixels	1,259	1,722	1,593
W/H Ratio	0.695	0.5975	0.54
Area in pixels	1,102,884	1,771,938	1,371,573

[2] Drawings can be found at
`http://profesores.chi.itesm.mx/~rcastell/vista_examples.html`.

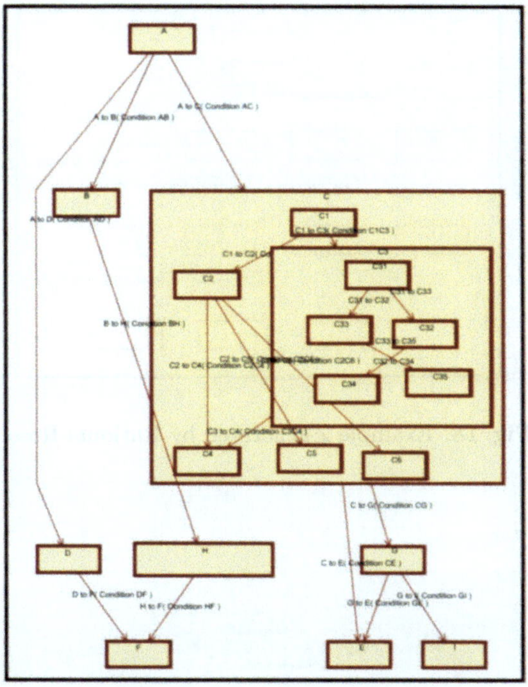

Fig. 16. Example 1 generated by Rational Rose.

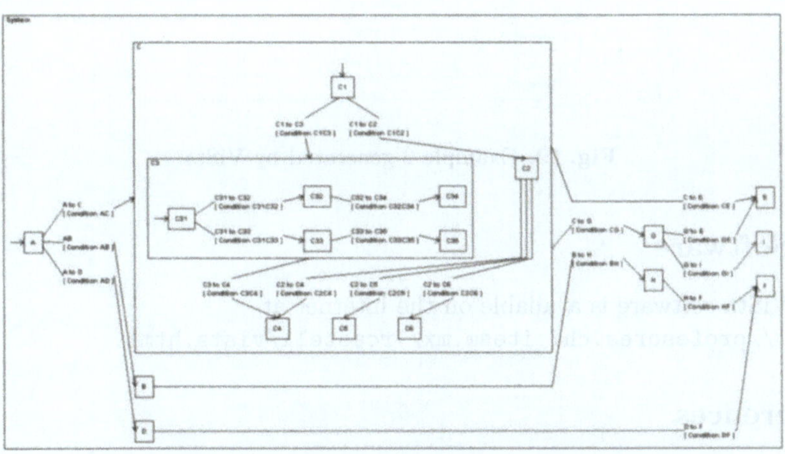

Fig. 17. Example 1 generated by ViSta.

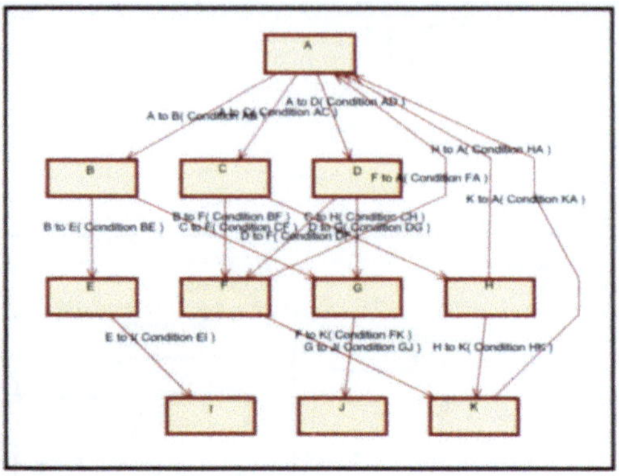

Fig. 18. Example 2 generated by Rational Rose.

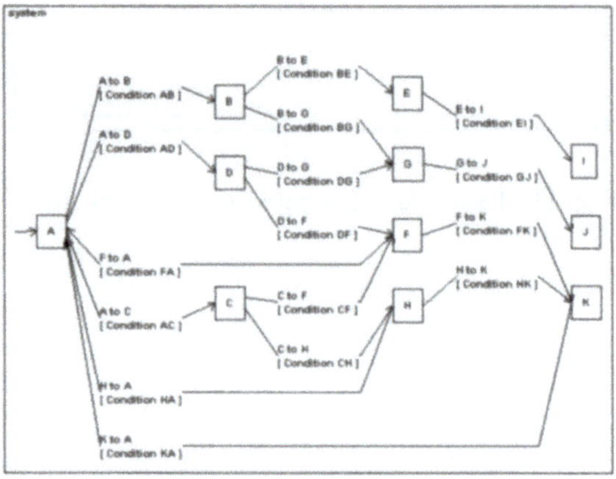

Fig. 19. Example 2 generated by ViSta.

6 Software

The ViSta software is available on the internet at
`http://profesores.chi.itesm.mx/~rcastell/vista.html`.

References

1. Artisan Software Tools. (accessed in April 1999) Real-time studio: The rational alternative. Available from Artisan Software Tools over the Internet. `http://www.artisansw.com/rtdialogue/pdfs/rational.pdf`

2. Di Battista, G., Eades, P., Tamassia, R., Tollis, I. G. (1994) Algorithms for drawing graphs: an annotated bibliography. Computational Geometry Theory and Application, (4), 235–282
3. Di Battista, G., Eades, P., Tamassia, R., Tollis, I. G. (1999) Graph Drawing: Algorithms for the Visualization of Graphs. Prentice Hall
4. Biedl, T., Kaufman, M. (1997) Area-efficient static and incremental graph drawings. In: Proceedings of the 5th. Annual European Symposium on Algorithms **1284**, Springer-Verlag, 37–52
5. Biedl, T. C., Madden, B. P., Tollis, I. G. (1997) The three-phase method: A unified approach to orthogonal graph drawing. In: G. Di Battista (ed.) Graph Drawing '97, Lecture Notes in Computer Science 1353, Springer-Verlag, 391–402
6. Castelló, R. (2000) From Informal Specification to Formalization: An Automated Visualization Approach. PhD thesis, The University of Texas at Dallas.
7. Castelló, R., Mili, R., Tollis, I. G. (2002) A framework for the static and interactive visualization of statecharts. Journal of Graph Algorithms and Applications **6** (3)
8. Castelló, R., Mili, R., Tollis, I. G. (2002) Vista: a tool suite for the visualization of behavioral requirements. The Journal of Systems and Software **62**, 141–159
9. Eades, P., Lin, T., Lin, X. (1993) Two three drawing conventions. International Journal of Computational Geometry and Applications **3** (2), 133–153
10. Eades, P., Feng, Q.-W. (1997) Drawing clustered graphs on an orthogonal grid. In: G. Di Battista (ed.) Graph Drawing '97, Lecture Notes in Computer Science 1353, Springer-Verlag, 146–157
11. Eades, P., Feng, Q.-W., Lin, X. (1997) Straight-line drawing algorithms for hierarchical graphs and clustered graphs. In: S. North (ed.) Graph Drawing '96, Lecture Notes in Computer Science 1190, Springer-Verlag, 113–128
12. Gansner, E. R., North, S. C., Vo, K. P. (1988) Dag—a program that draws directed graphs. Software Practice and Experience **18** (11), 1047–1062
13. Gansner, E. R., Koutsofios, E., North, S. C., Vo, K.-P. (1993) A technique for drawing directed graphs. IEEE Transactions on Software Engineering **19** (32), 214–230
14. Harel, D. (1987) Statecharts: A visual formalism for complex systems. Science of Computer Programming **8** (3), 231–274
15. Harel, D., Lachover, H., Naamad, A., Pnueli, A., Politi, M., Sherman, R., Shtull-Trauring, A., Trakhtenbrot, M. (1990) Statemate: A working environment for the development of complex reactive systems. IEEE Transactions on Software Engineering **16** (4), 403–414
16. Harel, D., Yashchin, G. (1990) An algorithm for blob hierarchy layout. In: Proceedings of International Conference on Advanced Visual Interfaces, AVI'2000, Palermo, Italy
17. Kakoulis, K. G., Tollis, I. G. (1997) An algorithm for labeling edges of hierarchical drawings. In: G. Di Battista (ed.) Graph Drawing '97, Lecture Notes in Computer Science 1353, Springer-Verlag, 169–180
18. Kakoulis, K. G., Tollis, I. G. (1997) On the edge label placement problem. In: S. North (ed.) Graph Drawing '96, Lecture Notes in Computer Science 1190, Springer-Verlag, 241–256
19. Kuh, E. S., Ohtsuki, T. (1990) Recent advances in VLSI layout. Proceedings of the IEEE **78** (2), 237–263

20. Lengauer, T. (1990) Combinatorial Algorithms for Integrated Circuit Layout. John Wiley & Sons
21. Messinger, E.B., Rowe, L. A., Henry, R. R. (1991) A divide-and-conquer algorithm for the automatic layout of large graphs. IEEE Transactions on Systems, Man, and Cybernetics **21** (1), 1–11
22. Misue, K., Eades, P., Lai, W., Sugiyama, K. (1995) Layout adjustment and the mental map. Journal of Visual Languages and Computing **6** (2), 183–210
23. North, S. C. (1996) Incremental layout in dynadag. In: F. J. Brandenburg (ed.) Graph Drawing '95, Lecture Notes in Computer Science 1027, Springer-Verlag, 409–418
24. O'Donnel, R., Waldt, B., Bergstrand, J. (accessed in April 1999) Automatic code for embedded systems based on formal methods. Available from Telelogic over the Internet. `http://www.Telelogic.se/solution/techpap.asp`
25. Papakostas, A., Tollis, I. G. (1998) Interactive orthogonal graph drawing. IEEE Transactions on Computers **47** (11), 1297–1309
26. Peterson, J. (accessed in July 2001) Overcoming the crisis in real-time software development. Available from Rational over the Internet. `http://www.objectime.com/otl/technical/crisis.html`
27. Purchase, H. (1997) Which aesthetic has the greatest effect on human understanding. In: G. Di Battista (ed.) Graph Drawing '97, Lecture Notes in Computer Science 1353, Springer-Verlag, 248–261
28. Rational. (accessed in November 1999) Rose java. Downloaded from Rational over the Internet. `http://www.rational.com`
29. Rowe, L. A., Davis, M., Messinger, E., Meyer, C. (1987) A browser for directed graphs. Software Practice and Experience **17** (1), 61–76
30. Ryall, K., Marks, J., Shieber, S. (1997) An interactive system for drawing graphs. In: S. North (ed.) Graph Drawing '96, Lecture Notes in Computer Science 1190, Springer-Verlag, 387–393
31. Seeman, J. (1997) Extending the sugiyama algorithm for drawing UML class diagrams: Towards automatic layout of object-oriented software diagrams. In: G. Di Battista (ed.) Graph Drawing '97, Lecture Notes in Computer Science 1353, Springer-Verlag, 415–424
32. Stockmeyer, L. (1983) Optimal orientations of cells in slicing floorplan designs. Information and Control, (57), 91–101
33. Sugiyama, K., Tagawa, S., Toda, M. (1981) Methods for visual understanding of hierarchical system structures. IEEE Transactions on Systems, Man and Cybernetics **11** (2), 109–125
34. Wimer, S., Koren, I., Cederbaum, I. (1988) Floorplans, planar graphs and layout. IEEE Transactions on Circuits and Systems, 267–278

visone

Analysis and Visualization of Social Networks*

Ulrik Brandes[1] and Dorothea Wagner[2]

[1] University of Passau, Department of Mathematics & Computer Science, 94030 Passau, Germany. brandes@algo.fmi.uni-passau.de
[2] University of Konstanz, Department of Computer & Information Science, 78457 Konstanz, Germany. Dorothea.Wagner@uni-konstanz.de

1 Introduction

We describe visone, a tool that facilitates the visual exploration of social networks. Social network analysis is a methodological approach in the social sciences using graph-theoretic concepts to describe, understand and explain social structure. The visone software is an attempt to integrate analysis and visualization of social networks and is intended to be used in research and teaching. While we are primarily focusing on users in the social sciences, several features provided in the tool will be useful in other fields as well.

In contrast to more conventional mathematical software in the social sciences that aim at providing a comprehensive suite of analytical options, our emphasis is on complementing every option we provide with tailored means of graphical interaction. We attempt to make complicated types of analysis and data handling transparent, intuitive, and more readily accessible. User feedback indicates that many who usually regard data exploration and analysis complicated and unnerving enjoy the playful nature of visual interaction.

Consequently, much of the tool is about graph drawing methods specifically adapted to facilitate visual data exploration. The origins of visone lie in an interdisciplinary cooperation with researchers from political science which resulted in innovative uses of graph drawing methods for social network visualization, and prototypical implementations thereof. With the growing demand for access to these methods, we started implementing an integrated tool for public use. It should be stressed, however, that visone remains a research platform and test-bed for innovative methods, and is not intended to become

* Many people have contributed directly or indirectly to the current state of our tool. We thank Sabine Cornelsen, Patrick Kenis, Jörg Raab, and Volker Schneider for many years of fruitful cooperation, and the participants of POLNET summer schools for their feedback and suggestions. We are indebted to Michael Baur, Marc Benkert, Marco Gaertler, Boris Köpf, and Jürgen Lerner for their implementation efforts, and gratefully acknowledge financial support from the Deutsche Forschungsgemeinschaft (DFG) under grant BR 2158/1-1 and the European Commission within FET Open Project COSIN (IST-2001-33555).

a standard tool with all due consequences such as extensive user-support and product marketing. Essentially all components are in development and therefore subject to change. In a nutshell, visone is a

- tool for interactive analysis and visualization of networks, in which
- originality is preferred over comprehensiveness, and that
- caters especially to social scientists.

The organization of the subsequent sections follows the common structure of all chapters in this book. In particular, we start with background information on the main area of application for visone, and give application examples in Section 5. While other interesting algorithms have been implemented, Section 3 focuses on those for graph drawing.

2 Applications

The main application area of visone is a methodological approach in the social sciences: *Social Network Analysis* uses graph-theoretic concepts to describe, understand and explain, sometimes even predict or design, social structure. The objects of interest are emergent patterns of relationships and their interplay with entity attributes.

To motivate the decisions made in the design of visone, we describe the data model on which we operate, types of analysis provided, and visualization principles governing our choice of graph drawing algorithms.

2.1 Model

A social network consists of *nodes* (often referred to as *actors*), i.e., entities such as persons, organizations, or simply objects that are *linked* by binary relations such as social relations, dependencies, or exchange. Both nodes and links may have additional *attributes*.

Relations constituting a social network may be directed, undirected, or mixed. Attributes can be of any type, and numerical link attributes may strengthen or weaken the tie between two nodes. Since data is often gathered by means of questionnaires, even the existence of a link is subject to interpretation because two respondents may have different perceptions regarding the presence of a specific type of tie between them, i.e., the link may be confirmed or unconfirmed. Rather typical examples of the kind of structures studied are given in Section 5.

To simplify usage, implementation, and documentation, visone operates on a single, unified network model (in essence, a labeled digraph) that is general enough to capture the essential features of a broad range of conceivable cases. Since the tool is interactive, objects may be selected to alter the subgraph to which an operation is applied. The rules on how particular network features are mapped to the uniform model are described in Section 6.

Definition 1 (visone network model). A *social network* is a labeled directed graph $G = (V, E = E_C \cup E_U; \delta, \omega)$,[1] where E_C and E_U are disjoint sets of *confirmed* and *unconfirmed* edges, $\delta : E \to \mathbb{R}_{\geq 0}$ is a non-negative edge *length*, and $\omega : E \to \mathbb{R}_{\geq 0}$ a non-negative edge *strength*.

A vertex or edge *attribute* is a (partial) function assigning values to vertices or edges. The values assigned by a *nominal* attribute are strings, while those of a *numerical* attribute are non-negative real numbers.

A crucial feature in many studies is the interrelation between structural properties of a social network and its attributes. We hence provide convenient mechanisms to handle an arbitrary number of vertex and edge attributes. These can be mapped to the visual appearance of the graph, or used to define length and strength labels and thus influence the outcome of an analysis.

Although there is no restriction on the class of graphs that constitute a social network, instances from social science projects tend to be sparse but locally dense, and to exhibit small average distances between vertices. Moreover, these graphs are frequently small to medium in size. We thus assume that, roughly, $|V| + |E| \leq 1000$ and consider algorithms running in time $O(|V| \cdot |E|)$ (for reasonable constants) to be acceptable. For significantly larger graphs, we recommend to try `Pajek`, a tool for the analysis of large networks also described in this book.

2.2 Analysis

The purpose of social network analysis is to identify important actors, crucial links, subgroups, roles, network characteristics, and so on, to answer substantive questions about structures.

There are three main levels of interest: the element, group, and network level. On the element level, one is interested in properties (both absolute and relative) of single actors, links, or incidences. Examples for this type of analyses are bottleneck identification and structural ranking of network items. On the group level, one is interested in classifying the elements of a network and properties of subnetworks. Examples are actor equivalence classes and cluster identification. Finally, on the network level, one is interested in properties of the overall network such as connectivity or balance.

Currently, the types of analyses provided in visone are almost exclusively on the element level (with corresponding network level statistics). More specifically, we have focussed on indices measuring structural importance of vertices. While there is no universally accepted definition of what makes a vertex important, a small collection of indices forms the basis of most studies. Several of these originally do not apply to our rather general network model (e.g., some only apply to connected undirected graphs), but we were able

[1] Recall that the definition in Section 2 of the Technical Foundations allows for multiple edges and self-loops.

to generalize and unify them. The complete list of currently implemented indices is given in Figure 1.

index	definition	reference
	local measures	
degree	$c_v = \sum_{e \in \text{instar}(v) \cup \text{outstar}(v)} \omega(e)$	–
in-degree	$c_v = \sum_{e \in \text{instar}(v)} \omega(e)$	–
out-degree	$c_v = \sum_{e \in \text{outstar}(v)} \omega(e)$	–
	distance measures	
betweenness	$c_v = \sum_{s \neq v \neq t \in V} \frac{\sigma_G(s,t\|v)}{\sigma_G(s,t)}$ where $\sigma_G(s,t)$ and $\sigma_G(s,t\|v)$ are the number of all shortest st-paths and those passing through v	[2,19,9]
closeness	$c_v = \frac{1}{\sum_{t \in V} \delta(v,t)}$	[7,32]
eccentricity	$c_v = \frac{1}{\max_{t \in V} \delta(v,t)}$	[21]
radiality	$c_v = \frac{\sum_{t \in V} (\text{diam}(G) + 1 - \delta(v,t))}{(n-1) \cdot \text{diam}(G)}$	[35]
	feedback measures	
status	$c_v = \alpha \cdot \sum_{(u,v) \in \text{instar}(v)} (1 + c_u)$ where $\alpha = \min\{\max_{v \in V} \text{indeg}(v), \max_{v \in V} \text{outdeg}(v)\}^{-1}$	[24]
eigenvector	$c_v = \mu^{-1} \sum_{(u,v) \in \text{instar}(v)} \omega(u,v) \cdot c_u$ where μ is the largest eigenvalue of $A(G)$	[8]
page-rank	$c_v = \gamma \cdot \frac{1}{n} + (1-\gamma) \sum_{(u,v) \in \text{instar}(v)} c_u$ where $0 < \gamma < 1$ is a free parameter	[15]
authority	$c_v = \mu^{-1} \cdot \sum_{(u,v) \in \text{instar}(v)} \omega(u,v) \cdot \sum_{(u,w) \in \text{outstar}(u)} \omega(u,w) c_w$ where μ is the largest eigenvalue of $A(G)^T A(G)$	[26]
hub	$c_v = \mu^{-1} \cdot \sum_{(v,w) \in \text{outstar}(v)} \omega(v,w) \cdot \sum_{(u,w) \in \text{instar}(w)} \omega(u,w) c_u$ where μ is the largest eigenvalue of $A(G) A(G)^T$	[26]

Fig. 1. Available vertex centralities. Note that most indices have been generalized with respect to the original references, and all are rescaled to percentages.

One particular consequence of our unification is that all vertex indices are non-negative and have unit sums, i.e., they can be viewed as probability distributions on the vertex set and interpreted as the share of importance a node assumes in its network.

Since the theory for edge indices is even less developed, we are currently investigating extensions to edges along the same lines. Moreover, support for graphic comparison of different vertex or edge indices and for some types of group level analysis is intended to be added in the future, but will require entirely different forms of visualization (cf. next subsection). A comprehensive, though non-visual, tool for social network analysis is UCINET [1].

Note that it is a long-standing debate whether unconfirmed edges should be considered for analysis. Typically, researchers decide to either treat all unconfirmed edges as if confirmed, or to exclude them completely. We leave this decision with the researcher, but add the freedom to make it on a per-edge basis (cf. Section 6). This way, the user has full control over the assumptions made, and the ability to experiment with different hypotheses and compare their consequences.

2.3 Visualization

Visualized information must neither be misleading nor hard to read. Hence there are two obvious criteria for the quality of social network visualizations:

1. Is the information manifest in the network represented accurately?
2. Is this information conveyed efficiently?

With these criteria in mind, the following three aspects should be carefully thought through when creating network visualizations [11]:

- the *substantive aspect* the viewer is interested in,
- the *design* (i.e., the mapping of data to graphical variables), and
- the *algorithm* employed to realize the design (artifacts, efficiency, etc.).

In addition to algorithms that try to produce what is often termed an "æsthetic" drawing of a graph (and thus are oblivious to the first aspect) we developed the following two types of visualization specifically for the vertex index analyses currently available in visone.

Depending on the context, actors of high structural importance are interpreted as a being *central* or as having *high status.* With this substantive aspect in mind, we designed visualizations that represent vertex indices by constraining vertex positions to fixed distances from the center or from the bottom of the drawing, in either case depending linearly on the vertex index. See Figure 2 for illustration and note that relative scores are difficult to determine from the straightforward representation based on vertex size.

The information can thus be represented accurately, and it is up to the (constrained) graph layout algorithm to optimize readability. To avoid user

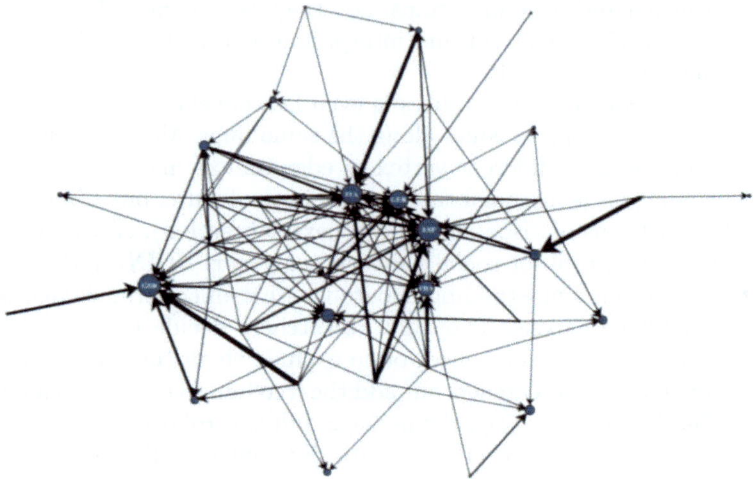

(a) vertex index represented by vertex size

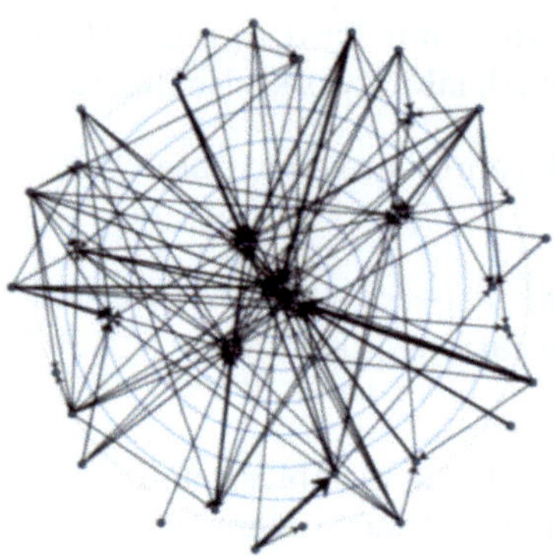

(b) interpreted as centrality

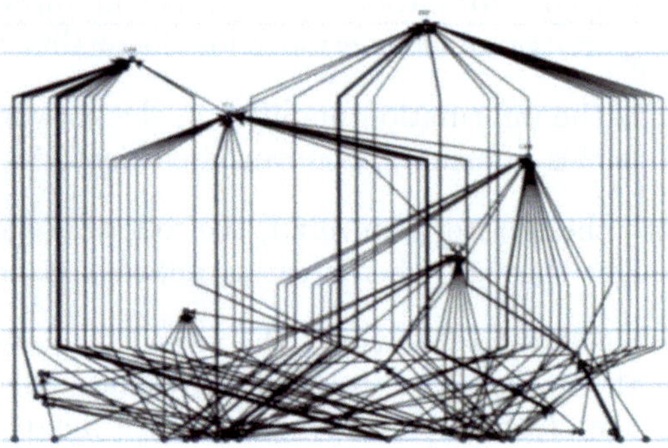

(c) interpreted as status

Fig. 2. Different means of visualizing a vertex index: most prestigious football leagues based on which ones the participants of the 1998 World Cup Final played in (network data courtesy of Lothar Krempel). Thickness of edges indicates number of players in foreign league. Like graph paper, background lines support determination and comparison of scores.

dissatisfaction with suboptimal drawings, we strive to find at least locally optimal layouts that are not obvious for users to improve. The algorithms used for status and centrality drawings are described in Sections 3.3 and 3.4.

3 Algorithms

From the computer science point of view, one of the main aspects of the visone project and software is that of a stimulus and test-bed for algorithmic research. Indeed, new and more efficient algorithms have been developed for many components of the tool.

For example, more efficient generators have been implemented to create graphs according to popular stochastic models such as random graphs [20], small worlds [36], and evolving graphs with preferential attachment [3]. Time and space complexity of these generators is linear in the size of the graph generated [4].

For vertex indices, not only unified definitions and normalizations, but also unified algorithms are introduced in visone. While all feedback measures are computed using variants of sparse-matrix power iteration, all distance measures are determined by solving an augmented single-source shortest path problem from each vertex. For betweenness centrality, in particular, this yields a substantial improvement over previous algorithms [9].

Though we are facing many more interesting algorithmic challenges during the course of this project, we focus here on some that arise in the context of visualization, the main topic of this book. In the subsections below we describe our approaches for the more involved types of layouts provided.

3.1 Uniform layouts

When exploring a network, spring embedder layouts are useful to catch a first glimpse of the overall structure of the graph. However, the algorithms' performance and layout quality tend to worsen significantly with increasing size of the graph.

A related, yet more reliable approach to draw very large graphs is introduced in [23], but limited to undirected graphs without tree-like substructures. We first describe the original approach and then sketch extensions we are currently implementing to take edge directions into account and alleviate the problems caused by low connectivity.

A high-dimensional embedding approach. Let $G = (V, E)$ be a simple and connected undirected graph with vertices $V = \{v_1, \ldots, v_n\}$. Similar to the spring embedder variant of Kamada and Kawai, the basic goal is to place every pair of vertices at a distance proportional to its graph-theoretic distance. Rather than placing vertices directly in two dimensions, first an n-dimensional layout is determined in which each dimension is contingent on a different vertex. In the dimension of a vertex $v \in V$, the coordinate of each vertex is its centered distance from v in the graph, $p_v^{(i)} = d_G(v, v_i) - \frac{1}{n}\sum_{w \in V} d_G(w, v_i)$. This high-dimensional drawing is projected down into two dimensions using principal component analysis. That is, a projection with maximum variance is determined from two eigenvectors associated with the largest eigenvalues of the covariance matrix $\Sigma = (\sigma_{ij})_{1 \leq i,j \leq n}$, where

$$\sigma_{ij} = {p^{(i)}}^T \cdot p^{(j)} .$$

With eigenvectors $e^{(1)}, e^{(2)}$, which can be computed using power iteration, the location $p_v = (x_v, y_v)$ of $v \in V$ is obtained from

$$x_v = \sum_{i=1}^{n} e_i^{(1)} \cdot p_v^{(i)} \quad \text{and} \quad y_v = \sum_{i=1}^{n} e_i^{(2)} \cdot p_v^{(i)} .$$

Note that, because of the size of the covariance matrix, the overall algorithm has running time $\Omega(d^2 n)$, where d is the number of dimensions of the high-dimensional embedding. Thus, if the number n of vertices is large, only a sample is used to determine the initial embedding. A simple heuristic for the k-center problem serves well to select that sample [23].

Modifications. The above approach cannot take into account the direction of edges. Likewise, it is not suitable for large graphs of low connectivity. Consider the block-cut-point tree of a non-biconnected graph. If a subtree contains none of the sample vertices, all vertices in the subtree will be placed at the same relative positions in every dimension, and thus in the projection.

We are therefore modifying the high-dimensional embedding approach in several ways: mainly, we reserve some of the dimensions of the initial embedding to display edge directions, and introduce dependencies between others to avoid strong correlations between substructure layouts. We also consider edge lengths in the computation of distances. Finally, we add dimensions in which only the subgraph induced by confirmed edges is considered to make it visually more dominant.

3.2 Spectral layouts

Let $G = (V, E; \omega)$ be an undirected graph with positive edge weights, e.g., obtained from the underlying undirected graph of a social network and its strength label ω. Consider the following weighted version of the minimization objective of Tutte's barycentric layout model (cf. Section 4.5 of the Technical Foundations)

$$\sum_{\{v,w\} \in E} \omega(e) \cdot \|p_v - p_w\|^2 = \sum_{\{v,w\} \in E} \omega(e) \cdot \left((x_v - x_w)^2 + (y_v - y_w)^2 \right) \qquad (1)$$

where $p_v = (x_v, y_y) \in \mathbb{R}^2$ is the location of vertex $v \in V$. Recall that optimum solutions place all vertices in the same location. In *spectral!graph layout*, first introduced by Hall [22], these undesirable solutions are avoided not by fixing the location of select vertices, but by putting more uniform constraints on the location vector $p = (p_v)_v \in V$ as follows.

In matrix notation, Tutte's objective (1) can be expressed as $p^T L(G)p$, where

$$L(G) = D(G) - A(G)$$

is called the *Laplacian matrix* of G, with $D(G)$ the diagonal matrix of vertex degrees and $A(G)$ the weighted adjacency matrix. To eliminate the dependency on the scale of p we divide this quadratic form by $p^T p = \|p\|^2$. Now observe that, if p is an eigenvector of $L(G)$, the associated eigenvalue is $\frac{p^T L(G)p}{p^T p}$, and that the trivial optima of (1) are multiples of $p = \mathbf{1}$, i.e., the vector with all components equal to one, and associated with eigenvalue 0.

The eigenvalues of the Laplacian are non-negative real numbers, and their eigenvectors are pairwise orthogonal. Two eigenvectors associated with the smallest non-zero eigenvalues of $L(G)$ therefore minimize

$$\sum_{\{v,w\}\in E} \omega(e) \cdot (x_v - x_w)^2 = \frac{x^T L(G)x}{x^T x} \qquad \text{subject to } \mathbf{0} \neq x \perp \mathbf{1}$$

and

$$\sum_{\{v,w\}\in E} \omega(e) \cdot (y_v - y_w)^2 = \frac{y^T L(G)y}{y^T y} \qquad \text{subject to } \mathbf{0} \neq y \perp \mathbf{1} \text{ and } y \perp x \ .$$

As a consequence of orthogonalization with $\mathbf{1}$, the resulting layouts are centered around the origin.

Symmetries are displayed well in spectral layouts, and structurally equivalent vertices (i.e., vertices with identical neighborhoods) are placed in the same location. If a graph is not balanced, however, most vertices are clustered in the center of the drawing, and only some loosely connected vertices are placed far away. To counter this effect, a slightly modified Laplacian $L_\rho(G) = (1 - \rho)D(G) - A(G)$ in which the diagonal is weakened by a constant factor ρ, $0 \leq \rho \leq 1$, is used. This can be viewed as pushing vertices out of the center by applying a radial force that depends on the degree of a vertex and is illustrated in Figure 3.

Since the graphs we deal with are of medium size, no sophisticated algorithm is needed. The eigenvalues are simply reversed using an upper bound Λ on the largest one, so that power iteration with re-orthogonalization yields the two desired eigenvectors. The current positions on the screen are used for initialization, and the *residual*, i.e., the squared distance of a vector from being an eigenvector, serves as convergence criterion. The entire layout algorithm is given in Algorithm 1. Note that $\rho = 0$ yields the standard spectral layout, whereas $\rho = 1$ yields two eigenvectors of the adjacency matrix.

With an additional fixed upper bound on the number of iterations, Algorithm 1 runs in time $O(|V| + |E|)$. Since the current positions on the screen

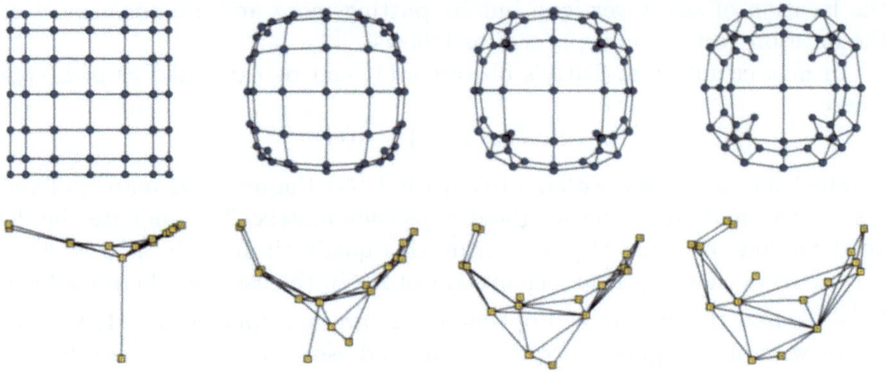

L_0 $L_{0.25}$ $L_{0.5}$ $L_{0.75}$

Fig. 3. Spectral layouts with modified Laplacian L_ρ. The graph in the lower row is from Figure 24 of the Technical Foundations.

Algorithm 1: Spectral layout with a modified Laplacian matrix

---

Input : Undirected graph $G = (V, E; \omega)$ with edge strengths, $n = |V|$
Initial layout $p_v = (x_v, y_v)$, $v \in V$
Parameter $0 \leq \rho \leq 1$

Output: Layout $p_v = (x_v, y_v)$, $v \in V$

$r \leftarrow 2$

while $r > 1$ **do**

$x' \leftarrow (\Lambda \cdot I - L_\rho(G)) \cdot x; \quad y' \leftarrow (\Lambda \cdot I - L_\rho(G)) \cdot y$

$x' \leftarrow x' - (\sum_{v \in V} \frac{x'_v}{n}) \cdot \mathbf{1}; \quad y' \leftarrow y' - (\sum_{v \in V} \frac{y'_v}{n}) \cdot \mathbf{1}$

$y' \leftarrow y' - \frac{y'^T x'}{x'^T x'}$

$r \leftarrow \max\{\|x' - \frac{x^T x'}{x^T x} x\|^2, \|y' - \frac{y^T y'}{y^T y} y\|^2\}$

$x \leftarrow \frac{n}{\max_{v \in V} x'_v} x'; \quad y \leftarrow \frac{n}{\max_{v \in V} y'_v} y'$

od

---

are used for initialization, more iterations can be performed simply by calling spectral layout again. Note that, using more elaborate multi-scale methods, spectral layouts can be computed efficiently even for very large graphs [27].

3.3 Layered layouts

To visually support status analyses of networks as described in Section 2, an algorithm for layered graph layouts is provided. The algorithm is a particular instance of the Sugiyama framework (cf. Section 4.2 of the Technical Foundations), with some rather unusual modifications induced by our special setting.

In particular, our layered layout algorithm does not modify relative vertical positions of vertices. This is because our visualization criteria demand that the vertex index be represented precisely. The purpose of the layout algorithm is therefore to make the drawing as readable as possible without changing y-coordinates. The algorithm is described along the three main phases of the Sugiyama framework and a refinement of what is outlined in [14]. Note that we treat each connected component separately.

Layer assignment. Fixed y-coordinates immediately induce a layering in which vertices with equal vertical position are placed in the same layer. However, typical status indices then yield layerings with many singleton layers and pairs of layers with tiny vertical distance so that edges running between them are almost indistinguishable.

Instead, we run a one-dimensional clustering algorithm on the set of y-coordinates assumed by vertices, and treat each cluster as a layer.

Crossing minimization. It is particularly difficult for crossing reduction procedures to untangle sparsely connected subgraphs. Since we strive for layouts that appear difficult to improve, we start by removing all dangling trees. Note that a layered tree is trivially ordered to have no crossing.

For crossing reduction we apply the barycenter heuristic, followed by a weighted variant of sifting [29]. While the barycenter heuristic is fast and good at separating biconnected components, a few rounds of subsequent sifting ensure that we end up with a layout that cannot be improved by moving a single vertex.

In our weighted variant, each crossing contributes the product of the two edge weights involved, where edges are weighted according to their thickness on the screen. Recall that a social network has two types of edges, confirmed and unconfirmed. Confirmed edges are considered to be more important, and it should be possible to recognize the subgraph induced by confirmed edges in the drawing of the overall graph. To discourage crossings between confirmed edges, their weight is doubled in the algorithm.

After vertex orderings have been determined for the reduced components, the temporarily removed dangling trees are re-inserted into the ordering.

Finally, we make sure that pairs of long edges do not cross at inner segments, so that they can be drawn with only two bends (at their extreme dummy vertices). Note that crossings can be moved up or down by swapping the order of dummy vertices on one layer. We move crossings downward, because the more important part of the drawing is the top – i.e., where the high status actors are (cf. Figure 2).

Coordinate assignment. Using the linear-time algorithm of [13] we obtain integer horizontal coordinates that are subsequently scaled to fit the entire graph on the screen.

3.4 Radial layouts

We provide an algorithm for radial graph layouts to support centrality visualizations as described in Section 2.3.

A radial layout is described in polar coordinates $p_v = (r_v, \varphi_v)$, $v \in V$, but since we use them to convey a structural vertex centrality index c, the first coordinate of vertices $v \in V$ with $c_v > 0$ is fixed at $r_v = \frac{c_v - \underline{c}}{\overline{c} - \underline{c}}$, where $\overline{c}$ and $\underline{c}$ are the maximum and the minimum non-zero score. If the two highest centrality scores differ only marginally, the range of radii is reduced by a fixed offset to avoid vertex overlap in the center. Vertices with zero centrality are placed on an outer orbit.

Similar to computing x-coordinates in layered layouts, the angular φ-coordinates are determined so as to increase the readability of the diagram. The main layout objectives are uniform distribution of vertices, and few edge crossings. While the three-stage force-directed method of [12] yields the most appealing layouts to date, it is too slow for an interactive tool. A faster, purely combinatorial algorithm is therefore used.

Note that, different from the layered case, the (cyclic) ordering of vertices in (circular) layers does not even determine the number of edge crossings. Instead of the radial layout problem we therefore restrict our attention to *circular layouts*, i.e., to the case $r_v = r_w > 0$ for all $v, w \in V$. Nevertheless, crossing minimization is $\mathcal{NP}$-hard even for circular layouts [28].

Similar to the approach taken for layered layouts in the previous subsection, we split the graph into its connected components and treat them individually. In fact, it is split into its biconnected components, because their layouts can be combined without introducing any additional crossings (see Figure 4).

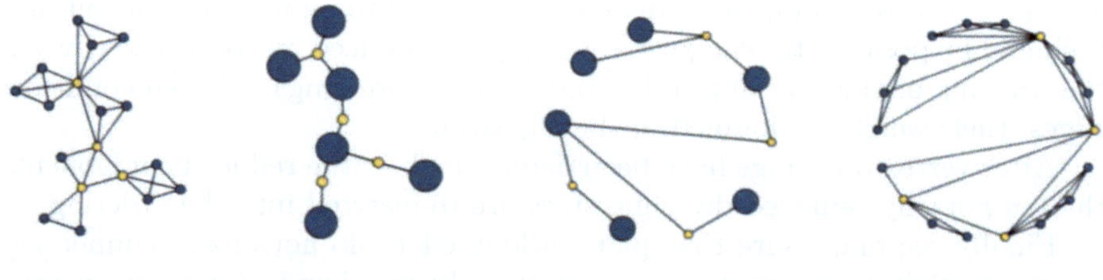

Fig. 4. Utilizing the tree of blocks and cut-vertices to avoid crossings between edges that belong to different blocks.

An efficient algorithm for circular layouts of biconnected graphs is introduced in [34,33] and experimentally shown to produce fewer crossings than previous approaches. A simpler algorithm [6] based on circular sifting yields even fewer crossings. Starting from the cyclic ordering given by current positions on the screen, the idea is to iteratively place a single vertex in its locally optimal position, i.e., where the number of crossings in which its incident edges are involved is minimized. To find this position, the vertex is moved around the circle, and each time the change in the number of crossings is recorded.

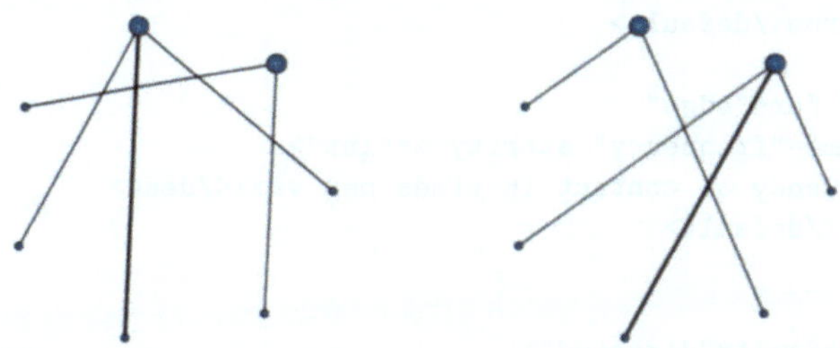

Fig. 5. After swapping two neighboring vertices v and w, an edge of v crosses exactly those edges of w that it didn't cross before.

Assume that all adjacency lists are cyclic and ordered according to the current cyclic ordering of vertices. This can be achieved using bucket sort in time $O(|E|)$. The vertex v to be placed optimally is moved clockwise, one position at a time. When swapping the vertex with a neighbor w, the resulting difference in the number of crossings is determined by merging the two sorted adjacency lists. For each edge incident to v, the change in crossings is the difference between the length of the prefix and suffix of the current position in the adjacency list of w. See Figure 5 for an illustration.

A single swap takes time $O(\deg(v)+\deg(w))$. Locally optimal positioning once for each vertex therefore takes amortized time $O(|V|\cdot|E|)$. Experimental evidence indicates that a few such rounds suffice, and that this algorithm consistently outperforms other heuristics.

4 Implementation

The visone software is implemented in C++ using LEDA, the *Library of Efficient Data Types and Algorithms* [30]. While the user interface is a customized version of LEDA's GraphWin class, all graph generation, analysis, and layout algorithms (except for LEDA's force-directed layout routine) have been implemented from scratch.

Starting with version 1.1, the main data format used in visone will be the XML sublanguage GraphML (Graph Markup Language) [10]. GraphML support is implemented in a LEDA extension package which will be made available for public use. It will hence be possible to administer project files with several social networks and any number of attributes. Figure 6 shows a self-explanatory fragment of a social network represented in GraphML. Data attributes can be mapped freely to graphical attributes like color, shape, and so on.

```
...
<key id="k0" for="edge"
     attr.name="visone:confirmed" attr.type="boolean">
  <default>true</default>
</key>
<key id="k1" for="edge"
     attr.name="frequency" attr.type="int">
  <desc>frequency of contact in times per week</desc>
  <default>1</default>
</key>
...
<graph edgedefault="directed">
  ...
  <edge id="e7" source="v0" target="v1"/>
  <edge id="e11" source="v0" target="v2">
   <data key="k0">false</data>
    <data key="k1">7</data>
  </edge>
...
```

Fig. 6. GraphML fragment representing two edges, one confirmed with a unit value and the other unconfirmed with a value of seven. The first edge label is a standard attribute stored by visone, the other is user-defined.

Besides GraphML, import and export in a number of simple formats and some formats customary in social network analysis and graph drawing are supported. To communicate results, visualizations can be exported in Scalable Vector Graphics (SVG) or PostScript format. Many conversion tools exist for both. The SVG export routine has been adopted into the core LEDA package.

There is neither a macro language nor an interface for third-party extensions, but limited support of command-line options for batch-mode operations is planned in the future.

5 Examples

We illustrate the intended usage of visone by three exemplary studies in which predecessors of the system have been used to explore and analyze network data.

Drug policy. This project [25] studies the presence of HIV-preventive measures for IV-drug users in nine selected German municipalities. The substantive question underlying this research is, why municipalities with comparable problem pressure differ significantly in the provision of HIV-preventive measures such as methadone substitution or needle exchange.

The policy networks under scrutiny comprise all local organizations directly or indirectly involved in the provision of such measures. In each of the nine municipalities, the 22–38 actors included in the study were queried about relations such as strategic collaboration, common activities, or informal communication with other organizations in the same municipality. None of the networks has more than 120 edges of the same type, and typically more than 50% of them are unconfirmed.

Figure 7 is a typical example of such a network visualized with visone. Note that centrality indices provide insight into the social and political structure of policy making and help understanding the policy outcomes produced.

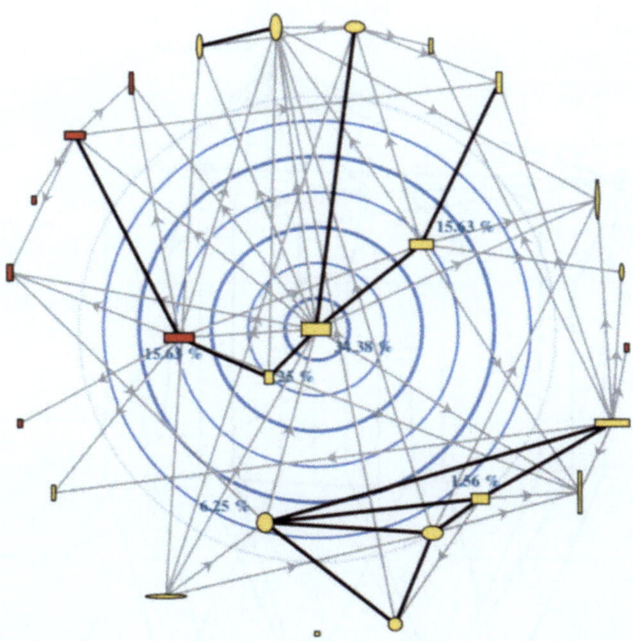

Fig. 7. Organizations involved in drug policy making. Radial visualization of betweenness centrality in network of informal communication. Organizations either have a supportive (yellow) or a repressive (red) attitude towards drug users, and they are public (rectangles) or private (ellipses). Height, width, and area indicate in-degree, out-degree, and degree when unconfirmed edges are counted as directed along the claim of existence.

Industry privatization. The second study [31] deals with networks of public, societal and private organizations that developed during the privatization of industrial conglomerates in East Germany as part of the economic transformation after German unification in 1990. Their privatization is understood as political bargaining processes between actors that are connected by ties such as exchange of resources, command, or consideration of interest.

The privatization was foreseen to be carried out by the Treuhandanstalt, a public agency of the federal government. Due to its institutional position and its ownership of all companies, it was generally assumed to be one of the most powerful actors in the transformation of East Germany.

As part of the analysis, status indices are used as indicators for the power or influence of actors. Since the specific index considered for these networks [16, p. 35ff] is not yet provided in visone, it was imported from another software tool (STRUCTURE [17]). Figure 8 gives a visualization example showing whose interests actors involved in the privatization of the ship-building industry claim that they considered.

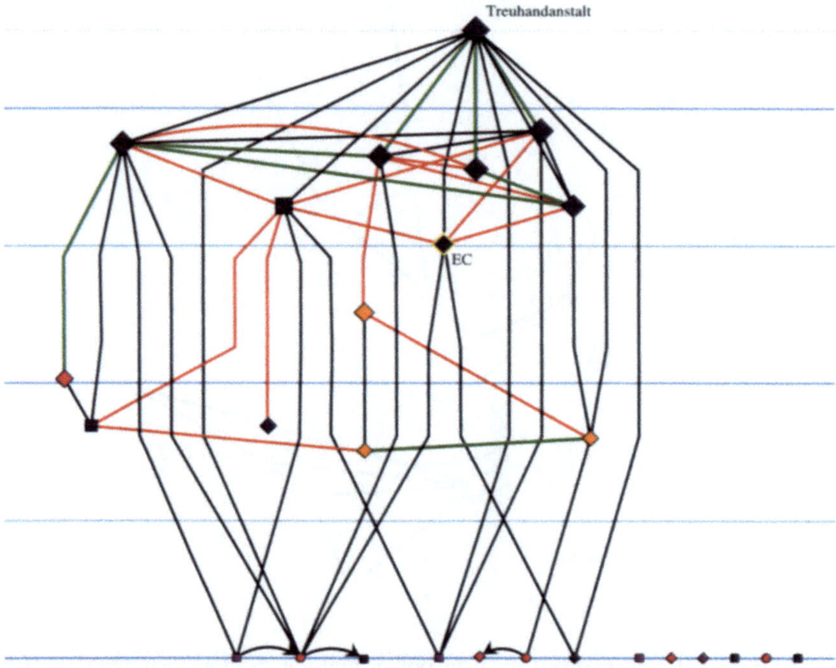

Fig. 8. Interest consideration among actors involved in privatization of the East German ship-building industry after German unification (redrawn from [14], for clarity black and red code edge directions up and down, while green edges are bidirected). Vertex color and shape code additional attributes.

Topic identification. Our third example illustrates the use of methods from social network analysis in another domain, namely topic identification in texts by centering resonance analysis [18]. The structure of texts is represented by graphs that have a vertex for each word occurring in a noun phrase and an edge for each pair of words that appear together in the same noun phrase or consecutively in the same sentence. It is argued that words corresponding to nodes with high betweenness centrality in such a graph are important for the structure of the text and thus a proxy for its topic.

This method was applied to Reuters news dealing with the terrorist attacks of September 11, 2001 [5] to identify, among other things, the main topics, topic changes, side stories, etc. in the news. Figure 9 shows the main topics identified for the very first day of media coverage.

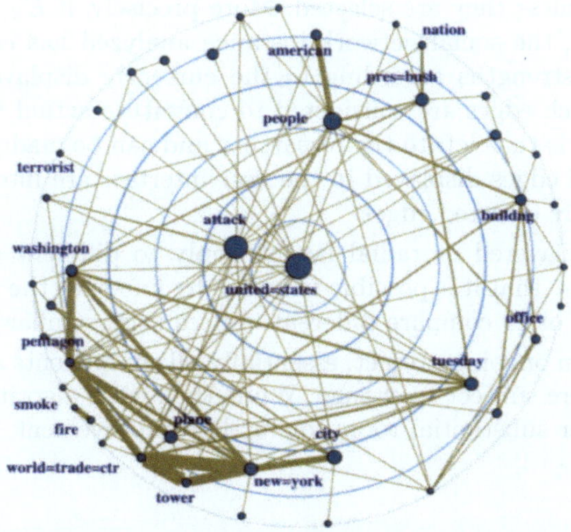

Fig. 9. Text structure in Reuters press releases following the 9/11 terrorist attacks. The news body of more than 46,000 words on the first day leads to a graph with more than 2,400 vertices, of which the 42 most central are shown. Thickness of lines indicates the number of co-occurrences (minimum of two).

6 Software

The visone software is provided as a stand-alone executable for systems running Linux, Solaris, or Windows, and is free for academic purposes.

Technically, the user interface inherits from LEDA's graph editor class `GraphWin`, though several internal modifications were necessary to address the needs of researchers and students in the social sciences. With application-specific terminology it comprises the usual drawing canvas with pull-down and context (pop-up) menus. Therefore, network data can be imported from a file but also input or edited graphically.

Aside from the analytic and layout procedures described above, we provide some non-standard user interaction facilities as shown in Figure 10. Most importantly, extensive attribute-based selection mechanisms facilitate exploration of data by hiding, adding, or altering objects. For example, users can select vertices based on labels, attributes, graphical attributes, or the selection status of incident edges. These criteria can be combined with an existing selection in various ways. Moreover, the attributes interpreted as strengths and lengths in our unified network model can be switched and modified interactively.

Analytic routines are always applied to the data currently seen by the user, except for unconfirmed edges which are shown for context, but disregarded in the analysis unless they are selected. More precisely, if $E_S \subseteq E$ is the set of selected edges, the social network instance analyzed has edges $E_C \cup E_S$ with lengths or strengths according to the currently displayed edge label. The decision which edges are considered to constitute actual ties and which edges are labeled is thus left to the researcher and can be made on a per-edge basis. Undirected edges displayed in the user interface are internally treated like two oppositely directed edges.

Analysis and layered or radial layout apply to different coordinates of vertex locations, so that it is possible to manually fine-tune the representation of a vertex index or to compare different indices using similar layouts.

Since this is an ongoing project, essentially all components are in development and therefore subject to change. While the layout algorithms currently implemented offer substantial room for further improvement, our long-term

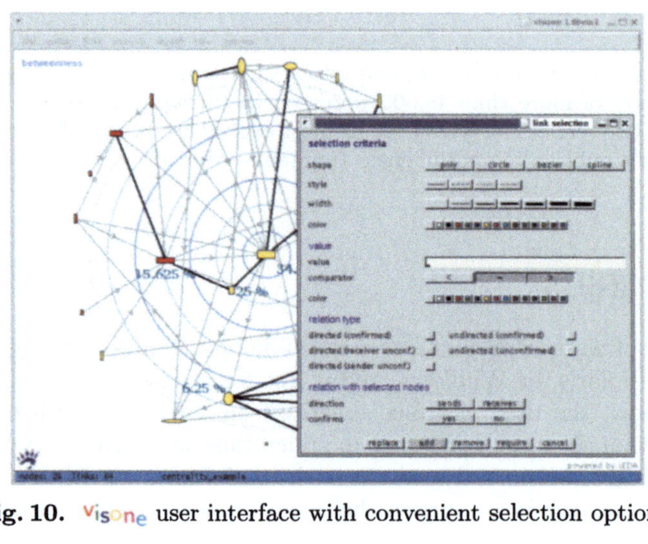

Fig. 10. visone user interface with convenient selection options.

goal is to extend visone with additional visualization modes facilitating, e.g., the comparison of different vertex or edge indices.

References

1. Analytic Technologies. *UCINET V*. Network analysis software. See `http://www.analytictech.com/`
2. Anthonisse, J. M. (1971) The rush in a directed graph. Technical Report BN 9/71, Stichting Mathematisch Centrum, Amsterdam
3. Barabási, A.-L., Albert, R. (1999) Emergence of scaling in random networks. Science **286** (5439), 509–512
4. Batagelj, V., Brandes, U. (2003) Efficient generation of random graphs. Working Paper
5. Batagelj, V., Brandes, U., Johnson, J. C., Kobourov, S., Krempel, L., Mrvar, A., Wagner, D. (2002) Analysis and visualization of network data. Special Session during *Sunbelt Social Network Conference XXII*, New Orleans
6. Baur, M., Brandes, U. (2003) An improved heuristic for crossing minimization in circular layouts. Working Paper
7. Beauchamp, M. A. (1965) An improved index of centrality. Behavioral Science **10**, 161–163
8. Bonacich, P. (1972) Factoring and weighting approaches to status scores and clique identification. Journal of Mathematical Sociology **2**, 113–120
9. Brandes, U. (2001) A faster algorithm for betweenness centrality. Journal of Mathematical Sociology **25** (2), 163–177
10. Brandes, U., Eiglsperger, M., Herman, I., Himsolt, M., Marshall, M. S. (2002) GraphML progress report: Structural layer proposal. In: P. Mutzel, M. Jünger, S. Leipert (eds.) Graph Drawing '01, Lecture Notes in Computer Science 2265, Springer-Verlag, 501–512. For up-to-date information see `http://graphml.graphdrawing.org/`.
11. Brandes, U., Kenis, P., Raab, J., Schneider, V., Wagner, D. (1999) Explorations into the visualization of policy networks. Journal of Theoretical Politics **11** (1), 75–106
12. Brandes, U., Kenis, P., Wagner, D. (2003) Communicating centrality in policy network drawings. IEEE Transactions on Visualization and Computer Graphics **9** (2), 241–253
13. Brandes, U., Köpf, B. (2002) Fast and simple horizontal coordinate assignment. In: P. Mutzel, M. Jünger, S. Leipert (eds.) Graph Drawing '01, Lecture Notes in Computer Science 2265, Springer-Verlag, 31–44
14. Brandes, U., Raab, J., Wagner, D. (2001) Exploratory network visualization: Simultaneous display of actor status and connections. Journal of Social Structure **2** (4)
15. Brin, S., Page, L. (1998) The anatomy of a large-scale hypertextual Web search engine. Computer Networks and ISDN Systems **30** (1–7), 107–117
16. Burt, R. S. (1982) Toward a Structural Theory of Action: Network Models of Social Structure, Perception, and Action. Academic Press
17. Burt, R. S. (1991) Structure, Version 4.2. Center for the Social Sciences, Columbia University, New York. See `http://gsbwww.uchicago.edu/fac/ronald.burt/teaching/`

18. Corman, S. R., Kuhn, T., McPhee, R. D., Dooley, K. J. (2002) Studying complex discursive systems: Centering resonance analysis of communication. Human Communication Research **28** (2), 157–206
19. Freeman, L. C. (1977) A set of measures of centrality based on betweenness. Sociometry **40**, 35–41
20. Gilbert, E. N. (1959) Random graphs. The Annals of Mathematical Statistics **30** (4), 1141–1144
21. Hage, P., Harary, F. (1995) Eccentricity and centrality in networks. Social Networks **17**, 57–63
22. Hall, K. M. (1970) An r-dimensional quadratic placement algorithm. Management Science **17** (3), 219–229
23. Harel, D., Koren, Y. (2002) Graph drawing by high-dimensional embedding. In: M. T. Goodrich and S. G. Kobourov (eds.) Graph Drawing '02, Lecture Notes in Computer Science 2528, Springer-Verlag, 207–219
24. Katz, L. (1953) A new status index derived from sociometric analysis. Psychometrika **18**, 39–43
25. Kenis, P. (1998) An analysis of cooperation structures in local drug policy in Germany. Unpublished Report.
26. Kleinberg, J. M. (1999) Authoritative sources in a hyperlinked environment. Journal of the Association for Computing Machinery **46** (5), 604–632
27. Koren, Y., Carmel, L., Harel, D. (2002) ACE: A fast multiscale eigenvectors computation for drawing huge graphs. In: Proceedings IEEE Symposium on Information Visualization (InfoVis '02), 137–144
28. Masuda, S., Kashiwabara, T., Nakajima, K., Fujisawa, T. (1987) On the $\mathcal{NP}$-completeness of a computer network layout problem. In: Proceedings IEEE International Symposium on Circuits and Systems, 292–295
29. Matuszewski, C., Schönfeld, R., Molitor, P. (1999) Using sifting for k-layer straightline crossing minimization. In: J. Katochvíl (ed.) Graph Drawing '99, Lecture Notes in Computer Science 1731, Springer-Verlag, 217–224
30. Mehlhorn, K., Näher, S. (1999) The LEDA Platform of Combinatorial and Geometric Computing. Cambridge University Press
31. Raab, J. (2002) Steuerung von Privatisierung. Westdeutscher Verlag
32. Sabidussi, G. (1966) The centrality index of a graph. Psychometrika **31**, 581–603
33. Six, J. M., Tollis, I. G. (1999) Circular drawings of biconnected graphs. In: M. T. Goodrich and C. C. McGeoch (ed.), Proceedings 1st Workshop on Algorithm Engineering and Experimentation (ALENEX '99), Lecture Notes in Computer Science 1619, Springer-Verlag, 57–73
34. Six, J. M., Tollis, I. G. (1999) A framework for circular drawings of networks. In: J. Katochvíl (ed.) Graph Drawing '99, Lecture Notes in Computer Science 1731, Springer-Verlag, 107–116
35. Valente, T. W., Foreman, R. K. (1998) Integration and radiality: Measuring the extent of an individual's connectedness and reachability in a network. Social Networks **20** (1), 89–105
36. Watts, D. J., Strogatz, S. H. (1998) Collective dynamics of "small-world" networks. Nature **393**, 440–442

Polyphemus and Hermes – Exploration and Visualization of Computer Networks*

Gabriele Barbagallo[1], Andrea Carmignani[2], Giuseppe Di Battista[2], Walter Didimo[3], and Maurizio Pizzonia[2]

[1] CASPUR c/o Università "La Sapienza", P. le A. Moro 5, 00185 Roma, Italy
[2] Università di Roma Tre, Dipartimento di Informatica e Automazione, Via della Vasca Navale 79, 00146 Roma, Italy
[3] Università degli Studi di Perugia, Dipartimento di Ingegneria Elettronica e dell'Informazione, Via G. Duranti 93, 06125 Perugia, Italy

1 Introduction

Computer networks are an endless source of problems and motivations for the Graph Drawing and for the Information Visualization research communities. Graphical representation of computer networks at different abstraction levels are interesting for different types of users. To give only some examples (an interesting survey can be found in [10]):

1. Application level: visualization of Web sites structures, Web maps [11,9], and Web caches [6] are important for designers and developers of Web sites and Web based systems.
2. Network level: visualization of interconnections among routers are interesting for Internet Service Providers (ISP) which need to manage large and complex networks. ISPs may be also interested in understanding the structure of the Internet at a higher level (connections among ISPs) in order to understand the position of their partners and/or competitors in the Internet. Visualization of such information is also interesting for content delivery companies to choose where to place their content servers with strategic ISPs for obtaining low delivery latency and high robustness.
3. Data Link level: visualization of interconnection of switches and repeaters in a local area network [2] is interesting for installers and maintainers of the local area.

Drawing graphs related with computer networks is a challenging activity. Such graphs may have a huge number of nodes and edges. Further, nodes of network-related graphs are often naturally grouped into clusters. As an

* Work partially supported by European Commission - Fet Open project COSIN – COevolution and Self-organisation In dynamical Networks – IST-2001-33555, by "Progetto ALINWEB: Algoritmica per Internet e per il Web", MIUR Programmi di Ricerca Scientifica di Rilevante Interesse Nazionale, and by "The Multichannel Adaptive Information Systems (MAIS) Project", MIUR Fondo per gli Investimenti della Ricerca di Base.

extreme example, the Web has been estimated to have about 800 millions of pages in 1999 [14] which are grouped into several millions of Web servers [18].

Plain application of standard graph drawing techniques for the visualization of large network-related graphs will easily lead to huge inefficiencies and useless results.

We present two systems, Polyphemus and Hermes, along with their graph drawing algorithms and user interaction techniques. The two systems permit to explore clustered graphs representing the internal topology of an ISP and large and dense graphs representing the topology of the Internet as reported by the Internet Routing Registries [13], respectively.

2 Applications

The software applications we present allow users to explore and visualize the Internet topology at two different abstraction levels. Namely, we consider interconnections of network devices (routers) inside a specific *Autonomous System* (also denoted by *AS*), and interconnections between Autonomous Systems (ASes).

In the Internet, each AS groups a set of networks under the same administrative authority (usually an Internet Service Provider). An AS is identified by an integer number, while each network is identified by its IP address. Intuitively, an AS can be seen as a portion of the Internet, and the Internet can be seen as the totality of its ASes.

2.1 Intra-AS routing: Polyphemus

Inside an AS, routing protocols especially tailored for intra-AS routing are used. The Open Shortest Path First protocol (OSPF) [16] is one of the most popular and efficient of these protocols.

The OSPF routing protocol groups networks into *areas*. Routers connect networks of one area and/or networks of different areas (see Figure 1(a)). Routers connecting networks of different areas are called *area border routers* (*ABR*). In an OSPF network there is one *backbone area*. In common OSPF configurations all non-backbone areas are directly connected to the backbone area. However, complex topologies can be obtained by using the *virtual links* capability of OSPF [16]. If we consider all the areas and their relations with the area border routers the graph is in general a bipartite graph (see Figure 1(b)).

Each OSPF router knows the topology of the area it resides in or of the areas it connects. However, such information is available to network maintainers only in tabular form and from each router only the part of the network it knows is available. Polyphemus permits to show the relations among all areas and to drill down in order to show the topology of each area.

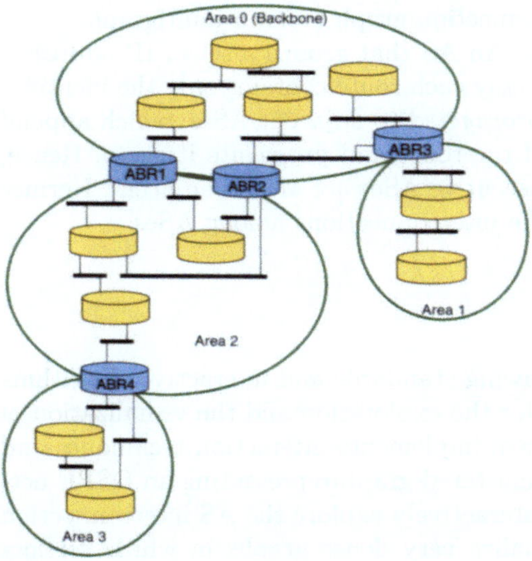

(a)

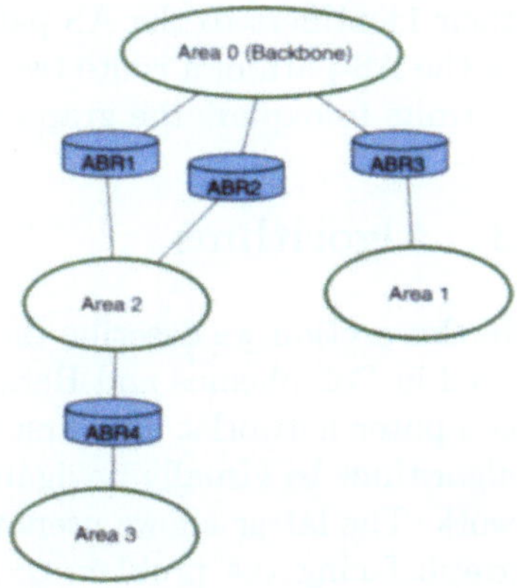

(b)

Fig. 1. (a) An example of *OSPF network*. Each *area* is represented by a green circle, *area border routers* are shown in blue while non-border routers are shown in yellow, horizontal thick lines represent local area networks interconnecting different routers. (b) Distinct areas are connected by area border routers forming in general a bipartite graph.

2.2 Inter-AS routing: Hermes

Let us now change the level of abstraction by looking at the whole Internet. Each AS exchanges routing information with other ASes by means of a routing protocol called Border Gateway Protocol (*BGP*) [19]. Such a protocol is based on a distributed architecture where *border routers* that belong to distinct ASes exchange the information they know.

A *route* is a (directed) path on the Internet that can be used to reach a specific set of (contiguous) IP addresses, representing a set of networks. A route is completely described by its destination IP addresses, its cost, and by the ordered set of ASes that it traverses (usually called *AS-path*). Routes can be seen as advertisements, from an AS to its adjacent ASes, meaning "through me you can reach a certain set of networks, with a certain cost and traversing a certain set of other ASes".

Two border routers that directly exchange information are said to perform a *peering session*, and the ASes they belong to are said to be *adjacent*. We define the *ASes interconnection graph* as the graph having one vertex for each

AS and one edge between each pair of adjacent ASes. Note that, according to our definition, the ASes interconnection graph is not a multigraph.

Routes are incrementally built. An AS that groups a set of IP addresses *originates* a route for this set. Initially each route contains only the identifier of the originating AS, then it is *propagated* to adjacent ASes, which append their identifiers to the AS-path of the route and propagate it again. Hence, in the AS-path of a route two consecutive ASes are always adjacent. Hermes permits to explore the graph of the interconnections among ASes.

3 Algorithms

In this section we describe the drawing standards and interactive algorithms used in Polyphemus and Hermes for the exploration and the visualization of computer networks. The first system implements interaction techniques and algorithms to visually navigate a clustered graph representing an OSPF network. The latter allows users to interactively explore the AS interconnection graph facing the problem to visualize very dense graphs in which vertices may have very high degree.

3.1 Interactive Models and Drawing Standards

Very often vertices of network-related graphs are naturally grouped into clusters. A cluster groups objects that are related from a technical and/or administrative point of view. Polyphemus visualizes OSPF networks which may be modeled as clustered graphs in which each OSPF area is a cluster. Routers are represented as vertices. A local area network that connects two routers is represented as an edge. A local area network that connects more than two routers is represented as a vertex adjacent to all the connected routers. Area border routers are represented by a particular kind of vertices called *border vertices* which are associated with more than one cluster. The *border* of a cluster is the set of border vertices associated with it. Vertices representing non-border routers and local area networks are always associated with only one cluster.

Suppose to have a drawing of a clustered graph in which each cluster is shown as a regular vertex and the inner details of the cluster are hidden (*overall map*). Information contained in each cluster can be shown by means of the following interaction primitive:

Drill down. A cluster c is selected among those displayed. A new map is created containing vertices and edges associated with c along with vertices associated with its border. In the new map the vertices that are the border of c are positioned on the border of the drawing.

In Polyphemus the overall map is drawn according to the basic Kandinsky drawing standard (see Section 4.4 in the Technical Foundations). When the

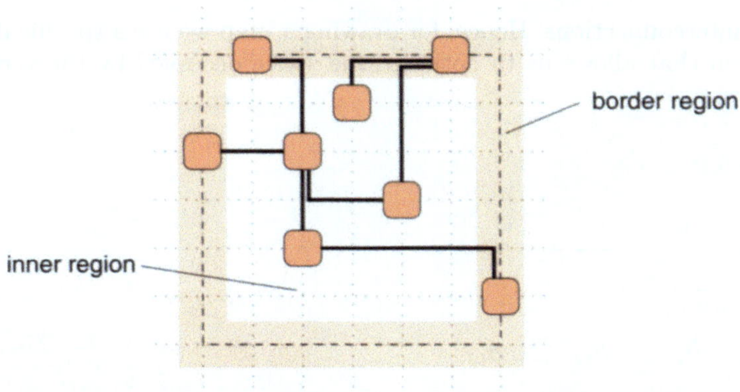

Fig. 2. Variation of the basic Kandinsky drawing standard used by Polyphemus for drawing a cluster. Border vertices are positioned on the border region.

user applies the drill down primitive to a cluster the map of the selected cluster is drawn according to a variation of the basic Kandinsky drawing standard as described below.

The grid used to place the vertices is divided into two regions: the *border region* and the *inner region* (see Figure 2), where the border region is a rectangular strip of grid points surrounding the inner region. Border vertices of the cluster are placed on the border region. All other vertices of the cluster are placed in the inner region. Edges cannot cross the border region but can run along it as shown in Figure 2.

A very different drawing problem is faced by Hermes. The ASes interconnection graph is very large (about 12 thousand vertices and about 30 thousands edges) and many vertices have a very high degree (up to 2 thousand).

To incrementally explore such a large graph G we define the following strategy. A map M is originally constructed visualizing a first node of G and all the nodes that are adjacent to it. The first node can be chosen by the user, for example, by means of some form of text based search. Then, the user can explore G and enrich the current map M, by using the following primitive:

Exploration. A node u among those displayed in M is selected. Map M is augmented with all the nodes that are connected to u. Further, for each node v connected to u an edge (u, v) is added. According to this definition, M is a subgraph of N but in general it is not an induced subgraph.

When the exploration primitive is applied on the current map M of G, the vertices of $G \setminus M$ added to M will have degree one in the new current map. Also, these vertices of degree one may be numerous, depending on the structure of G. This is, for example, the case of the Internet topology in terms of ASes interconnections. Hence, for drawing a map we use a specific drawing convention that allows us to optimize the space occupied by the vertices of degree one.

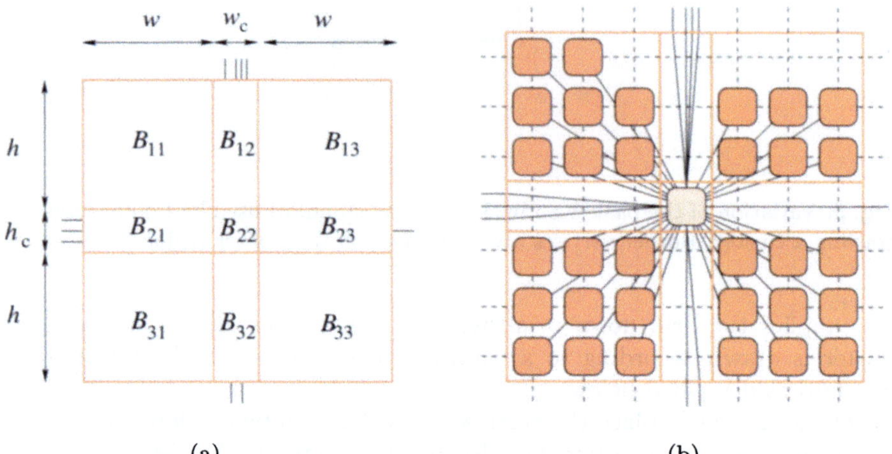

Fig. 3. Using a box to make room around a vertex. (a) The nine rectangles that partition the box. (b) Using the nine rectangles to place the degree-one vertices. Each vertex in the box is centered on an integer grid point.

Such a drawing convention is based on a variation of the Kandinsky model for orthogonal drawings (see Section 4.4 in the Technical Foundations). We modify the Kandinsky model as follows. Each vertex of degree one adjacent to a vertex v is appropriately positioned on an integer coordinate grid around v and connected to v with a straight-line edge. Namely, as shown in Figure 3, vertex v is associated with a box partitioned into nine rectangles arranged into three rows and three columns. Denote these rectangles as B_{ij}, $(i, j \in \{1, 2, 3\})$. Rectangle B_{22} is used for drawing v centered on a grid point. Rectangles B_{11}, B_{13}, B_{31}, and B_{33} are used for drawing the degree-one vertices adjacent to v. Their incident edges are represented by straight-line segments, possibly overlapping other degree-one vertices. Actually, they are drawn on the back of the vertices. Rectangles B_{12}, B_{21}, B_{32}, and B_{23} are used for hosting the connections of v to the other vertices.

The height h_c of the center row is equal to one grid unit as well as the width w_c of the center column. Rectangles B_{11}, B_{13}, B_{31}, and B_{33} all have the same width w and height h. The values of h and w are expressed in terms of grid units and must guarantee enough room for placing all the degree-one vertices. How w and h are computed will be detailed Section 3.4.

3.2 Drill Down Algorithm

Let G be a clustered graph representing an OSPF network as described in Section 3.1. Denote by G' the (non clustered) graph derived from G by turning each cluster into a single vertex. In G' border vertices are kept distinct from clusters (see Figure 1(b)). More formally, G' is a bipartite graph with vertices $C \cup B$ where C is the set of the clusters and B is the set of the border vertices. Say that the map M of G' is drawn within the basic Kandinsky standard, for example by modifying the topology-shape-metrics approach to handle high degree vertices (see Section 4.4 in the Technical Foundations). For each cluster c we call B^c_{north} the sequence of border vertices of M that are adjacent to the north side of c in clockwise order. Analogously we define sequences B^c_{east},B^c_{south}, B^c_{west}.

The technique we describe in this section implements the drill down primitive and computes a new map M_c for c with the following properties:

- M_c conforms to the drawing standard detailed in Section 3.1.
- vertices of B^c_{north}, B^c_{east}, B^c_{south}, B^c_{west} are positioned the north, east, south and west side respectively into the border region, in clockwise order.

We propose a variation of the topology-shape-metrics approach in order to obtain the properties we mentioned above.

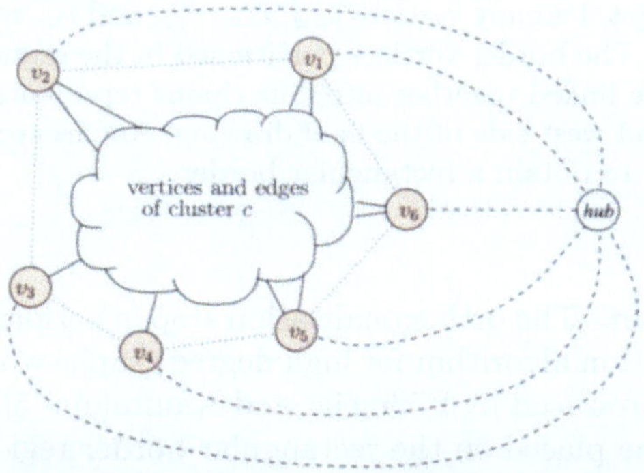

Fig. 4. The *wheel* gadget. Vertices $v_1, \ldots, v_6$ are the border vertices of cluster c. Dummy edges connect the border vertices in a prescribed circular order forming the *rim* of the wheel (dotted). Dummy edges called *spokes* (dashed) connect each border vertex with the *hub* of the wheel.

Planarization. The planarization step is performed by applying a modified version of the classical edge re-insertion algorithm described in Section 4.3 of the Technical Foundations. Since the border vertices of M_c must lay on the external face in a prescribed order, we build the *wheel* gadget shown in Figure 4, composed by a dummy vertex, called *hub*, and dummy edges which form the *rim* and the *spokes* of the wheel (shown respectively dotted and dashed in Figure 4). The border vertices of c are connected by the rim respecting the order they should have in the external face of M_c.

In performing the edge re-insertion we chose the initial planar subgraph P such that it contains hub, rim and spokes; this ensures that border vertices have the right order in M_c. Then, we delete the edges of the rim and perform edge re-insertion without crossing the spokes; this ensures that all the border vertices are on the external face of the final embedding. Finally, we delete the spokes and the hub.

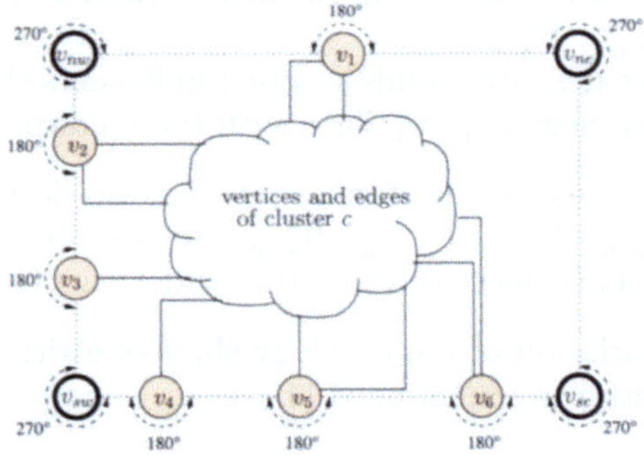

Fig. 5. The *box* gadget. Dummy vertices v_{nw}, v_{sw}, v_{se}, and v_{ne} represent the corners of the final drawing. The border vertices partitioned in the sequences B^c_{north}, B^c_{east}, B^c_{south}, and B^c_{west} are linked together into four chains representing respectively the north, east, south and west side of the final drawing. Angles around the border are constrained in order to obtain a rectangular border.

Orthogonalization. The orthogonalization step is performed by applying a bend minimization algorithm for high degree graphs which is a simplification of that introduced by Fößmeier and Kaufmann [5]. Since the border vertices must be placed on the rectangular border region of the drawing, we build the *box* gadget shown in Figure 5. Four dummy vertices are introduced to represent the corners of the drawing area: v_{nw}, v_{sw}, v_{se}, and v_{ne} (shown with bold circles in the figure). Vertices in sequence B^c_{north} (B^c_{east}, B^c_{south}, B^c_{west}) are linked together, according to the specified order, in a chain of dummy edges starting with v_{nw} (v_{ne}, v_{se}, v_{sw}) and ending with v_{ne} (v_{se}, v_{sw}, v_{nw}). Edges of the four chains are constrained to have no bend. Angles that such edges form on the external face are constrained: around v_{nw}, v_{sw}, v_{se}, and v_{ne} they must be 270 degree while around the border vertices they must be 180 degree (see Figure 5).

The bend minimization algorithm is realized by a reduction to a min-cost-flow problem where each unit of flow represents a 90 degree angle. The support for bends and angles constraints is a standard feature of that approach and it is implemented by setting upper bounds and lower bounds on specific arcs of the flow network. Details on the flow network and on the supported constraints can be found in Section 4.4 of the Technical Foundations and in [5].

Compaction. The compaction step can be performed by applying one of many compaction techniques available in literature (see Section 4.4 in the Technical Foundations).

3.3 Exploration Algorithm

Consider the maps constructed by the exploration primitive during a sequence of exploration steps. In this section we provide two different algorithms that compute drawings of these maps within the defined drawing convention. At each exploration step, we update the current map and we compute a new drawing for it by using one of the following algorithms.

`Static algorithm` The current map is completely redrawn, after the new vertices and edges have been added. The drawing of the previous map is not taken into account by this algorithm.

`Dynamic algorithm` The new vertices and edges are added to the current drawing while trying to preserve the shape of the existing edges and the coordinates of the existing vertices and bends.

The static algorithm usually constructs drawings that are more readable for the user. Indeed, the static algorithm allows each existing vertex or edge to completely change its position or shape with respect to the previous drawing, in order to optimize several global æsthetics, like for example the total number of bends and the drawing area. The drawback of the static algorithm however is that the user's mental map can be lost, because the new drawing can be significantly different from the previous one. To the opposite, the target of the dynamic algorithm is to preserve as much as possible the user's mental map. This implies that further constraints must be taken into account by the algorithm in the computation of the new drawing. These constraints make more difficult and less effective the optimization of the æsthetic parameters.

In the following we give some details about the static and the dynamic algorithms.

3.4 The Static Algorithm for Exploration

Let G be the network to be explored and let $M \subseteq G$ be the current map. Denote by v the vertex of M that is explored at the generic step. Map M is enriched with the vertices and the edges of G that do not belong to M and that are directly connected to v in G. The static algorithm completely redraws the new map, which we still call M for simplicity, according to the following steps:

Step 1 (Degree-one Vertex Removal) All vertices of degree one are temporarily removed from M. Denote by M' the new map. Each vertex u of M' is labeled by the number $\delta(u)$ of vertices of degree one that were attached to it.

Step 2 (Planarization) A well known planarization technique is applied to M' (see Section 4.3 in the Technical Foundations). In this phase a planar embedding of M' is computed. Crossings among edges are represented by dummy vertices, which will be removed later. We call these dummy vertices *cross vertices*.

Step 3 (Orthogonalization) A basic Kandinsky representation of M' is constructed within the computed embedding, by using a polynomial-time algorithm for the minimization of the bends [5].

Step 4 (Compaction) A drawing for M' is computed from its orthogonal representation by assigning coordinates to vertices and bends. Since for each vertex u, our drawing convention requires that $\delta(u)$ vertices of degree one are placed around u, we must guarantee enough room for them (see Section 3.1). To do that we compute a (non-basic) Kandinsky drawing using the algorithm described in [8] (see Section 4.4 in the Technical Foundations). Each vertex u is drawn as a box whose height h and width w depend on $\delta(u)$. Namely, we set $w = \lceil \sqrt{\delta(u)}/2 \rceil$. The height h is set equal to $= w - 1$ if this ensures enough room for all the vertices to be placed; else we set $h = w$. If $\delta(u) = 0$ then we set $h = w = 0$. We recall that w and h are expressed in terms of grid units. For example, referring to Figure 3, we have that $\delta(u) = 32$ (u is the vertex on the center of the box and has 32 vertices of degree one connected to it) and then $w = 3$. Also, $h = 2$ is not sufficient for hosting all the 32 vertices into the four rectangles B_{11}, B_{13}, B_{31}, B_{33} (in fact, if $h = 2$ we can place at most $w \times h \times 4 = 3 \times 2 \times 4 = 24$ vertices inside the box). Hence h is set equal to 3 (in this way we can place up to 36 vertices inside the box; we use 32 positions for placing vertices and 4 positions will be not used). Also, we must ensure that the edges that connect u to vertices with degree greater than one are incident to the middle points of the sides of the box. Although the algorithm described in [8] allows the edges to freely shift along the side they are incident to, it is easy to slightly vary this algorithm to guarantee the above property. Eventually, cross vertices are removed from the drawing.

Step 5 (Degree-one Vertex Re-insertion) For each vertex u such that $\delta(u) > 0$, the box representing u is replaced by a half unit square, and the edges that are incident to u are stretched. Also, the vertices of degree one that are incident to u are distributed in the rectangles B_{11}, B_{13}, B_{31}, and B_{33} and connected to u with a straight edge, according to the adopted drawing convention (see Figure 3(b)).

3.5 The Dynamic Algorithm for Exploration

We still denote by G the network to be explored and by M the current map. Also, let D be the current drawing of M, and let v be the vertex of M explored by the user at the generic step. The dynamic algorithm enriches M and D incrementally, by adding the vertices and the edges of G that do not belong to M and that are directly connected to v in G. This is done trying to preserve the user's mental map. Before describing the steps of the dynamic algorithms, we need to introduce some further notation.

Denote by ΔE_v and by ΔV_v the set of the edges and the set of the vertices that must be inserted when exploring v. We remark that all the edges in ΔE_v are incident to v and that the vertices in ΔV_v will be degree-one vertices attached to v in the final drawing. For simplicity, we always use the notation M and D to denote the intermediate maps and drawings computed throughout the execution of the dynamic algorithm. At the generic step of the dynamic algorithm, some of the vertices of M might be not explicitly represented in D. Namely, each vertex u of D might absorb all the degree-one vertices adjacent to it and implicitly represent the number of these vertices by a label $\delta(u)$, as in the case of the static algorithm. We call V_1 the set of degree-one vertices of M that are not explicitly represented in D, and V_2 all the vertices of M that are explicitly represented in D. Subsets V_1 and V_2 partition the set of vertices of M and initially V_1 is empty. Sets ΔV_v, V_1, and V_2 are modified throughout the algorithm.

The steps of the dynamic algorithm are described hereunder (refer to Figure 6):

Step 1 We temporarily remove from D all the degree-one vertices. Each vertex u of D is labeled with the number $\delta(u)$ of vertices of degree one that were attached to it (see Figure 6(b)). The deleted vertices are moved from V_2 to V_1. Note that D is now a basic Kandinsky drawing, where edge crossings are still replaced by cross vertices.

Step 2 We incrementally add to M the edges of ΔE_v and the vertices of ΔV_v. At the same time, specific subsets of edges and vertices of M are added to D, by applying on D a sequence of two primitives that modify the drawing within the basic Kandinsky standard. The two primitives are as follows:

- **New-Edge(u,z)** A new edge is added to the drawing between the two vertices u and z; vertices u and z must be already explicitly represented in D.
- **Attach-Vertex(u)** A new vertex z is added to D and connected to u with a new edge (u, z); vertex u must be already explicitly represented in D.

A detailed description of these two primitives is provided in Section 3.6. Vertices and edges are reinserted in M and D according to the following two rules:

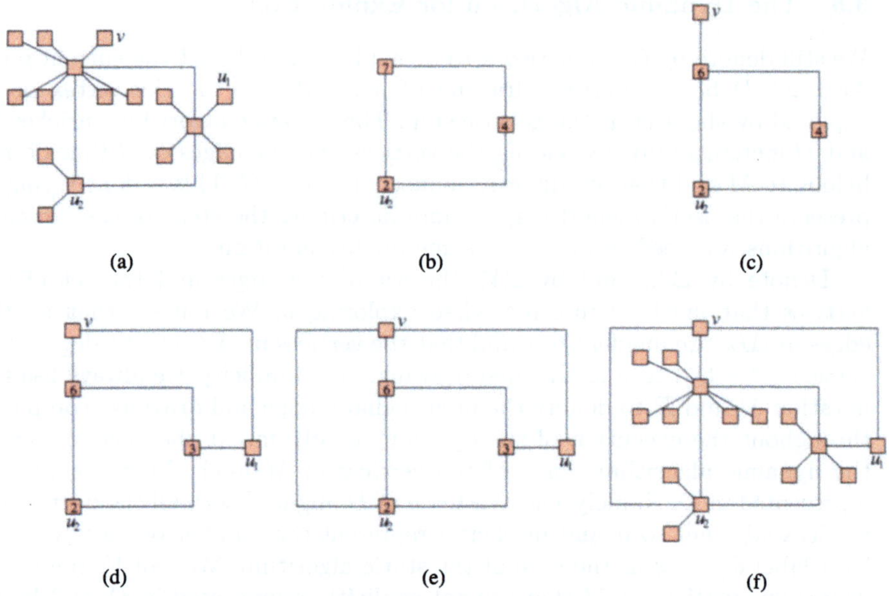

Fig. 6. An example of the dynamic algorithm. (a) The initial drawing of a map; the user chooses to explore vertex v; suppose that v is directly connected to u_1 and u_2 in the network. (b) All the degree-one vertices of the drawing are temporarily removed; the remaining vertices are labeled with the number of vertices of degree one that were connected to them. (c) Vertex v is reinserted by using the Attach-Vertex primitive. (d) Vertex u_1 is reinserted by using the Attach-Vertex primitive and edge (v, u_1) is inserted by using the New-Edge primitive. (e) Edge (v, u_2) is inserted by using the New-Edge primitive. (f) The compaction step is applied and the removed degree-one vertices are reinserted.

1. If the explored vertex v belongs to V_1 (that is, if v is a one-degree vertex in M), call w the vertex of V_2 that is connected to v in M. Reinsert v in D by performing primitive Attach-Vertex(w) (see Figure 6(c)). Consistently, decrease $\delta(w)$ by a unit, set $\delta(v) = 0$, and move v from V_1 to V_2.
2. For each edge $e = (v, u)$ of ΔE_v insert in M vertex u, if it is not already present in M, and edge e. Then, modify D according to the following three cases: (i) If u is in V_1, reinsert u in D by performing primitive Attach-Vertex(z), where z is the vertex of V_2 connected to u in M; then add e to D, by using primitive New-Edge(v,u) (see Figure 6(d)). Consistently, decrease $\delta(z)$ by a unit, set $\delta(u) = 0$ and move u from V_1 to V_2 . (ii) If u is in V_2, add edge e to D by using primitive New-Edge(v,u) (see Figure 6(e)). (iii) If u is in ΔV_v increase $\delta(v)$ by a unit, and move u from ΔV_v to V_1.

Once all edges in ΔE_v have been considered ΔV_v is empty, M is completely updated with the vertices and edges selected for insertion by the exploration of v, and the only vertices that remain to be added to D (those in V_1) are all the vertices (different from v) that have degree one in M.

`Step 3` We perform on D the `Compaction` step and the `Degree-one Vertex Re-insertion` step described for the static algorithm. The degree-one vertices reinserted are those in V_1 (see Figure 6(f)).

3.6 Dynamic Primitives

Primitives New-Edge and Attach-Vertex modify a basic Kandinsky drawing D preserving this drawing standard. They compute the position of the new vertices and edges trying to optimize, at the same time, the following measures: number of crossings, number of bends, and edge length. Each of these measures has a prescribed cost, which can be passed as a parameter to the primitives. In this way it is possible to decide the priority of each measure in the whole optimization. The primitives do not modify the shape of the part that the new drawing and the previous drawing have in common.

The two primitives use two auxiliary data structures to perform their actions. We now describe these data structures, and then describe how they are used by the primitives. Let H be the orthogonal representation of D.

First Data Structure. The first data structure is an orthogonal representation H' obtained from H in the following way:

- H is simplified in such a way that all vertices have degree less than or equal to four. This is done with a standard technique adopted in the basic Kandinsky model [5], where all the edges incident to the same vertex from the same side are collapsed into a chain of edges (see Figure 7). Each edge of the chain replaces a certain number of edges (possibly only one). With each edge we associate a *thickness* representing the number of edges replaced by it. The new vertices inserted by this operation are called *chain vertices.*
- Each face of H (including the external one) is decomposed into rectangles by adding a suitable number of dummy edges and vertices, with the linear time algorithm described by Tamassia (see Section 4.4 in the Technical Foundations). We call *dashed* the dummy edges and *solid* the edges of the original orthogonal representation.

Second Data Structure. The second data structure is a directed network N associated with H', which we call the *incidence network* of H'. It is used to implicitly describe all the orthogonal paths that a new edge can follow

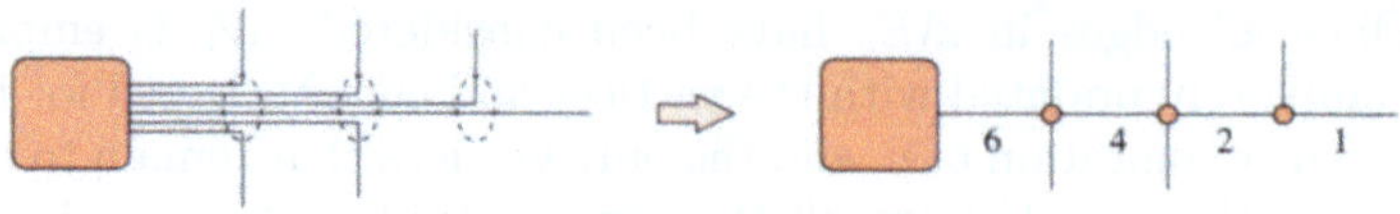

Fig. 7. Collapsing the edges incident to the same side of a vertex. The labels represent the thickness of the edges. The small circles are the chain vertices.

in H'. N is defined so that each path has an associated cost that reflects the cost of the new edge in terms of bends, edge crossings, and edge length. We denote by χ, β, and λ the costs of one crossing, one bend, and one edge length unit, respectively. Network N is defined as follows (see Figure 8(a)):

Nodes of the network. N has a node v associated with each edge e (solid or dashed) of H'. Also, v has a cost that represents the cost of crossing e. More in detail:

1. If e is a solid edge the cost of v is set-up equal to the thickness of e multiplied by χ (see Figure 8(a)). This reflects the fact that a path of N traversing v corresponds to a new edge of H' traversing edge e, and hence to a new edge of H that crosses a number of edges equal to the thickness of e.
2. If e is a dashed edge the cost of v is set-up equal to zero. This is because dashed edges of H' are dummy and will be removed in the final drawing. Hence, they do not really originate edge crossings.

Arcs of the network. N has an arc between every pair of nodes associated with two edges e_1 and e_2 in the same face f of H'. Such an arc represents an orthogonal path inside f, which can be used to reach e_2 from e_1 (or vice-versa) in H'. We distinguish three different kinds of arcs of N with respect to a face f of H' (refer to Figure 8):

1. An arc a between nodes associated with two horizontal (vertical) edges that lie on different sides of f (see, for example, arc a_1 in Figure 8(a)). In this case, a corresponds to a straight-line path p (a path with no bends) inside f, because it suffices to move from a side of f to its opposite in the orthogonal representation (see Figure 8(b)). Denoted by d_1 and d_2 (d_3 and d_4) the lengths (in terms of number of edges) of the two vertical (horizontal) sides of f, we assign cost $d\lambda$ to arc a, where $d = \max\{d_1, d_2\}$ ($d = \max\{d_3, d_4\}$). Such a cost is a lower bound on the length of p.
2. An arc a between a node associated with a horizontal edge e_h and a node associated with a vertical edge e_v of f (see, for example, arc a_3 in Figure 8(a)). In this case, a corresponds to an orthogonal path p with exactly one bend, as depicted in Figure 8(c). Denoted by s_v the side of f on which e_v lies, let d_v be the number of edges of s_v that are necessarily spanned (completely or partially) by the projection of p on s_v. Analogously, denoted by s_h the side of f on which e_h lies, let d_h be the number of edges of s_h that are necessarily spanned by the

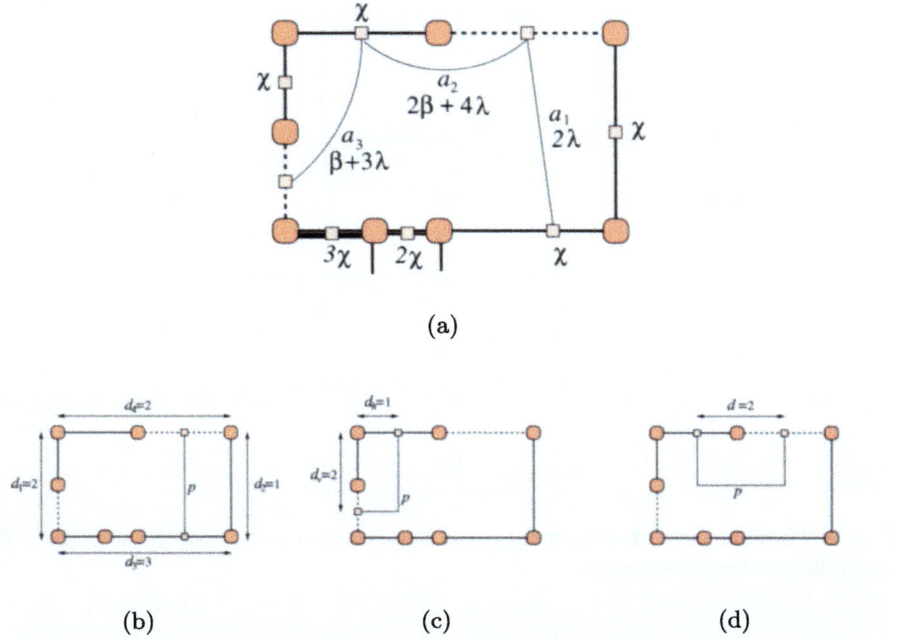

Fig. 8. (a) Example of construction of an incidence network. Nodes (little squares) and three arcs of the incidence network for a face of a simplified orthogonal representation. (b),(c),(d) Orthogonal paths corresponding to arcs a_1, a_2, a_3.

projection of p on s_h. The cost we assign to a is equal to $\beta+(d_v+d_h)\lambda$. In particular, $(d_v + d_h)\lambda$ still represents a lower bound on the length of p, while β is the cost for one bend.

3. An arc a between the nodes associated with two edges e_1 and e_2 that lie on the same side of f (see, for example, arc a_2 in Figure 8(a)). In this case, a corresponds to an orthogonal path p with two bends, as shown in Figure 8(d). Denoted by s the side of f in which lie the two edges, let d be the number of edges of s that are necessarily spanned (completely or partially) by p. Hence, the cost we assign to a is equal to $2\beta+(d+2)\lambda$. The two extra units for the length are due to the fact that p consists also of two (unit-length) segments having a direction (vertical or horizontal) orthogonal to the direction of s.

Primitive New-Edge(u,v). First, it computes from D the simplified orthogonal representation H' and the associated network N' above described. From the point of view of the primitive interface, H' and N are transparent. It just needs to know u, v and D. After that, two different cases are possible:

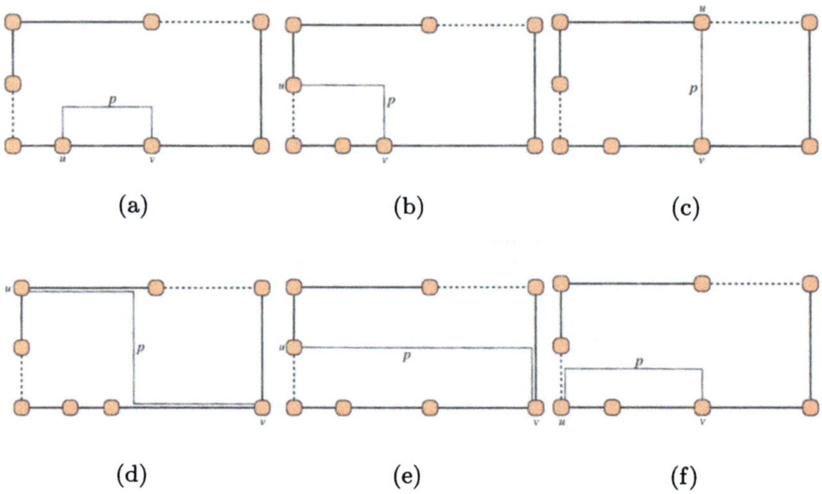

Fig. 9. Possible cases of orthogonal paths between two vertices of the same face of an orthogonal representation.

Case 1. Nodes u and v do not share a face of H'. In this case, the primitive completes network N by adding two extra nodes representing u and v. For simplicity we still refer to these extra nodes as u and v. Also, for each edge e of H' incident to u (resp. v) the primitive adds to N an arc between u (resp. v) and the node of N associated with e. All these extra arcs of N have zero cost. The primitive computes on N a shortest path between u and v, which determines the route and the shape of the new edge (u, v) in H', according to the rules illustrated in the construction of N. The new edge is added to H' following the arcs of the shortest path. The route and the shape of the new edge in H' uniquely induces the route and the shape of the same edge in H. Hence, the primitive adds edge (u, v) to H and computes the new drawing D by compacting H with a standard compaction algorithm for basic Kandinsky orthogonal representations (see Section 4.4 in the Technical Foundations).

Case 2. Nodes u and v share a face. In this case the shape of edge (u, v) is simply chosen according to the set of cases shown in Figure 9.

Primitive Attach-Vertex(u). It works much simpler than New-Edge. It adds a new edge e connecting a new node to u. The primitive looks in H' for a side s of u such that either no edge is incident to s or a dashed edge is incident to s. If such a side s exists, the primitive adds to H', and therefore to H, edge e as a straight edge incident to s. Otherwise, the primitive chooses an arbitrary side of u to insert edge e, and in this case edge e will have one bend in H.

Finally, the new drawing D is computed by compacting H with a standard compaction algorithm for basic Kandinsky orthogonal representations.

We briefly discuss the time complexity of the dynamic primitives. Primitive New-Edge requires the computation of the two auxiliary data structures described above. Denoted by n the number of vertices of H, the first data structure, that is, the orthogonal representation H', can be computed in $O(n)$ time (the number of edges of H is $O(n)$, since H is planar); the second data structure, that is, the network N, is computed in $O(n^2)$ time and has $O(n)$ nodes and $O(n^2)$ arcs. After that, Dijkstra's algorithm is run to find a shortest path on N. This algorithm takes $O(n^2)$ time. Finally, the compaction step is performed by means of a min-cost-flow algorithm, which takes $O(n^2 \log n)$ time. Although the time complexity is quite high, in practice the algorithm runs in a few seconds on a map that has a few hundreds of vertices. On the other hand, it is difficult for the user to take advantage of maps that have too many vertices. Usually, when a map becomes complicated, the user stops its exploration session and starts with a new one.

Primitive Attach-Vertex only requires the computation of H' and it works on simple local considerations. The time complexity is dominated by the time spent for the compaction algorithm, that is, $O(n^2 \log n)$.

In order to save time, when a sequence of consecutive dynamic primitives have to be applied before D is displayed, the compaction step is delayed until the end of the sequence, and applied only one time. In this case, H' and N are kept up to date after each primitive is executed instead of reconstructing them each time.

4 Implementation

In this section we describe the features and the architecture of Polyphemus and Hermes. Polyphemus permits the exploration of the topology inside a specific AS. Hermes makes possible, for the user, to explore the Internet at the level of interconnections among ASes. Because of their different targets, the two systems have different architectures and functionalities.

4.1 Polyphemus

Polyphemus is an application that supports discovery and visualization of the topology of an OSPF network. Since Polyphemus needs to access information stored by the routing devices inside an AS, the users are usually technical persons of the organization that runs the network. Polyphemus obtains information about the OSPF topology by accessing a Management Information Base [3] stored by the routers. Access is performed by means of the Simple Network Management Protocol (SNMP) [7]. Few hints should be provided to Polyphemus in order to start the discovery. The discovery process is driven by a wizard in which the user specifies the IP address of the first router

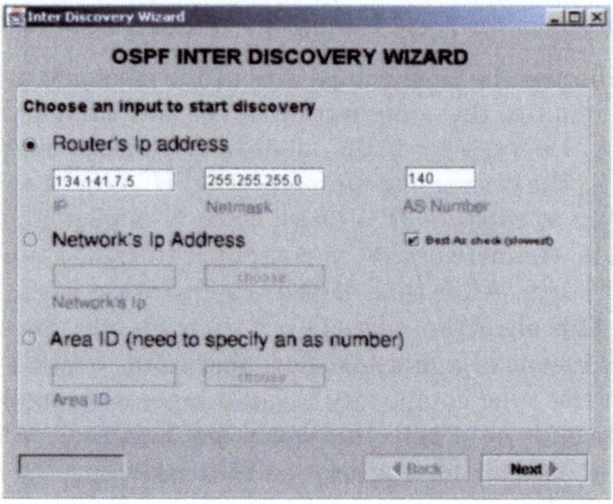

(a)

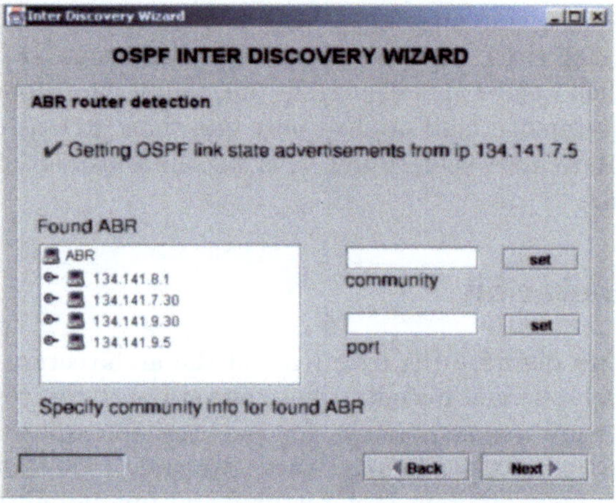

(b)

Fig. 10. Polyphemus discovery process is driven by a wizard in which the user specifies IP addresses and SNMP community names for the routers.

(see Figure 10(a)) and the SNMP community name to access the OSPF MIB information. Since newly discovered routers may have different community names these can be specified (see Figure 10(b)). The discovery process stores data about the topology in a database. We used a lightweight DBMS that does not require a specific installation procedure since it is embedded into the application.

At the end of the discovery process the map of the network can be visually explored by means of the drill down navigation primitive. At each navigation step the drawing engine computes a drawing of the current map. The drawing engine is based on the GDToolkit graph drawing library [12]. Since GDToolkit is written in C++ the Java Native Interface technology [20] is adopted to integrate GDToolkit into Polyphemus. Examples of maps displayed during navigation sessions are shown in Section 5.1.

4.2 Hermes

Hermes is a three-tiered client/server service accessible on the Web. The user interacts with a top-tier client which is in charge of collecting user requests and showing results. The requests are forwarded by the client to a middle-tier server which is in charge to process the raw data extracted from a repository (bottom-tier).

The client is a multi-document GUI-based application. It allows the user to carry-on multiple explorations of the ASes interconnection graph at the same time. The Java technology has been used to ensure good portability.

In Hermes the middle-tier server maintains the state of the session, that is the current map, for each connected user. The client communicates with the server opening a permanent connection for each user. This permits to amortize the inefficiency of the connection set up over all the requests of session. The protocol transported by such connections is specifically tailored for our application. In particular, the server sends its reply in the form of serialized software objects describing ASes, links, and related geometric information. The Java run-time environment transparently encodes objects into bytes on the middle-tier server and consistently decodes them on the client side.

The repository is updated off-line from a plurality of sources. At the moment we access the following databases adopting, for representing data, the RPSL language [1]: ANS, APNIC, ARIN, BELL, CABLE&WIRELESS, CANET, MCI, RADB, RIPE, VERIO. Further, we access the routing BGP data provided by the Route views project of the Oregon University [15]. However, the repository is easily extensible to other data sources.

Data are filtered so that only the information used by Hermes are stored in the database, but no consistency check or ambiguity removal is performed in this stage. The overall size of the repository is about 50 MB. The adopted DBMS technology is currently MySQL [17].

The crucial part of the system is mainly located in the middle-tier. The top-tier requests two types of service to the middle-tier.

General info services the top-tier queries about ASes, routes, and path properties.

Topology services the top-tier queries for a new exploration and gets back a new map.

Info services requests are independent of each other and hence are independently handled by the middle-tier. On the contrary, topology services requests are always part of a *drawing session*. Each client may open one or more drawing sessions. Each drawing session is associated with a map that can be enriched by means of exploration requests. Examples of drawing sessions are shown in Section 5.2.

Info services requests are directly dispatched to a *mediator*. The mediator module is in charge to retrieve the data from the repository and to remove ambiguities on-the-fly (e.g., when the polices of an AS are encountered more than once).

Topology services requests are handled by the kernel of the middle-tier. It gets information from the mediator and inserts new edges and vertices into the map. The drawing is computed by the *drawing engine* module, which implements the static and the dynamic algorithms described in Section 3.3. The drawing engine uses the facilities of the GDToolkit [12] library.

5 Examples

In this section we give some examples of maps displayed during navigation sessions in Polyphemus and Hermes.

5.1 Polyphemus

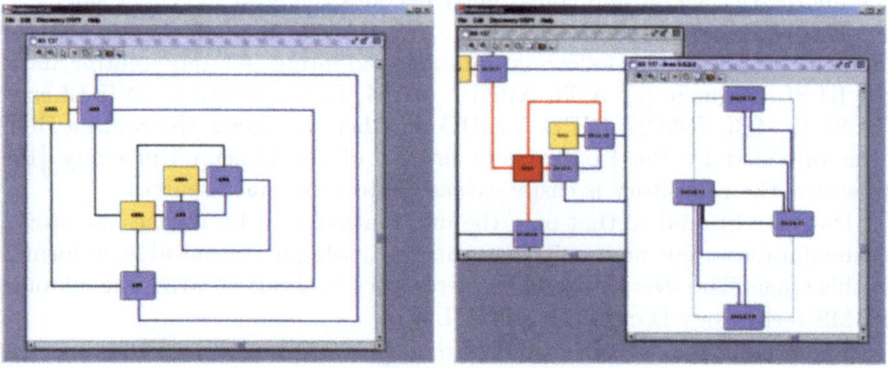

(a) (b)

Fig. 11. (a) At the end of the discovery process the overall map is displayed. (b) The user can interactively explore the content of each area. Area border routers are correctly placed on the border of the drawing.

In Polyphemus, at the end of the discovery process, the overall map is displayed (see Figure 11(a)) showing interconnections between areas and area border routers. Topologies stored into the database can be visually explored by means of the drill down interaction primitive described in Section 3.1. The user interactively selects an OSPF area and obtains a new map in which the routers of the area are placed on the border of the drawing, according to the drawing standard described in Section 3.1 (see Figure 11(a) and 11(b)).

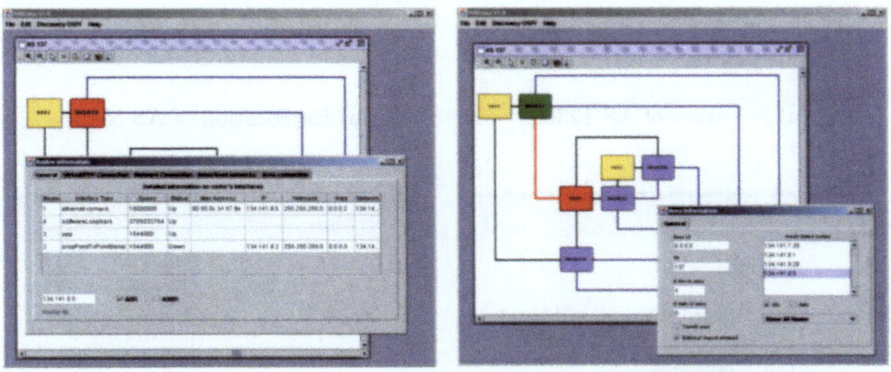

(a) (b)

Fig. 12. The user can ask detailed information about objects shown in each map.

The user can ask detailed information about objects shown in each map. For example, for each router it is possible to show configuration information like point-to-point and transit network connections (see Figure 12(a)). Other details can be shown for the backbone area like the list of the area border routers (see Figure 12(b)).

5.2 Hermes

The user interacts with Hermes through a map that represents a portion of the ASes interconnection graph. A map is initially constructed by selecting a first AS either numerically or by a text based search on the database. The user can explore and enrich the map by using the exploration primitive presented in Section 3.1. By selecting a specific AS all the interconnections of such an AS are displayed possibly introducing new ASes into the current map. Figure 13 shows a sequence of explorations starting from AS 12300 and consecutively selecting ASes 5583, 5484 and 6715.

Hermes can construct new drawings either using a static or a dynamic graph drawing algorithm. The drawing of Figure 13(b) has been constructed

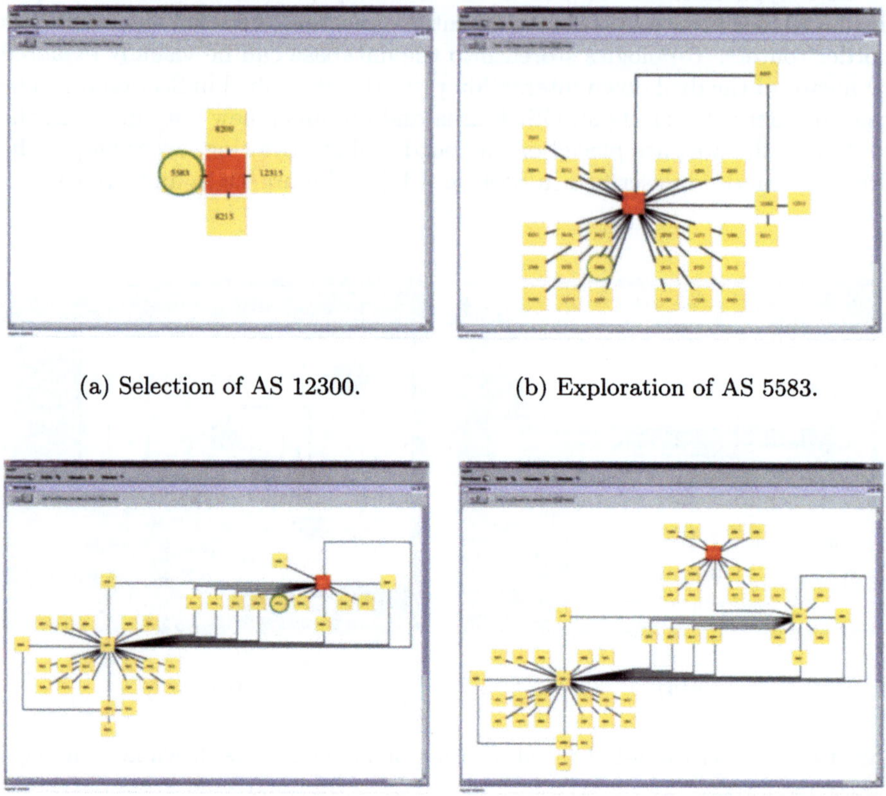

(a) Selection of AS 12300.

(b) Exploration of AS 5583.

(c) Exploration of AS 5484.

(d) Exploration of AS 6715.

Fig. 13. Exploration steps in the ASes graph. The selected AS or the AS that was just explored is always drawn red while the AS which is about to be explored is highlighted by a green circle.

with a dynamic algorithm starting from the drawing of Figure 13(a), and the drawing of Figure 13(d) has been constructed with the same algorithm starting from the drawing of Figure 13(c). Conversely, the drawing of Figure 13(c) is obtained with a static algorithm. The choice of the algorithm to be applied can be done by the system or forced by the user. Since the ASes degree can be large, we implement the drawing convention described in Section 3.1 for representing vertices of degree one in a small rectangular area. Figure 13 shows how the vertices of degree one are placed around their adjacent vertices. A complex map with more than 150 ASes is shown in Figure 14.

Working on a map, independently on the way it has been obtained, the user can get several information on any AS.

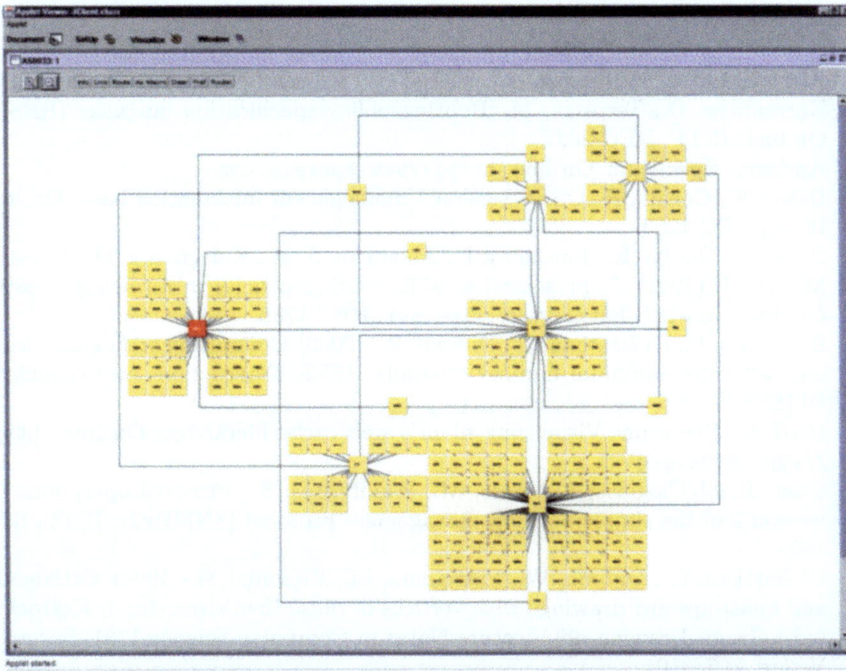

Fig. 14. A map with more than 150 ASes, obtained with several exploration steps.

General Info name, maintainers, and description of the AS.

Routing Policies For each connected AS, an expression describing the policy and its cost. This is possible both for in and for out policies. The default AS is also displayed.

Internal Routers List of the known border routers with the IP-numbers of the interfaces. Peering sessions with other routers are displayed.

Routes List of the routes originated by the AS. It is also possible to visualize the propagation of a given route in the ASes composing the map.

AS Macros List of the macros [4] including the AS.

6 Software

Hermes is a service publicly available over the Web at `http://www.dia.uniroma3.it/~hermes`.

Polyphemus is available for download at `http://www.dia.uniroma3.it/~polyph` or you can obtain it by directly contacting the authors.

References

1. Alaettinoglu, C., Villamizar, C., Gerich, E., Kessens, D., Meyer, D., Bates, T., Karrenberg, D., Terpstra, M. Routing policy specification language (RPSL). On line. IETF, RFC 2622
2. Aprisma. Spectrum. On line. `http://www.aprisma.com`
3. Baker, F., Coltun, R. OSPF version 2 management information base. On line. IETF, RFC 1253
4. Bates, T., Gerich, E., Joncheray, L., Jouanigot, J. M., Karrenberg, D., Terpstra, M., Yu, J. (1994) Representation of IP routing policies in a routing registry. On line. ripe-181, `http://www.ripe.net`, RFC 1786
5. Bertolazzi, P., Di Battista, G., Didimo, W. (2000) Computing orthogonal drawings with the minimum number of bends. IEEE Transactions on Computers, 49 (8)
6. CAIDA. Plankton: Visualizing nlanr's web cache hierarchy. On line. `http://www.caida.org`
7. Case, J., McCloghrie, K., Rose, M., Waldbusser, S. Protocol operations for version 2 of the simple network management protocol (SNMPv2). IETF, RFC 1905
8. Di Battista, G., Didimo, W., Patrignani, M., Pizzonia, M. (1999) Orthogonal and quasi-upward drawings with vertices of prescribed sizes. In: J. Kratochvil (ed.) Graph Drawing '99, Lecture Notes in Computer Science 1731, Springer-Verlag, 297–310
9. Di Battista, G., Lillo, R., Vernacotola, F. (1998) Ptolomaeus: The web cartographer. In: S. H. Whitesides (ed.) Graph Drawing '98, Lecture Notes in Computer Science 1547, Springer-Verlag, 444–445
10. Dodge, M. An atlas of cyberspaces. On line. `http//www.cybergeography.org`
11. Eades, P., Cohen, R. F., Huang, M. L. (1997) Online animated graph drawing for web navigation. In: G. Di Battista (ed.) Graph Drawing '97, Lecture Notes in Computer Science 1353, Springer-Verlag, 330–335
12. Graph drawing toolkit. On line. `http://www.dia.uniroma3.it/~gdt`
13. Internet routing registry. On line. `http://www.irr.net`
14. Lawrence, S., Giles, C. L. (1999) Accessibility of information on the web. Nature **400**, 107–109
15. Meyer, D. University of oregon route views project. On line. `http://www.antc.uoregon.edu/route-views`
16. Moy, J. OSPF version 2. IETF, RFC 2328
17. MySQL documentation. On line. `http://www.mysql.com`
18. Netcraft web server survey. On line. `http://www.netcraft.com`
19. Rekhter, Y. A border gateway protocol 4 (BGP-4). IETF, RFC 1771
20. Java native interface specification 1.1. On line, 1997. `http://java.sun.com`

Index

Printing: Druckhaus Berlin-Mitte GmbH
Binding: Buchbinderei Stein & Lehmann, Berlin

MIX
Papier aus verantwortungsvollen Quellen
Paper from responsible sources
FSC® C105338

If you have any concerns about our products,
you can contact us on
ProductSafety@springernature.com

In case Publisher is established outside the EU,
the EU authorized representative is:
Springer Nature Customer Service Center GmbH
Europaplatz 3, 69115 Heidelberg, Germany

Printed by Libri Plureos GmbH
in Hamburg, Germany